US Army
Physician Assistant
Handbook

Second Edition

Borden Institute
US Army Medical Center of Excellence
Fort Sam Houston, Texas

Office of The Surgeon General
United States Army
Falls Church, Virginia

2021

"All Gave Some, Some Gave All"

In Memoriam to Our Fallen Physician Assistants . . .

CPT Sean Grimes
04 March 2005—Ramadi, Iraq—Operation Iraqi Freedom
1st Infantry Battalion, 9th Infantry Regiment,
2nd Brigade Combat Team, Camp Hovey, Korea

CPT Anthony R. Garcia
17 February 2006—Tikrit, Iraq—Operation Iraqi Freedom
Headquarters and Headquarters Company, 1st Battalion,
101st Aviation Regiment, 101st Aviation Brigade,
101st Airborne Division, Fort Campbell, Kentucky

CPT Kafele H. Sims
16 June 2009—Mosul, Iraq—Operation Iraqi Freedom
18th Engineer Brigade, Schwetzingen, Germany

CPT Barry A. McGowan
10 August 2009—Greene Mountain Falls, Colorado
HHC 1-68 AR, 3rd Brigade, 4th Infantry Division,
Colorado Springs, Colorado

CPT Corey Jenkins
25 August 2009—Sha Wali Kot, Afghanistan—Operation Enduring Freedom
1st Battalion, 17th Infantry Regiment, 5th Stryker Brigade, 2nd Infantry Division, Fort Lewis, Washington

CPT Michael Cassidy
17 June 2010—Mosul, Iraq—Operation Iraqi Freedom
1st Battalion, 9th Field Artillery Regiment, 2nd Heavy Brigade Combat Team, 3rd Infantry Division, Fort Stewart, Georgia

CPT Jonathan Muniz
8 January 2015—Fort Hood, TX
Headquarters and Headquarters Company, 1st Air Cavalry Brigade, 1st Cavalry Division, Fort Hood, Texas

. . . From the Line, For the Line.

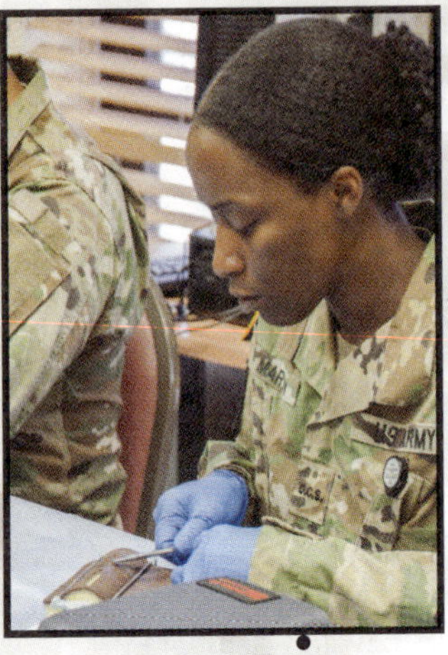

Officer Candidate Jessica Martin, an Interservice Physician Assistant Program (IPAP) Phase 2 student from William Beaumont Army Medical Center, Fort Bliss, Texas, participates in a suture and wound closure training at WBAMC's Simulation Center on March 9, 2018. Photo by March Sanchez. https://www.dvidshub.net/image/4241463/revamped-curricula-wbamcs-sim-center-aims-increase-safety-readiness

Lieutenant Colonel Avery Carney, the IPAP Phase 2 Clinical Coordinator at Evans Army Community Hospital, Fort Carson, Colorado, gives Captain Nelson Liuzzo his diploma during their graduation on October 5, 2018. Photo by Alexandra Shea. https://www.fortcarsonmountaineer.com/2018/10/ipap-graduation/

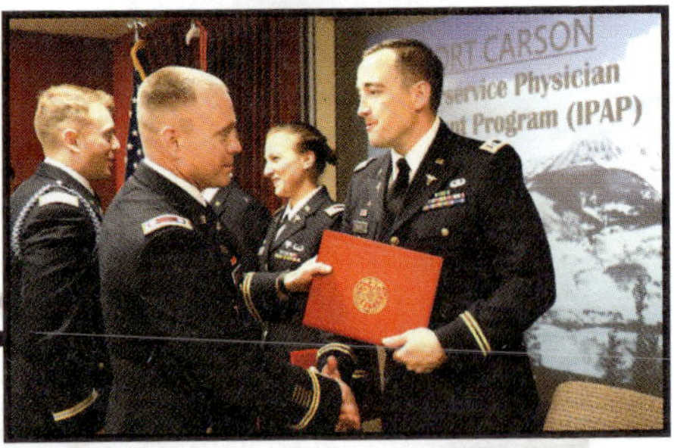

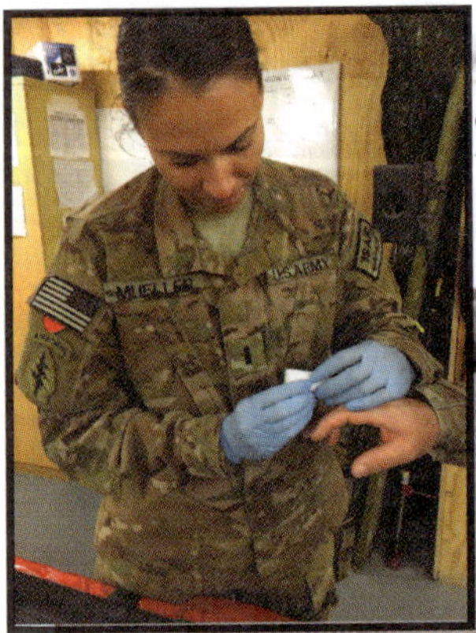

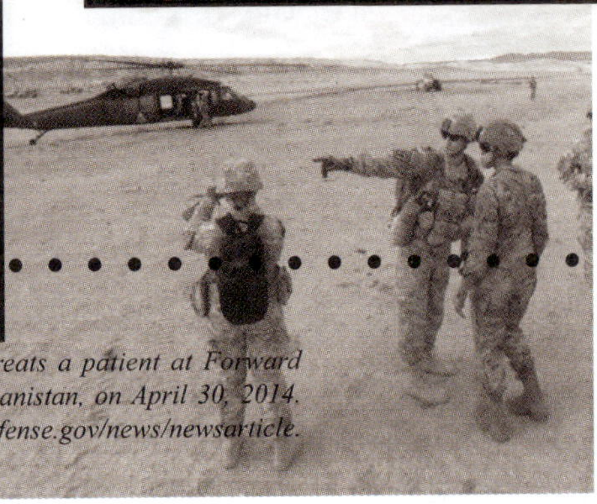

First Lieutenant Jamie Mueller treats a patient at Forward Operating Base Spin Boldak, Afghanistan, on April 30, 2014. US Army photo. https://archive.defense.gov/news/newsarticle.aspx?id=122192

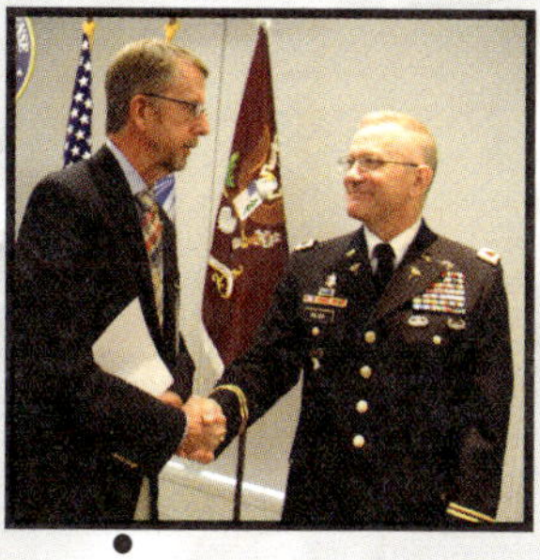

Colonel (Retired) Louis H. Smith, III, the third Chief of the PA Section from 1998 to 2002, congratulates Colonel John Balser during COL Balser's swearing in ceremony as the 19th Army Medical Specialist (SP) Corps Chief on March 30, 2017. COL Balser is the first PA selected as the SP Corps Chief and he was the Chief of the PA Section from 2010 to 2014. Photo courtesy of Colonel Jeffrey Oliver.

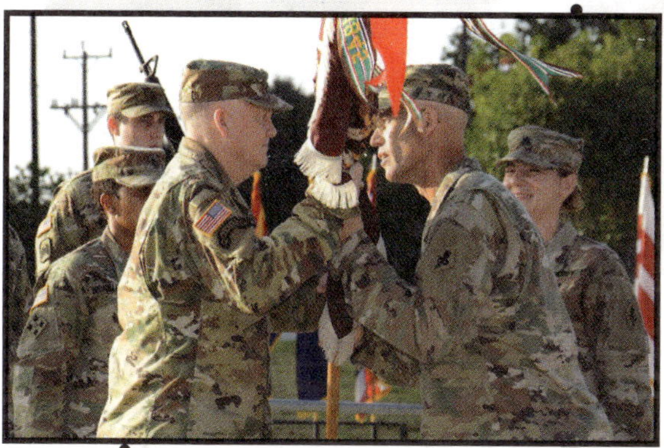

Lieutenant Colonel John F. Detro, the incoming commander of the 187th Medical Battalion, accepts the guideon from Colonel Scott Drennon, commander of the US Medical Department Center and School Academy Brigade (P), while Lieutenant Colonel Jodi Dugai, the outgoing commander, looks on; September 12, 2016. Photo courtesy of MEDCoE PAO.

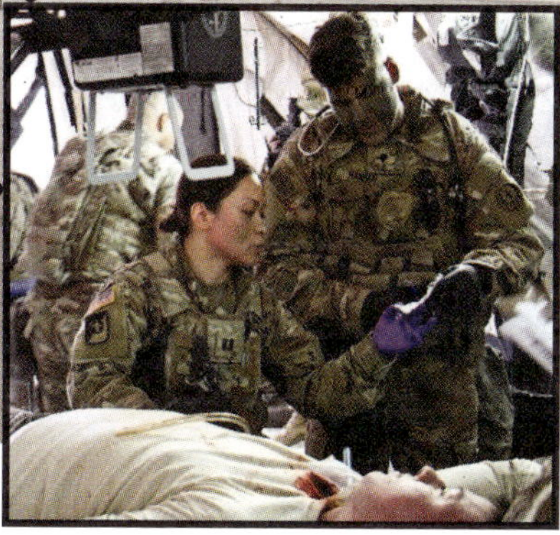

Captain Christine Cabal, 2nd Cavalry Regiment, Vilseck, Germany, takes care of a patient during a training exercise in September 2019. Photo by Wesley Elliott. https://www.dvidshub.net/image/5790944/army-physician-assistants-embrace-continued-front-line-roles-midst-transitions

Borden Institute
Edward A. Lindeke
Colonel (Retired), MS, US Army
Director

Dosage Selection: The authors and publisher have made every effort to ensure the accuracy of dosages cited herein. However, it is the responsibility of every practitioner to consult appropriate information sources to ascertain correct dosages for each clinical situation, especially for new or unfamiliar drugs and procedures. The authors, editors, publisher, and the Department of Defense cannot be held responsible for any errors found in this book.

Use of Trade or Brand Names: Use of trade or brand names in this publication is for illustrative purposes only and does not imply endorsement by the Department of Defense.

Neutral Language: Unless this publication states otherwise, masculine nouns and pronouns do not refer exclusively to men.

The opinions or assertions contained herein are the personal views of the authors and are not to be construed as doctrine of the Department of the Army or the Department of Defense. For comments or suggestions on additional contents in forthcoming editions, please contact the publisher (https://medcoe.army.mil/borden).

Published by the Office of The Surgeon General
Borden Institute
Army Medical Center of Excellence
Fort Sam Houston, Texas
2021

Library of Congress Cataloging-in-Publication Data

Names: Jackson, Amy L., editor. | Duran-Stanton, Amelia M., editor. | Paul, Johnny (Johnny Wayne), editor. | Auchincloss, P. Jason E. E. (Paul Jason E. E.), editor. | Borden Institute (U.S.), issuing body.
Title: US Army physician assistant handbook / senior editors, Amy L. Jackson, Amelia M. Duran-Stanton ; editors, Johnny Paul, P. Jason E. E. Auchincloss.
Other titles: U.S. Army physician assistant handbook
Description: Second edition. | Fort Sam Houston, Texas : Borden Institute, US Army Medical Center of Excellence ; Falls Church, Virginia : Office of The Surgeon General, United States Army, 2021. | Includes bibliographical references and index. | Summary: "The Army physician assistant (PA) has an important role throughout Army medicine. This handbook will describe the myriad positions and organizations in which PAs play leadership roles in management and patient care. Chapters also cover PA education, certification, continuing training, and career progression. Topics include the Interservice PA Program, assignments at the White House and the Old Guard (3d US Infantry Regiment), and roles in research and recruiting, as well as the PA's role in emergency medicine, aeromedical evacuation, clinical care, surgery, and occupational health"-- Provided by publisher.
Identifiers: LCCN 2021014140 (print) | LCCN 2021014141 (ebook) | ISBN 9780160955228 (hardback) | ISBN 9780160955976 (epub) | ISBN 9780160958229 (mobi)
Subjects: MESH: Military Medicine | Physician Assistants | Health Workforce | Military Medicine--education | Military Personnel--education | Professional Role | United States
Classification: LCC RC971 (print) | LCC RC971 (ebook) | NLM W 21.5 | DDC 616.9/8023--dc23
LC record available at https://lccn.loc.gov/2021014140
LC ebook record available at https://lccn.loc.gov/2021014141

Printed in the United States of America
26, 25, 24, 23, 22, 21 5 4 3 2 1

Contents

The following chapters are available online only at the Borden Institute *Army PA Handbook* link:

https://medcoe.army.mil/borden-pa-handbook

We dedicate this handbook to past Physician Assistants who forged the path that shaped our current environment. This second edition commemorates their legacy and achievements; may they never be forgotten. This handbook is also dedicated to the Physician Assistants stationed worldwide who are currently serving our nation.

The handbook propagates the illustrious narrative of the US Army Physician Assistant. Our hope is that this handbook will be worn and tattered from use, displayed prominently, and esteemed as a useful resource. We are honored to have had the pleasure and privilege to lead this literary effort, and we look forward to what the future generation of Physician Assistants will produce for the follow-on editions of the handbook.

"From the Line . . . for the Line."

Senior Editors

Amelia M. Duran-Stanton, PA-C, PhD, DSc, MPAS
LTC, SP, US Army
Chief, Ready and Resilient Integration Branch/Deputy Surgeon/
Deputy PA Consultant
Headquarters, Installation Management Command
JBSA-Fort Sam Houston, Texas

Amy L. Jackson, PA-C, MPAS
COL, SP, US Army
Commander, Keller Army Community Hospital
West Point, New York

Editors

Johnny Paul, APA-C, DMSc, MPAS
COL, SP, US Army
Branch Chief and Department Chair
68W (Combat Medic) Advanced Individual Training
METC Department of Combat Medic Training
JBSA-Fort Sam Houston, Texas

P. Jason E.E. Auchincloss, APA-C, MPAS
MAJ, SP, US Army
Deputy Surgeon for Clinical Services
Special Operations Command-Africa
Stuttgart, Germany

Administrative Support

Timothy Pekari, APA-C, DSc
MAJ, SP, US Army
Interservice Physician Assistant Program Clinical Coordinator &
Orthopedic Physician Assistant, Evans Army Community Hospital
Fort Carson, Colorado

Robert Gipson, PA-C, MPAS
CPT, SP, US Army
Battalion Physician Assistant, 2nd Battalion, 377th Parachute Field
Artillery Regiment
4th Airborne Brigade Combat Team, 25th Infantry Division
Fort Richardson, Alaska

Contributors

Curtis Aberle, RN, MSN; CIV
Victor Acevedo, PA-C, MPAS; CPT, SP, US Army
Jason C. Adams, PA-C, MPAS; MAJ, SP, US Army
Lucas Allmon, PA-C, MPAS; MAJ, SP, US Army
Mitchell R. Andreas, PA-C, MPAS; 1LT, SP, US Army
J. Brandon Atkins, PA-C, MPAS; MAJ, SP, US Army
P. Jason E.E. Auchincloss, APA-C, MPAS; MAJ, SP, US Army
John E. Balser, PA-C, MPAS, MSS; COL, SP, US Army
George Barbee, PA-C, DSc, MPAS; LTC, SP, US Army
William Paul Barras, CRNA, MSN, MS; COL, AN, US Army
David Bauder, PA-C, MPAS; LTC (Ret), SP, US Army
Jim Beecher, PA-C, MPAS, MPH; LTC (Ret), SP, US Army
Robert D. Blume, APA-C, MPAS; MAJ, SP, US Army
Stephanie Bocanegra, PA-C, MPAS; MAJ (Ret), SP, US Army
W. Joseph Bowman, PA-C, DSc; MAJ (Ret), SP, US Army
R. Scott Bradshaw, PA-C, MPAS; MAJ, SP, US Army
David W. Broussard, PA-C, MPAS; LTC (Ret), SP, US Army
Diane Bruessow, PA-C, MPAS; CIV
Jason Bruno, APA-C, MPAS; CPT, SP, US Army
Thomas A. Bryant, APA-C, MPAS; COL, SP, US Army
Alan Bucholz, PA-C, MPAS; CPT, SP, US Army
Leah Bucholz, PA-C, MPAS; CPT, SP, US Army
Pamela Budda, BSW, MEd; CIV
Brian E. Burk, PA-C, PhD, MEd; COL, SP, US Army
Craig Buss, PA, MBA, BS; CIV
Christine C. Cabal, PA-C, MPAS; MAJ, SP, US Army
Brandon M. Carius, PA-C, DSc, MPAS; MAJ, SP, US Army
Avery J. Carney, PA-C, MPAS; LTC, SP, US Army
James A. Carroll, APA-C, DMSc, MPAS; LTC, SP, US Army
Peter Carroll, PA-C, MPAS; MAJ (Ret), SP, US Army
Monica Casmaer, PA-C, DSc; MAJ (Ret), SP, US Army
Robyn L. Chalupa, PA-C, DSc, MPAS; MAJ, SP, US Army
Antonio F. Chang, PA-C, MPAS, MSHS; MAJ, SP, US Army
Terry Lee Clark Jr, PA-C, MPAS; LTC, SP, US Army
Donna Clouse, MS, CEAP; CIV
Christopher B. Cordova, PA-C, DSc, MPAS; MAJ (Ret), SP, US Army

Robert Cornfeld, MD; LTC, MC, US Army
Mary J. Coy, PA-C, MPAS, MSHS, MBA; LTC, SP, US Army
F. Eddie Criss, APA-C, MPAS; MAJ, SP, US Army
Colt Crutchfield, PA-C, MPAS; MAJ SP, US Army
Ryan Curtis, PA-C, DSc, RDMS; LTC, SP, US Army
Rolands J. Dale, APA-C, MPAS; MAJ, SP, US Army
Andrew Darrah, PA-C, MPAS; LT, US Navy
Michael A. Davidson, PA-C, MPAS; LTC (Ret), SP, US Army
Charles (Charlie) Day, PA-C, MPAS; LTC, SP, US Army
Margie Deck, PA-C, MPAS; MAJ (Ret), SP, US Army
Stephen M. DeLellis, PA-C, MPAS; LTC (Ret), SP, US Army
Susan Delozier-Hooks, PA-C, MPAS, MEd; CPT, SP, US Army
Sharon D. Denson, PA-C, DMSc, MPAS; LTC, SP, US Army
Patrick D. DePriest, PA-C, MPAS, MPH; MAJ, SP, US Army
Gonzalo de Taboada, PA-C, DSc, MPAS; MAJ, SP, US Army
John F. Detro, APA-C, MPAS, MSS, MEd; COL, SP, US Army
Sean M. Donohue, PA-C, MPAS; MAJ, SP, US Army
J. Scott Donoughe, PA-C, MPAS; MAJ (Ret), SP, US Army
Matthew S. Douglas, PA-C, DSc, MPAS; LTC, SP, US Army
Erin Driver, PA-C, DSc; LTC, SP, US Army
Amelia M. Duran-Stanton, PA-C, PhD, DSc, MPAS; LTC, SP, US Army
Joseph (Buck) Eddins, APA-C, MPAS; MAJ, SP, US Army
William H. Edmonds, PA-C, DHSc, MSHS; MAJ (Ret), SP, US Army
Craig J. Edwards, PA-C, MPAS; CPT, SP, US Army
John T. Elliott, APA-C, MPAS; LTC, SP, US Army
Walter Engle, PA-C, MPAS; LTC (Ret), SP, US Army
Gail A. Evans, PA-C, MPAS; LTC (Ret), SP, US Army
Derek Ferrell, MSM, MHA; CIV
Andrew D. Fisher, MD, PA-C, MPAS, LP; MAJ, SP, US Army
Colin Frament, APA-C, MPAS; LTC, SP, US Army
Larry France, PA-C, MPAS; COL (Ret), SP, US Army
Donald R. Frazee, PA-C, MPAS; MAJ, SP, US Army
David Freel, PA-C, MPAS; LTC (Ret), SP, US Army
Darron Fritz, PA-C, MPAS; MAJ, SP, US Army
Felipe Galvan, PA-C, MPAS; MAJ (Ret), SP, US Army
Maureen Giorio, PA-C, MPAS, MHA; LTC, SP, US Army
Robert Gipson, PA-C, MPAS; CPT, SP, US Army
Brian Gomez, APA-C, MPAS; MAJ, SP, US Army
Andrea N. Gonzalez, APA-C, MPAS; MAJ, SP, US Army

Christopher Gonzalez, PA-C, MPAS; MAJ (P), SP, US Army
Robert K. Greener, PA-C, MPAS; CPT, SP, US Army
Pauline V. Gross, PA-C, MPH; COL (Ret), SP, US Army
Seth A. Grubbs, APA-C, DMO, MPAS; MAJ, SP, US Army
Kelly A. Guerra, PA-C, MPAS; MAJ, SP, US Army
Edwin X. Gutierrez, APA-C, MPAS; LTC, SP, US Army
Jonathan R. Haller, APA-C, MPAS; MAJ, SP, US Army
David L. Hamilton, PA-C, MPAS, MPH; COL, SP, US Army
Daniel J. Hankes, PA-C, MPAS; LTC, SP, US Army
Keith D. Harris, APA-C, DMSc, MPAS; MAJ, SP, US Army
R. Scott Harrison, PA-C, MPAS; LTC, SP, US Army
Robert S. Heath, APA-C, MPAS; COL, SP, US Army
Sean Hermick, APA-C, MPAS; LTC (Ret), SP, US Army
Owen T. Hill, PA-C, PhD, MPAS; LTC (Ret), SP, US Army
Seth Holland, PA-C, DSc, MPAS; MAJ (Ret), SP, US Army
Michael Holloway, APA-C, MPAS; MAJ (Ret), SP, US Army
James Huang, PA-C, DSc, MPAS; MAJ, SP, US Army
Amy L. Jackson, PA-C, MPAS; COL, SP, US Army
Paul V. Jacobson, APA-C, MPAS; LTC (Ret), SP, US Army
Keary Johnston, PA-C, MPAS; LTC (Ret), SP, US Army
James J. Jones, PA-C, PhD, MPAS; COL, SP, US Army
Stephen A. Karagosian, PA-C, MPAS; CPT, SP, US Army
Travis Kaufman, PA-C, DMSc, MPAS; MAJ, SP, US Army
Scott A. Kavan, PA-C, MPAS; MAJ, SP, US Army
Jimmie E. Keller, PA-C, MPH; MAJ (Ret), SP, US Army
Matthew H. Kemm, MD; MAJ, MC, US Army
Drew Kennedy, PA-C, MPAS; MAJ, SP, US Army
Todd P. Kielman, PA-C, MPAS; MAJ (Ret), SP, US Army
John E. King, APA-C, DSc, MPAS; LTC, SP, US Army
Benjamin K. Kocher, PA-C, DSc, MPAS; LTC, SP, US Army
Michael Korczykowski, APA-C, MPAS; LTC, SP, US Army
Margaret Kucia, PA-C, MPAS; MAJ, SP, US Army
Maura Lappin, DO; CIV
Garrett Larson, APA-C, MPAS, MS; MAJ, SP, US Army
Courtney D. Legendre, PA-C, MPAS; MAJ, SP, US Army
Robert M. Levesque, PA-C, MPAS; MAJ, SP, US Army
Jay M. Lloyd Sr, PA-C, MPAS; MAJ, SP, US Army
Lakeshia T. Logan, PA-C, MPAS; MAJ, SP, US Army
Elizabeth Lopez, PA-C, DSc; MAJ, SP, US Army

James S. Lorenz, PA-C, MPAS; MAJ, SP, US Army
Alixandra M. Mackey, PA-C, DMSc, MPAS; CPT, SP, US Army
Roberto E. Marin, PA-C, DHSc, DMSc, MPAS; COL, SP, US Army
Daniel C. Martens, PA-C, MPAS; MAJ, SP, US Army
Gail A. Martin, APA-C, MPAS; LTC (Ret), SP, US Army
Robyn L. Mason, APA-C, MS; LTC, SP, US Army
Kevin C. Mayberry, APA-C, DSc; MAJ, SP, US Army
Jon C. McBride, APA-C, MPAS; CPT, SP, US Army
Kory McCullah, MSLA; SSG, US Army
Hugh S. McLeod, APA-C, MPAS; MAJ, SP, US Army
Frances Measells, DSW, LCSW, CEAP; CIV
Manuel Menendez, APA-C, MPAS; LTC, SP, US Army
Christopher G. Metcalf, PA-C, MPAS; MAJ (Ret), SP, US Army
Christopher Montoya, PA-C, MPAS; CPT (Ret), SP, US Army
Jeffrey D. Morgan, APA-C, MPAS; MAJ, SP, US Army
Kane D. Morgan, APA-C, MPAS, MPH; LTC, SP, US Army
D. Alan Nelson, PA-C, PhD, MPAS; MAJ (Ret), SP, US Army
Jeffrey E. Oliver, APA-C, MPAS, MSS; COL, SP, US Army
Dawn Orta, APA-C, MPAS; COL, SP, US Army
James G. Pairmore, APA-C, MPAS; COL, SP, US Army
Christopher Pase, APA-C, MPAS; LTC, SP, US Army
Johnny Paul, APA-C, DMSc, MPAS; COL, SP, US Army
Mandy L. Pears, PA-C, MPAS; CPT, SP, US Army
Timothy Pekari, APA-C, DSc; MAJ, SP, US Army
Eric W. Pelkey, BS, NRP, FP-C; SFC, US Army
John Joe Peña, APA-C, MPAS, MSIR; LTC, SP, US Army
Tiffany L. Pittman, PA-C, MPAS; CPT, SP, US Army
Michael Plotkowski, PA-C, MPAS; CPT, SP, US Army
David Polston, APA-C, MPAS; MAJ (Ret), SP, US Army
Joshua Randles, PA-C, DSc, MPAS; CPT, SP, US Army
Manish Rawat, PA-C, MPAS; MAJ, SP, US Army
Michael A. Robertson, OTR/L; COL, SP, US Army
Christopher Rogers, APA-C, MPAS; MAJ, SP, US Army
Sharon Rosser, PA-C, DSc, MPAS; LTC, SP, US Army
Jacob W. Rouse, PA-C, MPAS; CPT, SP, US Army
Christopher Sacheli, APA-C, MPAS; LTC (Ret), SP, US Army
Adam R. Sahlberg, APA-C, MPAS; CPT, SP, US Army
Joanna G. Sanford, PA-C, MPAS; CPT (Ret), SP, US Army
Jonathan Saxe, PA-C, DSc, MPAS; LTC (Ret), SP, US Army

Sarah E. Scott, BA; CIV
Dennison S. Segui, PA-C, MPAS; LTC, SP, US Army
Barry Seip, PA-C, BS; MAJ (Ret), SP, US Army
Patrick A. Sherman, APA-C, DSc, MHA; LTC (Ret), SP, US Army
Christopher R. Smith, PA-C, MPAS; MAJ, SP, US Army
Megan L. Smith, PA-C, MPAS; CPT, SP, US Army
Paul Smith, MBA, MA; CIV
Bill A. Soliz, APA-C, MPAS; COL, SP, US Army
Denise Souza, APA-C, MPAS; MAJ, SP, US Army
Erin Stibral, APA-C, MPAS; LTC, SP, US Army
Heather Sultemeier, MS; MAJ, MS, US Army
Cleve Sylvester, PA-C, DSc, MPAS; LTC, SP, US Army
Bradley Tibbetts, PA-C, MPAS; LTC, SP, US Army
Christopher L. Torres, PA-C, MPAS; CPT, SP, US Army
Jeremiah Tyler, PA-C, MPAS; 1LT, SP, US Army
Vince vanderMaarel, PA-C, MPAS; MAJ, SP, US Army
Luis Vidal, APA-C, MPAS; MAJ, SP, US Army
Richard A. Villarreal, APA-C, PhD, MPAS; COL, SP, US Army
Patrick Walsh, PA-C, MPAS; LTC, SP, US Army
Carolynn M. Warner, MD; CIV
Christopher H. Warner, MD; COL, MC, US Army
Bradley J. Warr, PA-C, PhD, MPAS; MAJ (Ret), SP, US Army
Geoffrey Washburn, APA-C, MPAS; MAJ, SP, US Army
Larry A. Wyatt, APA-C, MPAS; LTC, SP, US Army

Foreword

The Army's priorities have expanded and are comprised of people, readiness, modernization, and reform. Accordingly, the Military Health System transformation is a critical time for Army Medicine to ensure there are no gaps or decreases in the quality of healthcare provided to our Soldiers, Families, Civilians, and Soldiers for Life—because people matter. Army Physician Assistants (PAs) are key enablers of Army Medicine's provision of sustained health services at home and in combat operations, and as such, are inevitably present from the "Foxhole to Fixed Facility." Army PAs serve in operational units on the front lines with our troops in every country our forces are deployed. They work in our clinics to provide the full spectrum of care for patients, spearhead preventive healthcare and performance optimization initiatives, and are pivotal in the design and transformation of the Military Health System. PAs command our clinics and field hospitals, and serve as senior staff in all of our formations.

The history of the modern PA profession is rooted in military tradition. In 1965, Dr. Eugene Stead announced the Nation's first "physician assistant program" at Duke University and accepted four Vietnam Veteran Navy Medical Corpsmen to the inaugural class. In 1971, the Army began the Medical Field Service Physician Assistant Program at Fort Sam Houston, Texas—and to this day, Army PA candidates selected primarily from currently serving Soldiers are educated through rigorous graduate-level programs such as the Interservice Physician Assistant Program (IPAP) at the Medical Center of Excellence.

It is with tremendous honor that I present the second edition of the *US Army Physician Assistant Handbook*. The second edition not only updates content from the previous edition, but also expands upon the information available to the Army PA. This handbook is the collaboration of PAs past and present and enhances shared understanding, learning, and decision-making; a sharing of knowledge.

Army PAs are the face of the Army Medicine provider to the line and will continue to serve as members of our cohesive team taking care of Soldiers. Army PAs are agile, adaptable, versatile, and innovative in their ability to meet the ever-changing challenges of today and tomorrow. I'm proud of Army PAs and their work to take care of the Nation's greatest treasure: the men and women of the Armed Services, their Families, and our retirees.

Army Medicine is Army Strong!

TSG 45

VR

R. SCOTT DINGLE
Lieutenant General, US Army
The Surgeon General and
Commanding General, USAMEDCOM

Preface

The US military is approaching a milestone no one predicted when America was attacked on September 11, 2001. As the 20-year mark of the Nation's longest war nears, one of the most commendable achievements is the extraordinary care our medical teams have provided Soldiers, Marines, Sailors, and Airmen, on and off the battlefield. While our education and training, advanced technology, and enhanced techniques certainly factor in, it's the devotion of our medical teams that is the foundation of our improved outcomes. Physician Assistants have never served a more important role on those teams.

Deploying as a general surgeon in the Kosovo, Iraq, and Afghanistan theaters, I've had hundreds of experiences with casualties, most of them Soldiers and Marines wounded in combat and in need of surgical intervention. There's no doubt in my mind we have the highest survival rates and limb salvage rates in history because of our medics and corpsmen on the battlefield. They're the best in the world. The largely untold story is why they're so good.

The truth of the matter is, the best medics came from units with the best PAs. And the best PAs were not only superb practitioners, they were also great teachers; attentive to their responsibility to provide sustainment training for their medics. I saw it over and over again. When a Soldier or Marine came in with devastating injuries, those that had the best chance for survival almost invariably were treated by medics who had done everything right. They had the best chance of returning home to their families because the PAs in those units were always helping their medics. We owe nothing less to our warfighters, the best America has to offer.

I saw the extraordinary partners PAs were to all of the doctors, and in particular the surgeons, when I was the Chief of Surgery then Deputy Commander of Landstuhl Regional Medical Center early in the Afghanistan and Iraq wars. This was never more obvious than when casualties markedly increased patient loads. The general practice PAs were the combat multipliers of the MTF, treating everything from anxiety disorder to gastroenteritis. Specialty PAs were the physician extenders we needed, providing a significant amount of direct patient care, freeing up physicians to be where we needed them the most; carrying out the evaluations and procedures only they could perform.

I've served with hundreds of PAs during my 30+ years as an Army surgeon. As a former Military Medical Treatment Facility Commander, Regional Commander, and now as the Director of the Defense Health Agency, I appreciate the competence, commitment, and compassion you bring to the military medical profession. For these reasons and so many more, I'm extremely grateful for the privilege to present the second edition of the *US Army Physician Assistant Handbook*. Thanks for your continuing service to the men and women of our Armed Forces, and the Families who support them!

RONALD J. PLACE, MD
Lieutenant General, US Army
Director, Defense Health Agency

Prologue

The medical readiness of the force now and in the future is paramount. The US Army Medical Center of Excellence (MEDCoE) is responsible for envisioning and designing the responsive Army Medicine capabilities and structure that support the fielded force and the future force. As one of the US Army Training and Doctrine Command (TRADOC)'s ten Centers of Excellence, MEDCoE trains, educates, and inspires medical personnel to conduct medical operations in unified land operations and the multi-domain operational design of the future. Battle-focused training is the most crucial activity MEDCoE Soldiers and trainees do to achieve readiness. US Army physician assistants (PAs) have played an essential role in ensuring readiness since they first began serving in the 1970s. The PA initially met a need for healthcare providers which greatly expanded during the Iraq and Afghanistan conflicts of the 21st century. As the PA profession continued to grow, a need for a mentorship program developed, which led a group of PAs to write the first *US Army Physician Assistant Handbook*.

This second edition of the *US Army Physician Assistant Handbook* takes into account the changes in military medicine since the first edition was published in 2018. A comprehensive transformation occurred with the move of Army medical training to TRADOC, the transition of military medical treatment facilities to the Defense Health Agency, and research activities aligning with Army Futures Command. Army PAs are essential in this time of transition, using their clinical, educational, research, leadership, and management skills to maintain the highest quality of medical training as the command structure changes.

Today, Army PAs are integral to training activity in numerous positions and roles at MEDCoE: Interservice PA Program Director/ Associate professors, combat medicine training instructors, and commanders of training companies and battalions. Army PAs are contributing to readiness of the force by training Soldiers in tactical and technical competencies to build and sustain operational capabilities. Army PAs are critical to Army Medicine's ability to ensure the health of the maneuver element during competition, preserve Soldier lethality in conflict, and facilitate a return to competition. By leading their profession in meeting the changing mission and training demands in the 21st century and beyond, Army PAs are a true embodiment of their motto, "From the Line … For the Line."

DENNIS P. LEMASTER
Major General, US Army
Commanding

19th Army Medical Specialist Corps Chief Message

This second edition is an expansion on a very successful first edition launch of a handbook that, while intended as a guide for Physician Assistants, has touched on many aspects of Army Medicine. We will see significant changes when the Defense Health Agency (DHA) fully assumes the role of managing all the military medical treatment facilities, but PAs and the Specialist Corps will continue as the backbone of soldiers' medical care.

As Corps Chief, my job was to ensure that all components of the Corps (Occupational Therapists, Physical Therapists, Dietitians, and Physician Assistants) deliver the capabilities that the Army expects from these experts. The newest initiative is the Specialist Corps-driven Holistic Health and Fitness (H2F) program. These H2F providers are assigned to maneuver units working alongside the Physician Assistants already embedded in these units. This marriage shows what can be accomplished when the strength of the entire Corps works together. Working with the line as a collective group maintains the significant fighting strength the Army needs in any operational theater.

What about the future? Physician Assistants are popular and will continue to be a vital component of operational units. The DHA is the way forward, and as time goes by, we will likely see more collaboration between the various branches of the military, cementing our place in operational medicine. Likewise, many talented individuals have opened the door for leadership opportunities and proved that a PA is a capable leader at all echelons of command. There will always be a need for leaders in our various medical units, and this is a place where all those coming up through the ranks can take advantage of previous efforts and excel where others have paved the way. Rank opportunities have increased, and so it is up to those future individuals to carry the torch and forge new frontiers.

We are in an exciting time, and the future script is unwritten. I hope that the time and effort that has gone into this handbook is helpful and appreciated. Feel free to share it with others in the medical community because initiatives like this set us apart. Keep the machine moving!

Colonel John Balser, PA-C, MPAS, MSS
19th Army Medical Specialist Corps Chief

20th Army Medical Specialist Corps Chief Message

"Reading is to the mind what exercise is to the body." – Joseph Addison

The mission of the Army Medical Specialist (SP) Corps is to develop Corps leaders who enhance Soldier health and readiness in garrison and throughout multi-domain operations (MDOs). The Army PA Handbook, now in its second edition, provides an amazing resource to help our Corps reach our vision: to lead the advancement of Soldier health and readiness.

As the 20th Army Medical Specialist Corps Chief, I am honored and humbled to have witnessed the impact of Army PAs on the health and readiness of the force. Since joining the SP Corps in 1992, PAs have enhanced Corps capabilities in support of the total force. I have been fortunate to have worked with our best PAs in garrison and in deployed settings. This second edition of the PA Handbook highlights the value of Army PAs, which I have had the luxury of experiencing firsthand.

Gustave Flaubert stated, "The art of writing is the art of discovering what you believe." The Army PA serves a fundamental role in supporting Army Medicine's priorities in taking care of our people, enhancing battlefield medicine, and streamlining early identification and treatment of illness and injuries. Army PAs leverage their clinical, research, and force development expertise in ensuring the SP Corps delivers solutions in garrison, across MDOs, and in large-scale combat operations; in writing this handbook, they have shown the breadth and depth of their mission. Benjamin Franklin once stated, "Either write something worth reading or do something worth writing." This handbook exemplifies both. The number of Army PAs who leveraged their experiences to contribute is impressive and clearly demonstrates their tradition of sharing the roles and responsibilities of Army PAs. This edition has been expanded to include collaborative efforts with Compos 2 and 3, new roles, and lessons learned and tips for success. Additionally, our Army PAs have proven themselves at strategic, operational, and tactical environments; this second edition highlights the holistic impact of the Army's PAs on readiness. As the table of contents shows, this handbook is not just for Army PAs; it is also worth reading by anyone interested in military professional and personal development.

I am proud of our team's collaboration. The future of Army PAs remains bright. Stay fit!

Colonel Deydre S. Teyhen, DPT, PhD
20th Army Medical Specialist Corps Chief

Introduction and Acknowledgements

For almost 50 years, Army Physician Assistants (PAs) have supported the US Army by ensuring the military force is both ready to fight today and prepared for the challenges of tomorrow. Since the inception of the PA profession, military PAs have demonstrated that they are versatile and adaptable force multipliers, performing essential work in a variety of environments ranging from combat outposts to clinics and command suites. The role of the Army PA has evolved since the early 1990s when they first became commissioned officers. Over the years, the PA position has been tailored according to changing needs of the Army. Army PAs provide a wide range of care at each level, or echelon, of care, from emergency and life-saving treatment at the point of injury, to routine care or wellness visits, to specialty services such as orthopedics, emergency medicine, general surgery, and behavioral health, as well as serving in staff roles at various levels and organizations throughout the Department of Defense. Vast changes in the role of the PA, and in the opportunities for PA development, necessitated a dedicated resource; hence the initiation of a handbook to guide PAs: the *US Army Physician Assistant Handbook*.

The Borden Institute published the first edition of the *US Army Physician Assistant Handbook* in May 2018. The first edition originated from the need to understand the diverse positions and roles of the Army PA and prescribed PA-specific guidance for career development. This second edition of the handbook continues the legacy of the first edition in providing information on career development, current opportunities, and important lessons learned. The second edition also incorporates new roles and topics of interest that have emerged since 2015. It has been a "labor of love" to showcase PA foundations and recognize the advancements of the PA profession. This handbook serves as a chronological time capsule; a portrait in space and time. It depicts a thriving Army PA, a ready medical force multiplier who stands prepared to answer the call, whenever and where ever the nation has a need.

A literary work such as this handbook is no small feat. It requires extraordinary effort on the part of a dedicated and faithful team of collaborators. We are sincerely grateful for the contributions of so many of our colleagues and leaders in support of the second edition of the *US Army Physician Assistant Handbook*.

This handbook exists due to the support of the Borden Institute staff, namely Mr. Ed Lindeke (Director), Ms. Joan Redding (Senior Production Editor), Dr. Lisa O'Brien (Editor), Mr. Robert Dredden (Illustrator), and Mr. Ernest Barner (Public Affairs). We are forever indebted to them for their coaching and guidance in the arduous process of charting the path to produce the PA Handbook.

The PA Handbook working group was instrumental in ushering the completion of this project. We would like to thank COL Johnny Paul and MAJ Paul (Jason) Auchincloss for performing first draft chapter reviews, and MAJ Timothy Pekari and CPT Robert Gipson for their administrative support. This endeavor was made possible due to their devotion and commitment.

To the numerous contributing authors who dedicated their time and energy in sharing their knowledge and experience, we wholeheartedly thank you. These authors took precious time to capture and portray their expertise to ensure that others may benefit from their lessons learned and tips for success.

To the military and civilian leaders, thank you for your mentorship and confidence in PAs. Your trust and faith have enabled us to contribute to a medically ready force and a ready medical force. Army Medicine is Army Strong!

Amelia M. Duran-Stanton, PA-C, PhD, DSc, MPAS
Amy L. Jackson, PA-C, MPAS

Section 1

The Army Physician Assistant Profession

Chapter 1

FROM VIETNAM TO AFGHANISTAN: THE HISTORY OF THE ARMY PHYSICIAN ASSISTANT

John F. Detro, APA-C, MPAS, MSS, MEd; John E. Balser, PA-C, MPAS, MSS; David W. Broussard, PA-C, MPAS; Amelia M. Duran-Stanton, PA-C, PhD, DSc, MPAS; Pauline V. Gross, PA-C, MPH; Robert S. Heath, APA-C, MPAS; Amy L. Jackson, PA-C, MPAS; James J. Jones, PA-C, PhD, MPAS; Jimmie E. Keller, PA-C, MPH; and Sarah E. Scott, BA

> As the face of the AMEDD [Army Medical Department] provider to the line, Army PAs [physician assistants] will continue to serve as a key healthcare link between the Warfighter and the AMEDD. Army PAs fulfill the mission and vision of being agile, adaptable, versatile, and innovative to meet the ever-changing challenges of today and tomorrow. Army PAs are proud to take care of the Nation's greatest treasure: the men and women in uniformed service, their Families and beneficiaries. Army PAs are truly part of "One Team. One Purpose! Conserving the Fighting Strength!"
>
> *—Lieutenant General Nadja West*
> *The Surgeon General & Commanding General,*
> *Office of The Surgeon General/US Army Medical Command, 2016–2019*
> *2016 National Physician Assistant Week Email Message*

Introduction

The physician assistant (PA) community and the US military have been connected since the founding of the PA profession. Currently, National PA Week is celebrated annually from October 6 to 12. Initially, National PA Day was celebrated once a year, on October 6. This date is significant for two reasons: (1) it is the date three former Vietnam-era Navy corpsmen graduated from Duke University's PA program in 1967, and (2) it is the birthday of Dr Eugene Stead Jr, the founding father of this prestigious program and of the PA profession.[1]

The 1960s: Origins of the Profession

The PA profession's past can be traced to an article written in 1961 by Dr Charles L. Hudson. Titled "Expansion of Medical Professional Services with Nonprofessional Personnel," it was published in the *Journal of the American Medical Association*.[2] Due to a shortage of physicians and allied health care professionals, Dr Hudson's vision was to create two new groups of providers to assist doctors in performing supervised primary care support to the public.[3] During the 1961 American Medical Association (AMA) conference, he described the two groups.[4] The first group would be interns who lacked formal medical education but would undergo on-the-job training like physicians of the past, and would serve in medical and surgical inpatient settings, including operating and emergency rooms. The second group was to be called externs. These individuals were to undergo formalized medical training somewhere between the level of a physician and that of a technician. The graduates would then work as primary care physician extenders. For this group, Dr Hudson proposed a 2-year college program followed by a 2-year clinical rotation leading to a Bachelor of Science in Medicine (BSM) degree. He felt that these "assistants to doctors" could be employed to handle routine care, allowing doctors to manage more complex procedures and care for increased patient populations.[2]

Three physicians took Dr Hudson's vision to heart. Dr Eugene Stead Jr, at Duke University, Dr Richard Smith from the University of Washington, and Dr Hu C. Myers at Alderson Broaddus College all bought into the idea of creating a program to address the national primary care physician shortage and began to develop the curricula.[3] Dr Stead and Dr Smith were aware of the plight faced by discharged medics after serving in the Vietnam conflict. These individuals had developed exceptional medical skills while serving in the military, but much of their training failed to translate into civilian education or health care professions. Both physicians felt that these former military medics could be trained to meet the primary care void.[4]

As early as 1964, Dr Stead and others used the term "physician assistant" to describe this new health care provider.[4] In 1965, Dr Stead was the first to create a PA program. Originally, he had hoped to convince the nursing community that his development of a nurse clinician program was a worthy cause. Unfortunately, the National League for Nursing, on three separate occasions, declined to accredit the program. Disillusioned by their rejection of his proposal, Dr Stead enlisted former Navy corpsmen into his PA program. His idea was to develop a curriculum based on clinical versus didactic training, an approach that would produce results much more quickly than traditional academic programs.[5] The PA medical training model ultimately utilized was similar to a program developed during World War II that fast-tracked the training of physicians.[4]

This was not a totally new concept even during World War II. Peter the Great introduced a group of medical assistants called "fel'dshers" into the Russian army around 1721.[6] By the 1790s, over 500,000 fel'dshers were providing care in rural areas of Russia. "Loblolly boys" were used by the British and US navies to assist surgeons as early as the 1800s.[6] Their job description was "to do anything and everything that was required—from sweeping and washing the deck and saying 'amen' to the chaplain, down to cleaning the guns and helping the surgeons to make pills and plasters and to mix medicine."[6] Loblolly boys were predecessors of today's Navy corpsmen.[6]

According to Dr James Mau, first administrator of the Duke PA Program, he and Dr Stead traveled to Fort Bragg, North Carolina, to observe the Army Special Forces medic training program in 1965. The physicians noted that these medics were trained well beyond the level of Navy corpsmen. The Special Forces medics were equipped to operate independently, supporting units in austere environments without the presence of a physician. Dr Stead was impressed by this course, and the experience influenced his development of the PA program at Duke University.[5]

Though it was not easy to implement, Dr Hudson's original 1961 proposal to train former military medics as PAs made sense as a cost-efficient way to meet the growing health care needs of the country and to employ veterans returning from Vietnam.[3] To further help cover the costs of the PA program, Dr Stead tied the educational curriculum into an existing grant for training hyperbaric chamber specialists.[7]

In 1965 Dr Mau also visited with Dr Amos Johnson in Garland, North Carolina. Dr Johnson regularly interacted with the Duke University medical community.[5] In the 1940s Dr Johnson had employed a young African American man, Henry Lee "Buddy" Treadwell, who he trained as his assistant. Treadwell performed physical exams, made diagnoses, and treated patients. By 1960, Treadwell was traveling regularly with patients to Duke University Medical Center and interacting with students and physicians. This was significant given the South remained segregated into the late 1960s. His role in the medical community was well known and respected. On the recommendation of Dr Mau, Duke eventually made Treadwell an honorary PA.[8]

During this period, Dr Smith, who had made a separate visit to Fort Bragg's Special Forces medic course, started his "MEDEX" (medicine extension) model, focusing on development and employment of graduates in medically underserved communities around the world, with 14 former military medics making up the first cohort. This program was not about creating a new health profession, but rather constituted a strategy to transform health care. Both Dr Stead and Dr Smith were greatly influenced by the Special Forces medic curriculum in creating their programs.[9]

On October 6, 1967, three of the four original Duke students graduated from the PA program with certificates of completion. These men were Victor H. Germino, Kenneth F. Ferrell, and Richard J. Scheele. Due to the fledgling nature of the profession, all three were hired by and remained at the Duke University Medical Center.[10]

Dr Myers disagreed in part with the educational philosophy of his counterparts Dr Stead and Dr Smith. Dr Myers believed that a degree was necessary to confer a sense of professionalism on this new career field. In 1968, he established the first baccalaureate degree-producing program at then Alderson Broaddus College (now a university) in Philippi, West Virginia. It quickly became clear that the federal government favored degree-producing schools, and the majority of new programs followed Dr Myers' lead.[3]

From 1968 to 1972, Duke hosted the first of four conferences to promote the PA profession, develop and standardize the curricula, and promote related legislation. The first graduates of Duke University's PA program established the American Academy of Physician Assistants (AAPA) in 1968 and incorporated the organization in North Carolina.[7] Its purpose was to serve as a national professional society to represent PAs in all areas of practice and promote the profession.[7] AAPA is now headquartered in the Carlyle area near Old Town Alexandria, Virginia.[7]

The 1970s: Beginnings

In 1971, the AMA passed a resolution to recognize PAs and began to develop national certification standards.[3] The same year, Dr Marvin

Gliedman, Dr Richard Rosen, and Clara Vanderbilt, Registered Physician Assistant–Certified (PA-C), established the first postgraduate residency in general surgery at Montefiore Medical Center, Bronx, New York. Later that year, Congress passed the Comprehensive Health Manpower Training Act of 1971, which included $4 million to establish PA educational programs.[7] At the same time, cartoonist Dick Moores' popular comic strip *Gasoline Alley* first introduced PAs to the public when leading character and former Vietnam-era Navy corpsman Chipper Wallet decided to become a PA.[11]

To garner support for the program, Dr Stead collaborated with AMA to develop an advertisement that ran in the July 30, 1971, issue of *Life Magazine* (Figure 1-1). Showing a young African American Vietnam veteran washing a car's windshield, the copy read: "This man belongs in a hospital. Or a doctor's office. Working alongside doctors, helping to care for patients." The advertisement copy related how for 2 years, this man was the first one on the battlefield to make decisions that could save the arms, legs, and lives of wounded service members in action. After serving his country, he could not get a job in medicine, like others with his skills. Not only did the advertisement describe the story of military medics, but it also informed the public of PA educational opportunities. The publicity effort was a powerful reminder to members of Congress about the sacrifices of America's medics, and led to support for educational funding of PA programs.

Also in 1971, Colonel Dwight F. Morse Jr wrote his US Army War College research paper on the initiation of an Army PA program. He based his concepts on the civilian programs, recognizing the shortage of physicians within the nation and military: "During recent years, the Army Medical Department has been progressively plagued with increasing losses of career medical officers by resignation or retirement."[12] His article described the impetus for the first military PA class, which was scheduled to begin the following year. At the time, Lieutenant Colonel Henry A. Robinson Jr, Medical Corps, was the acting program manager of the former Medical Field Service School at Fort Sam Houston, Texas (now the Medical Center of Excellence). Lieutenant Colonel Robinson led efforts to develop student prerequisites, curriculum, and utilization tours for those who graduated from the PA program. According to Morse, the PA was meant to fill a need to provide medical care to soldiers in their respective field units and to allow nurses to continue providing care within military medical treatment facilities (MTFs),

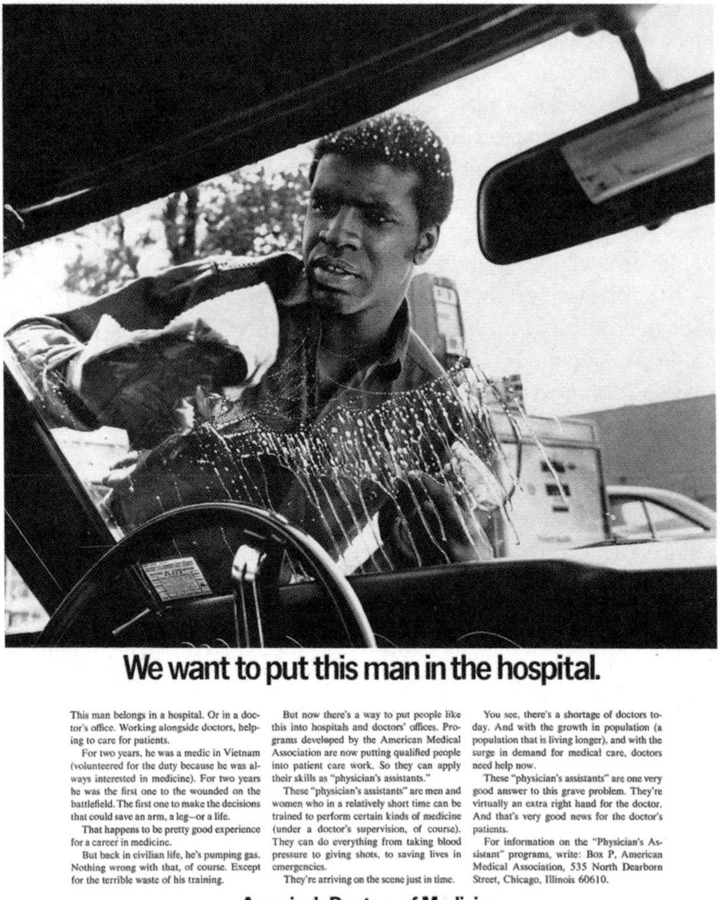

Figure 1-1. *Life Magazine* advertisement, July 30, 1971.

stating, "No plans exist at present for the assignment of the Army PA to duties in a hospital setting."[12] He concluded his paper by providing six recommendations to Army medical leaders:

(1) continual monitoring of civilian PA programs;
(2) involving all hospital staff at inpatient medical facilities in the education requirements of the Army PA program to maximize benefits;
(3) developing a marketing plan to ensure all involved understood the importance of PAs to Army medicine;
(4) urging physicians to utilize PAs in appropriate roles based on training and patient populations;
(5) developing further studies on the role of PAs within Army medicine; and
(6) conducting recurrent reviews to determine future extensions in the PA scope of practice.[12]

Up to this point, all the work of development and training in the profession had been conducted through universities with former US Army and Navy personnel. In 1971, the Air Force, under the direction of its surgeon general, Lieutenant General Alonzo A. Towner, was the first service to create a military PA program. Towner realized that the Air Force was not meeting medical needs in general and family medicine, and shortages could not be addressed through physician recruitment alone. To look into possible solutions to this problem, Towner created the Air Force Medical Services Health Manpower Utilization Study Committee. For the first time since 1966, the Air Force submitted a request to draft 150 medical professionals to cover this gap in active duty officers. Towner then requested that the committee establish a curriculum to train PAs to help fill the acute shortage in family medicine (email from John Heitz, US Air Force Medical Services History Office, Houston, TX, September 17, 2016).

The Navy and Army quickly followed suit. In 1973, the first Army PA class graduated (Figure 1-2), and its students became warrant officers. This initial class of Army PAs consisted of fifty-eight men and two women. Upon assignment, these graduates were designated "battalion surgeons" because of the lack of military physicians (general medical officers) within these units, therefore becoming first-line medical officers. Through their expertise, proximity to the troops, and respect earned within garrison and operational environments, they earned the affectionate designation of "doc."[5] Sergeant First Class Louis Rocco was a member of this first class. Rocco had gained fame in Vietnam while participating in a medevac mission as an Army medic. During

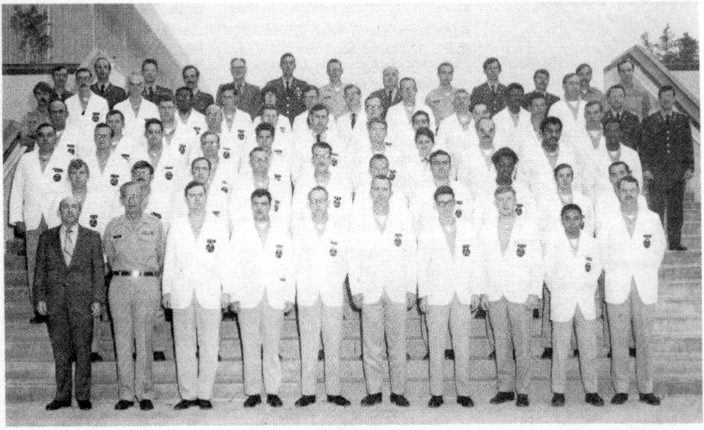

Warrant officer candidates attending the first class of the Physicians' Assistant Course, staff and faculty members include (from left, front) Dr. William G. Toland, Dean, Graduate School, Baylor University; Major General Kenneth D. Orr, Commanding General of Brooke Army Medical Center and Superintendent of AHSUSA; WOC's James O. Tanner, Benjamin N. Stewart, Dennis J. McCullough, De Leon Gunter, Roy D. Arian, Ray Barger Jr., Vincent Tenorio, David H. Jenkins, (second row) Hugh P. Hughes, Richard L. Curtis, Harold E. Slusher, Gerald E. Hults, Robert G. Hood, Joseph E. Swarts, Arthur Kyliavas, Harold B. Tyler Jr., William D. Long, Gary R. Herron, (third row) Daryl D. Butler, Harold W. Ward, David F. Duncan, James F. Madison, Louis R. Rocco, Harry M. Matthews Jr., Phillip O. Kerns, Ramona F. Deliz, George G. Strickler, Marvin H. Bruce, Milton Johnson, (fourth row) Don A. Johnson, Lawrence R. Williams Jr., Truman O. Thompson, Gilbert W. Coates, Howard L. Wells, Alvin R. Baccus, William H. Reinkins, Darvin D. Thomas, Jerry A. Massa and James L. Mountcastle; (fifth row) CPT Jerry J. Noren; WOC's John W. Hunt, Gordon E. Greentree, Clarence L. Thomas, Marshall E. Walker, Jo Ann E. Nick, Donald L. Edwards, Donald L. Spidel, Ernest C. Chastain, Walter E. Schofield, Johnny M. Brown Jr. and Joseph G. Obermire; CPT Joseph M. Long; CPT John Geesbreght; (back row) MAJ John Craig; MAJ Roger L. Christian; MAJ Dean Smith; CPT Peter B. Engber; Dr. Alton B. Lee, Baylor University; COL Henry A. Robinson Jr., Chief, Physicians' Assistant Branch, Medicine and Surgery Division, AHSUSA; COL Thomas C. Birk Jr.; LTC Joseph McNaney; CPT Stephen R. Uhlin; CPT Charles P. Cole; CPT Mark Langenfeld; MAJ George K. McMullan and CPT Henry S. Eden. Not shown is WOC Kurt M. Wyson.

Figure 1-2. Warrant officer candidates attending the first class of the Physician Assistant Course pose along with staff and faculty members. The photo appears to have been taken on the northern steps of the causeway between Willis and Aabel Halls.
US Army photo courtesy of the Medical Center of Excellence History Office.

a casualty evacuation mission, the UH-1H "Huey" helicopter Rocco was traveling in was shot down. Despite a fractured wrist, severe burns to his hands and body, and a badly injured hip and back, he carried several wounded crewmembers to safety while under enemy fire and was credited with saving their lives. For his bravery, Sergeant First Class Rocco received the Medal of Honor.[13]

In April 1972, the National Board of Medical Examiners (NBME) agreed to oversee development of the examination to certify PAs at the national level. The same year, the National Commission on Certification of Physician Assistants (NCCPA) was founded by 14 national health care organizations to oversee eligibility and standards for the NBME examination. Formally recognized as a nonprofit group, NCCPA's purpose was and continues to be providing certifying examinations for new PA graduates and recertifying examinations for licensed PAs. The NBME appointed an advisory committee and task force to construct a blueprint for test committees, which eventually became the examination administered by the NCCPA.[14] During early versions of the testing, the candidate was required to perform hands-on testing in addition to a challenging written exam. PA programs varied in recognition from awarding certificates to conferring college degrees. The first civilian PAs to receive baccalaureate degrees graduated in 1972.[15] The first Army PAs graduated in 1973, earning certificates, and in 1985 the first Army PAs received baccalaureate degrees from University of Oklahoma Health Science Center.

In 1975, the Army determined that enough PAs were on active duty to fulfill primary care requirements and terminated its program. Within 3 years, another shortage ensued, and the Army surgeon general ordered the program restarted. Due to a lack of funding, however, the Army contracted with the Air Force to send students to Sheppard Air Force Base, Texas, for training. In September 1979, the Army resumed its program at Fort Sam Houston.[15]

In 1976, a group of former Army PAs stationed at Fort Hood, Texas, started a civilian organization to represent Army PAs. The first recorded meeting for the Society of Army Physician Assistants (SAPA) was held on September 24, 1976. In 1980, the first annual SAPA PA refresher course was held in Fayetteville, North Carolina. The annual conference continues to be held in Fayetteville, and today the organization has an average active membership of around 466.[16]

The 1980s: Combat Tested and Valued Members of the Army Medical Team

In 1980 and 1981, the Army began specialty programs for PAs in orthopedics, cardiovascular perfusion, emergency medicine, occupational medicine, and aviation medicine.[5] These programs continue today, with the addition of general surgery training. The first Army PAs deployed into combat with the 82nd Airborne Division (ABN DIV) and the 1st and 2nd Ranger battalions, proving their worth during fierce fighting in support of Operation Urgent Fury. Though operations in Grenada were brief, several medical units that included PAs provided critical care to soldiers and civilians, treating their wounds and getting them safely away from the battlefield (email from Major [Retired] Jimmie E. Keller, former PA consultant to the Army surgeon general, Highlands Ranch, CO, November 17, 2015).

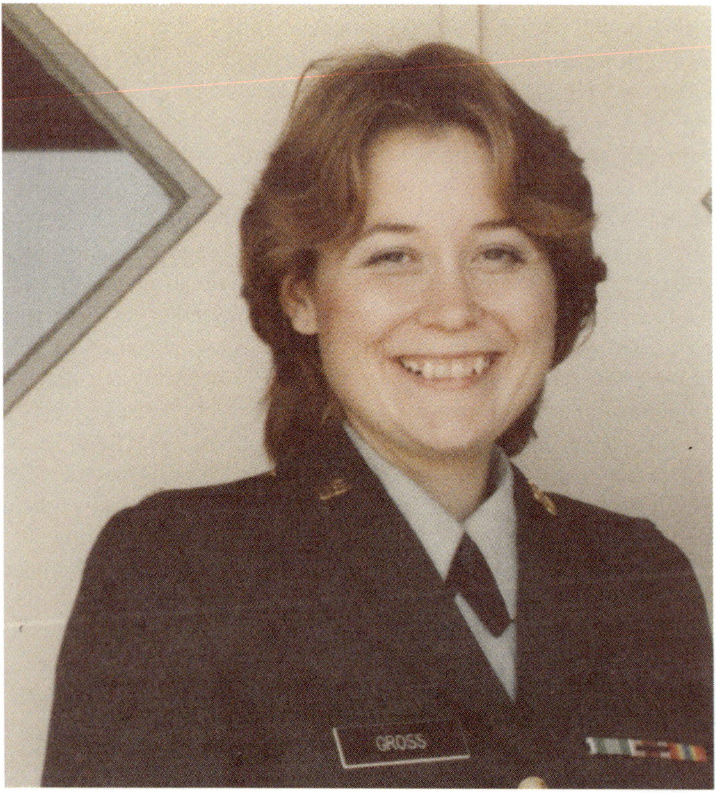

Figure 1-3. Chief Warrant Officer 2 Pauline Gross deployed to Palmerola Air Force Base in Honduras with the Joint Task Force-Bravo Medical Element as a physician assistant and surgical technician. As of this writing, now Colonel (Retired) Gross is the longest serving PA in the US Army Medical Department. She was appointed the Army Installation Management Command Surgeon in 2015. Photograph courtesy of Colonel (Retired) Pauline Gross.

On Mother's Day in 1986, Chief Warrant Officer 2 Pauline Gross (Figure 1-3) was deployed to Palmerola Air Force Base in Honduras to support Operation Golden Pheasant with the Joint Task Force (JTF)-Bravo Medical Element. The purpose of this operation was to disrupt the Contra supply chain during the Iran-Contra affair. The JTF-Bravo Medical Element included veterinarians, dentists, public health nurses, force protection officers, orthopedic surgeons, general surgeons, and family practice/internal medicine physicians, who traveled to different villages, providing sick call and sexually transmitted disease clinics for the troops as well as providing care for the local population outside the gates. Because of her prior operating room experience, PA Gross also worked in the surgical suite assisting the surgeons with emergency procedures. She previously served in the Women's Army Corps. In 2018 Colonel Gross retired as the Installation Management Command surgeon (Figure 1-4), earning the distinction of being the longest serving active duty PA in the Army,

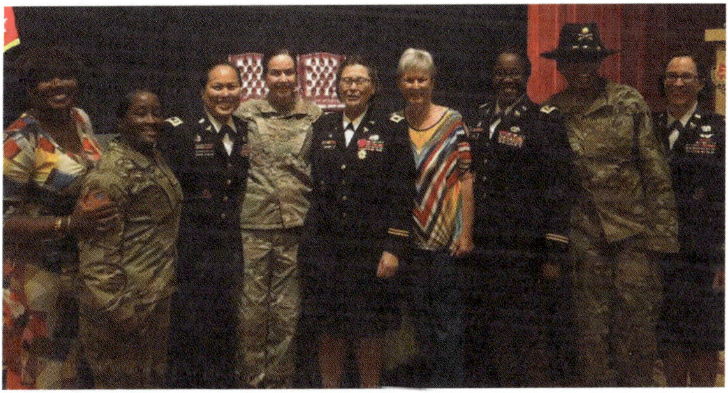

Figure 1-4. On June 15, 2018, Colonel Pauline Gross celebrated her retirement with fellow female Army physician assistants (left to right): Lieutenant Colonel (Retired) Rhonda Wynder, Lieutenant Colonel Sharon Denson, Lieutenant Colonel Amelia Duran-Stanton, Lieutenant Colonel Lauris Trimble, Colonel (Retired) Pauline Gross, Colonel (Retired) Sherry Morrey, Major Lakeshia Logan, Major Adhana McCarthy, and Colonel Dawn Orta.
Photograph courtesy of Lieutenant Colonel Amelia Duran-Stanton.

having served as an enlisted soldier, noncommissioned officer, warrant officer, and commissioned officer.

In 1984, Major (then Chief Warrant Officer 3) Jimmie Keller (Figure 1-5) became the first Army PA assigned to the White House Medical Unit. During his 4-year tour, he traveled to 35 states and 22 foreign countries to prepare for and support presidential and vice presidential travels. This included the travel of families, staff, Secret Service, and the traveling press corps. Military PAs remain the primary care providers within the White House clinic and support the staff and government workers in the White House compound (see Chapter 60 for information on the White House Medical Unit). Major Keller said his most memorable event was planning for and supporting the summits between President Ronald Reagan and Soviet General Secretary Mikhail Gorbachev in Geneva, Iceland, Moscow, and Washington, DC (email from Major [Retired] Jim E. Keller, PA-C, former PA consultant to the Army surgeon general, Highlands Ranch, CO, November 20, 2015).

In December 1989, in support of Operation Just Cause, several PAs deployed once again with the 82nd ABN DIV and the 75th Ranger Regiment to Panama in order to remove General Manuel Noriega from power. They parachuted into a hot Panamanian swamp in the middle of the night a few kilometers from the target, Torrijos International Airport, which was held by the Panamanian Defense Forces. While parachuting and upon landing, the paratroopers could see green tracer rounds coming at them from three different directions. Working through the marsh, then Chief Warrant Officer 3 Bob Oyler, PA-C, of the 82nd ABN DIV, finally hit solid ground and crawled out onto dry land. Under the light of a half-moon, he saw a fence. Reaching underneath, he found an 18-inch gap. Sliding his rucksack through the hole, Oyler began to crawl under the fence. Unfortunately, he had forgotten to remove his pistol belt, and his ammunition pouches got caught in the fence. As he struggled to get free, he heard voices speaking Spanish right above him. With the enemy virtually standing over him, Oyler managed to undo his belt and pull his weapon. The enemy failed to notice him and talked for a few moments but moved away in the other direction, and into a Ranger ambush. Oyler freed himself and proceeded to the assembly area. He was the first medic to arrive on the scene, and it had taken him 93 minutes to get there (email from Captain [Retired] Robert J. Oyler, PA-C, Headquarters

Company, 307th Medical Battalion, 82nd Airborne Division, Saint Pauls, NC, December 21, 2015).

The 1990s: Finally Commissioned

Though one of the first services to produce graduates from PA training, the Army was the last to commission them. Air Force PAs were first

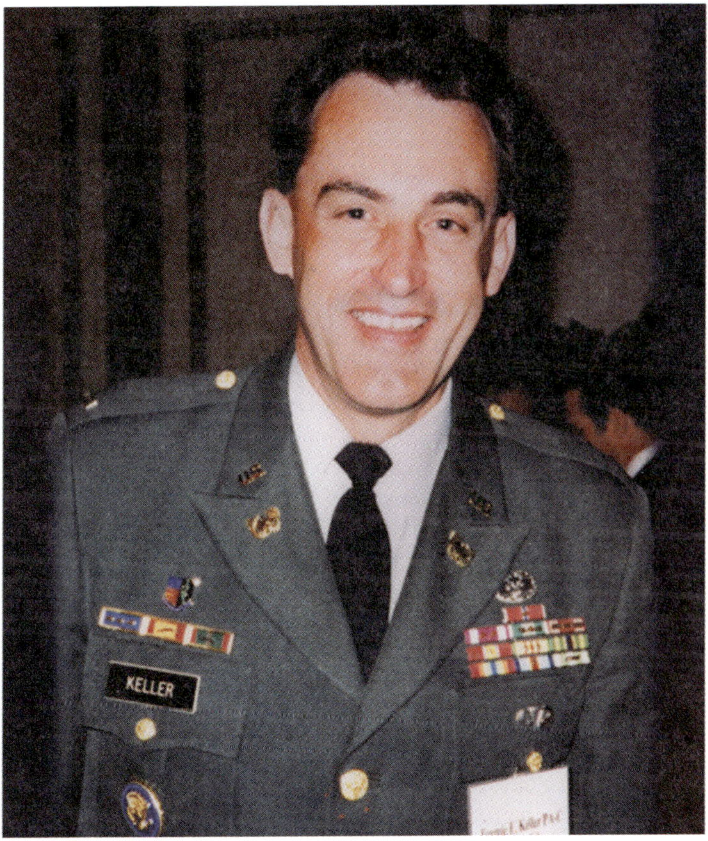

Figure 1-5. Then-Major Jimmie Keller, first Army physician assistant assigned to White House Medical Unit.
Photograph courtesy of Major (Retired) Jimmie Keller.

commissioned in 1978 and Navy graduates were commissioned in 1989.[17] A 1984 study found that PAs provided care to 79% of patients seen by primary care physicians at half the cost. The Defense Audit Task Force on Non-Physician Health Care Providers recommended to Congress that all military PAs be commissioned officers.[17] The SAPA was critical to the lobbying effort for commissioning. Despite Congress' desire to commission Army PAs, it was not until 1990 that a proposal to do so was approved by the Army chief of staff. A year later the defense authorization bill included funding for commissioning PAs, authorized the inclusion of Army PAs in the Army Medical Specialist Corps (AMSC), and created a fourth assistant chief of the AMSC to supervise the PA section.[18]

Through diligent staff work, SAPA and AAPA involvement, and congressional influence, senior PA leadership garnered the support of Lieutenant General (Retired) Frank Ledford, the Army surgeon general, for PA commissioning (Figure 1-6). Ledford and others (including PA consultant Major [Retired] Jimmie Keller) convinced key Army leaders, including the chief of staff of the Army, General Carl Vuono, future chief of staff General Gordon Sullivan, and the deputy chief of staff for personnel, Al Ono, to persuade Secretary of the Army Michael P.W. Stone to commission Army PAs. Despite ongoing officer force reductions, given the need for midlevel providers to support readiness of the force, the first Army PA commissioning ceremony occurred on February 4, 1992.[18] Across the globe, the Army commissioned 257 PAs, changing their rank from warrant officers to second lieutenant through major. In 2007, the US Public Health Service was the first, and remains the only, federal service organization to promote PAs to the rank of flag officer with the promotion of Captain Michael Milner to the rank of rear admiral.[19]

In December 1990, during Operation Desert Storm, eight physicians and four PAs were attached to the regimental clearing station for the 2nd Armored Cavalry Regiment (ACR). The job of the 2nd ACR was to spearhead the VII Corps' end-run deep into the Iraqi Republican Guard's Tawakalna Division, which ended with US forces decimating the Iraqis in the famed Battle of 73 Easting. The operation required quick movement and a mobile facility to treat casualties. The PAs also needed options for evacuating casualties from the battlefield. With air evacuation and ground options unsupported, medical staff had to be creative. Medics acquired two old Saudi National Guard buses and,

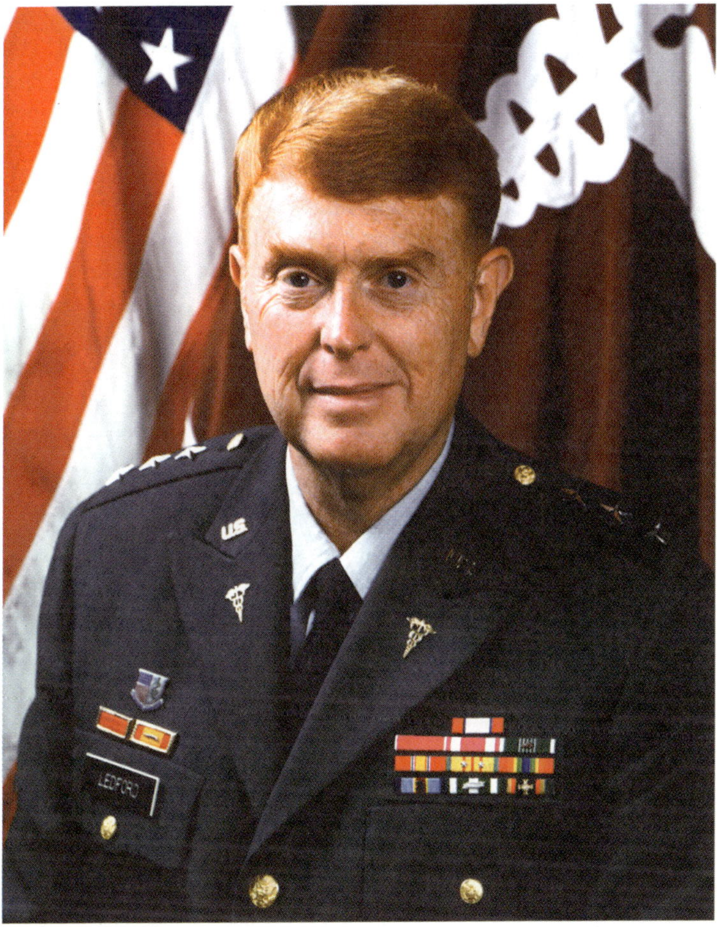

Figure 1-6. Lieutenant General (Retired) Frank F. Ledford Jr, 37th surgeon general of the US Army. Lieutenant General Ledford died on May 15, 2019.

with the help of maintenance troops and some scrap metal, converted these buses into mobile MTFs that would, supposedly, follow the battle and treat and remove casualties as needed. The buses were named the *Comfortless* and the *Merciless* after the Navy's medical ships, the USS *Comfort* and USS *Mercy*. On February 24, 1991, the buses crossed into Iraq. Unfortunately, just a few miles across the border, the brake line ruptured on the *Merciless* and it had to be abandoned. The *Comfortless* continued on, and in the course of the next 4 days, PAs treated approximately 60 wounded soldiers and civilians as the bus made its way across the desert. On February 28, the day the cease-fire went into effect, the *Comfortless* crossed the border back into Kuwait. Ingenuity and teamwork made this mission a success (Figure 1-7).[20]

Chief Warrant Officer 2 Thomas F. Haigler, who was assigned to the 2nd ACR, stated that the biggest concern early on was the estimated casualty count. "It was estimated that 220 casualties would come from a squadron of 1,200, including 40 men who were expected to die. We were expecting to lose one of our tanks for every four of theirs. We faced not only conventional weapons but also the very real threat of chemical weapons."[21] However, there were few American or coalition casualties during the conflict, and the 2nd ACR (like the majority of US medical personnel) spent most of its efforts treating enemy prisoners of war.[21]

In support of Operations Desert Shield and Desert Storm, over 230 PAs saw action in 1991; of these, 12 were women, and they deployed

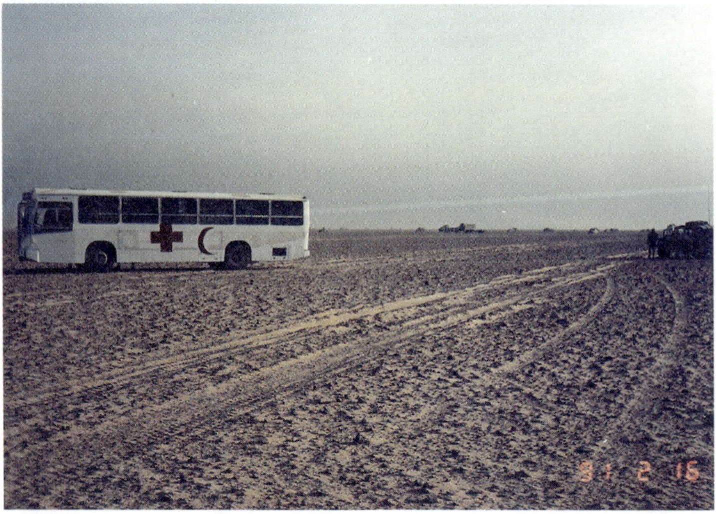

Figure 1-7. The *Comfortless*, in the Kuwaiti desert, 1991.
Photograph courtesy of Colonel John Balser.

across the battlefield. Chief Warrant Officer Karen K. Kelso deployed with the 3rd ACR. At the time, she was a 49-year-old grandmother; her second grandchild was born during her deployment. About a career spent supporting soldiers, Kelso remarked, "I fell in love with soldiers . . . It was amazing to me that they were willing to give their lives."[22] To meet the large number of PAs needed to support these operations, the Army recalled retired PAs to active duty for the first time, including Vietnam veteran Chief Warrant Officer 2 Louis Rocco.[13]

PAs continued serving with distinction throughout the 1990s. Chief Warrant Officer 3 William "Doc" Donovan was a legend in both the PA and Special Operations communities. In 1980, Donovan served as chief medic during the failed attempt to rescue the hostages in Iran. Among the hostages was Don Hohman, an Army medic on the embassy staff, who later went on to graduate from the PA program in 1984 (personal communication, Chief Warrant Officer 3 [Retired], William "Doc" Donovan, Atlanta, GA, August 25, 2015).

In 1991, Chief Warrant Officer 3 Louis "Lou" Smith III (Figure 1-8) was assigned to the 5th Special Forces Group when the 1st Battalion, 75th Ranger Regiment, conducted a combat parachute training mission into Kuwait. According to Smith, during high winds, the unit "evacuated some 40 guys off the drop zone." Two days later, "Doc" Donovan hobbled into Smith's aid station with a broken foot. Donovan had been blown off course during the jump and walked over 20 miles on his injured foot (personal communication, Colonel [Retired] Louis H. Smith III, Andrew Rader US Army Health Clinic, Fort Myer, VA, January 5, 2016).

In 1992, Donovan earned the Soldier's Medal for Heroism after he and two others rowed a Zodiac boat continuously for 4 hours in near-freezing weather to save fellow Rangers from drowning after a helicopter crash during a training mission in Utah. In 1999, Donovan, who had served in Vietnam and as well as multiple operations including Eagle Claw, Urgent Fury, Just Cause, Desert Storm, and Restore Hope, became the first PA to be inducted into the US Army Ranger Hall of Fame.[23]

After the Gulf War, the federal government began mandatory force reductions, which led to the consolidation of the military's PA programs. In 1995, the Army PA program was renamed and reflagged as the Interservice PA Program (IPAP), based at Fort Sam Houston, with an effective date of May 1996. Today, this program matriculates

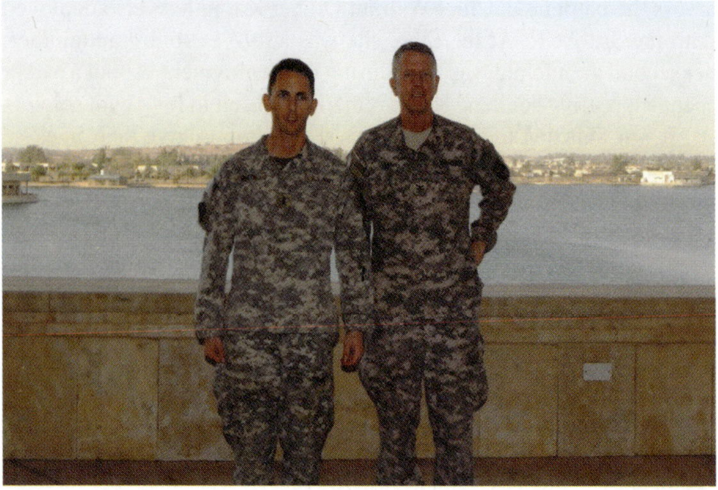

Figure 1-8. Colonel Louis H. Smith III, the third physician assistant chief, and son then-First Lieutenant Chris Smith at former Iraqi President Saddam Hussein's palace in Baghdad, Iraq. Chris was serving as a field artillery officer and Louis was present to promote him to captain. Then-Captain Chris Smith later also became a physician assistant through the Interservice Physician Assistant Program.
Photograph courtesy of Major Chris Smith.

students from the Army, Air Force, Navy, and Coast Guard, with the majority of IPAP students being Army active duty, Reserve, and National Guard. Recently the program was lengthened from 24 to 29 months. Currently, students attend a 16-month didactic phase (Phase 1) followed by a 13-month clinical phase (Phase 2) at one of 23 military MTFs (see Chapter 38 for more information on IPAP). The program's vision is "to be recognized as the world-class leader in physician assistant education,"[24] and in 2019 the IPAP was ranked 10th out of 170 US PA programs by *US News and World Report*.[25]

On October 2, 1995, Sergeant First Class Robert Howes, who was attending the Special Forces Advanced Noncommissioned Officer Course, helped prevent further deaths during a dawn sniper attack at Fort Bragg that resulted in the death of one officer and wounding of 18 soldiers. Sergeant First Class Howes, along with three other Special

Forces noncommissioned officers, was doing a physical training run nearby and heard the shots. They diverted to help subdue the shooter, and Howes was wounded in the foot. While at Womack Army Hospital, he was visited by the Fort Bragg senior PA, Major Michael Robertson, and asked what he wanted to do in the Army. Howes stated he wanted to go to PA school. He applied and was admitted to the IPAP, and served as a PA in the 1st Battalion, 36th Infantry Regiment, in Friedberg, Germany, and in Iraq, then attended training to become an orthopedic PA. He retired from military service at Brooke Army Medical Center (BAMC), on November 10, 2011, culminating his military career as the Army orthopedic PA residency director, and retired from BAMC as a civilian orthopedic PA in 2016 (email from Lieutenant Colonel David L. Hamilton, commander, Public Health Command District–Fort Bragg, Fort Bragg, NC, November 20, 2015, and personal conversation, Lieutenant Colonel Amelia Duran-Stanton, deputy chief, Thermal and Mountain Medicine Division, Natick, MA, October 4, 2016).

Early 21st Century: Battle Hardened

Army PAs remain the backbone of soldier readiness and frontline care. Following the attacks of September 11, 2001, and the beginning of the conflicts in Iraq and Afghanistan, Army PAs found themselves overworked and understrength. The Army PA became the most deployed AMEDD officer. Demand for the total force of PAs continues to outstrip inventory. Today, the Army has 778 active duty PA authorizations with an inventory of 683 active duty PAs, including those in the process of retiring and those attending graduate-level education. The significant delta in inventory versus authorizations is being addressed with a multipronged approach including mentorship, use of talent management principles, increased active duty accessions, increased IPAP starts, and reinstitution of the health professions officer retention bonus. The Army's PA total force also includes 393 Reserve 65Ds (the PA area of concentration), 942 National Guard 65Ds, and 352 civilian PAs. With the active duty force, this totals 2,461 PAs serving the nation. Collectively, Army PAs have conducted 1,129 combat tours for a total of 9,278 months. The average combat tour is 12 months. Individually, Army PAs averaged 21.6 months, or 1.75 combat tours per PA. Many PAs in these conflicts have been deployed for a total of 3 to 4 years (email communication, Major Nicholas Bradley, PA-C,

65D assignment officer, Human Resource Command, Fort Knox, KY, February 9, 2017).

In February 2001, Lieutenant Colonel (Retired) Donald Parsons, a retired Army PA (Figure 1-9) and combat medical specialist training instructor at AMEDD Center and School, became concerned that Regular Army units were not following the guidance developed by the Committee on Tactical Combat Casualty Care (CoTCCC) on the training of first responders and Army medics despite the success of this training and implementation seen within the special operations community. Before the establishment of CoTCCC, military medicine had employed training doctrine that was more in line with care of

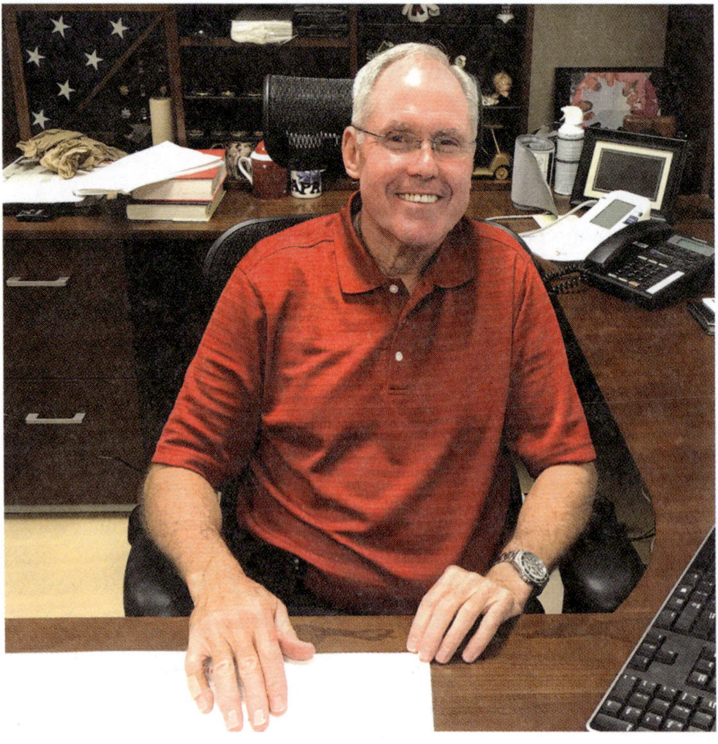

Figure 1-9. Lieutenant Colonel (Retired) Donald Parsons. Photograph courtesy of Don Parsons.

civilian trauma patients. This doctrine failed to fully recognize the unique challenges of providing care within austere environments, with medical personnel caring for injured at night or under enemy fire, while moving patients through long evacuation corridors. Parsons participated in numerous discussions with special operations medical personnel and became a member of the Committee on Tactical Combat Casualty Care (CoTCCC). The CoTCCC had been established in 2001 as a US Special Operations Command biomedical research effort to ensure that emerging technology and information is incorporated into the TCCC guidelines on an ongoing basis. The membership of the CoTCCC includes combat medics, corpsmen, pararescue jumpers, physicians, and PAs.[26]

As a former 18D (Special Forces medic), Parsons understood the training of Special Operations medics and was intrigued by the 75th Ranger Regiment's success at treating combat injuries, including a successful bleeding (hemorrhage) control kit that was attached to every Ranger's body armor. The kit was developed by a team that included then-Captain John F. Detro, an Army Ranger PA, who provided an example of the kit to Parsons. The original Ranger kit included a tourniquet, trauma dressing, a nasopharyngeal airway, a 14-gauge catheter for needle decompression, an oral antibiotic/analgesic pill pack, an intravenous starter kit, surgical tape, and gloves. This kit evolved into today's Individual First Aid Kit (IFAK), which has been issued to every soldier during Operation Enduring Freedom, Operation Iraqi Freedom, and other overseas contingency operations. The IFAK's contents, like the Ranger's kit, are focused on the three leading causes of preventable death: airway compromise, tension pneumothorax, and extremity exsanguination (personal conversation, Lieutenant Colonel John F. Detro, physician assistant consultant to the surgeon general, Falls Church, VA, January 5, 2016).

In 2003, Captain James Rice and fellow PAs developed a rough draft for a predeployment trauma course designed to prepare frontline PAs for combat. Eventually called the Tactical Combat Medical Care (TCMC) Course, the training was developed using principles of Tactical Combat Casualty Care to teach PAs the techniques required to treat preventable causes of battlefield death. The TCMC gained the Army surgeon general's approval and was first offered in April 2004. Shortly afterward, other medical providers began to attend the course. Today, the priority for attendance includes providers deploying to Roles 1 and 2 combat assignments.[27]

The United States again invaded Iraq in 2003, commencing Operation Iraqi Freedom. Many PAs stationed at military MTFs across the United States were deployed to support operations in theater, and many of these facilities were left without critical support. To provide adequate coverage for dependents, retired PAs were recalled to active duty for the second time. Recall was restricted to those still actively practicing medicine and included fill for 30 to 60 positions, with plans to recall more if the situation deteriorated (email from Major [Retired] Jim E. Keller, former PA consultant to the Army surgeon general, Highlands Ranch, CO, November 20, 2015).

On March 4, 2005, the first Army PA was killed in combat. Six months after Captain Sean Grimes deployed to Iraq, an improvised explosive device detonated near his convoy outside Ramadi, killing Grimes and three others. Grimes was the first PA killed on the battlefield in Iraq. At Fort Campbell, his home post, a training center at Blanchfield Army Community Hospital has been named for Grimes. His family used part of Grimes' life insurance money to establish an educational scholarship award through SAPA (email from Major Shawn Lockett, deputy division surgeon, 2nd Infantry Division, Beijing, China, September 27, 2016). SAPA provides three annual $1,000 Grimes scholarships to SAPA members and their beneficiaries (Figure 1-10).

In 2006, then-Major Leonard Gruppo, director of the Army's emergency medicine PA (EMPA) residency program, proposed a doctorate-level clinical training program for specialty PAs. The goal was to produce specialized PAs with a substantially higher level of clinical competency. This increased capability could then be forward deployed with units on the battlefield. The EMPA program, which had started in July 2005, was expanded from 12 to 18 months, and the first class graduated with a Doctor of Science in Physician Assistant Studies–Emergency Medicine from Baylor University on December 15, 2007. These PAs became the first in the nation to earn clinical doctorate degrees. Since this first graduation, the Army has developed similar doctorate programs in clinical orthopedics and clinical general surgery/intensivist.[28]

As the US footprint in Afghanistan began downsizing in 2009, Combat Outpost (COP) Keating was one of many forward operating bases being closed. The enemy was anticipating the closure, and on October 3, 400 Taliban troops launched a brutal attack on COP

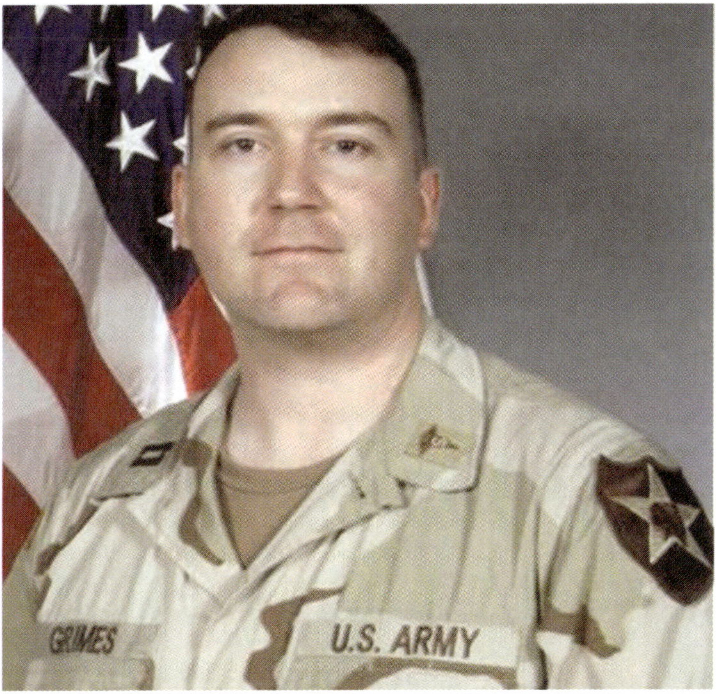

Figure 1-10. Captain Sean Grimes.

Keating. Intense fighting continued for more than 12 hours. A team of medics, led by PA Captain Christopher Cordova, Headquarters Troop, 3rd Squadron, 61st Cavalry Regiment, 4th Brigade Combat Team, 4th Infantry Division, cared for the injured and helped defend the COP. Under heavy fire and with medevac support unavailable, Cordova and his team treated traumatic battle wounds and evacuated 16 Afghan soldiers and US personnel while providing aid to another 27 "walking wounded." In an event that continued for 84 hours, Cordova successfully led his team and provided continuous medical support to soldiers at the base. In recognition of his actions over those long days, Cordova earned the Silver Star for gallantry in action against an armed enemy (Figure 1-11).[29]

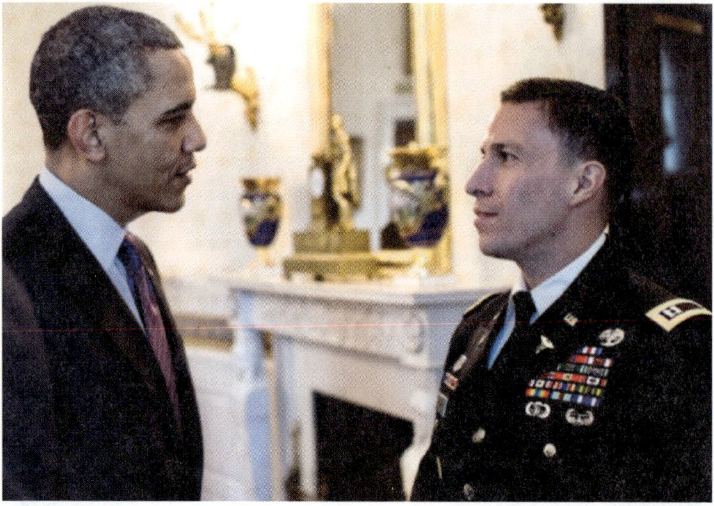

Figure 1-11. Then-Captain Christopher Cordova meeting with President Barack Obama.
Photograph courtesy of Major (Retired) Christopher Cordova.

Continuing Progress

In 2015, Major Saibatu Mansaray-Knight, PA-C, was designated as the Army military aide to the vice president of the United States (Figure 1-12). "This prestigious position is usually held by a line officer, such as an infantry officer or pilot," said Lieutenant Colonel James J. Jones, PhD, PA-C, deputy director and chief of protective medicine, White House Medical Unit. "It's not a medical role at all—which makes her appointment unique."[30] Another historic first was when Colonel John Balser (Figure 1-13) became the first PA to be selected as chief of the AMSC (email from Colonel Nikki Butler, Human Resources Command, Fort Knox, KY, January 19, 2016).

Many assignments traditionally limited to male PAs have now been opened to women. Several women have served in civil affairs units: Major Charisse Gonzalez served as the company commander for the Joint Special Operations Medical Training Center, and recently Major Katrina Monti became the senior PA, 1st Special Forces Group (email from Lieutenant Colonel John Elliott, US Special Operations Command, Fort Bragg, NC, March 15, 2020).

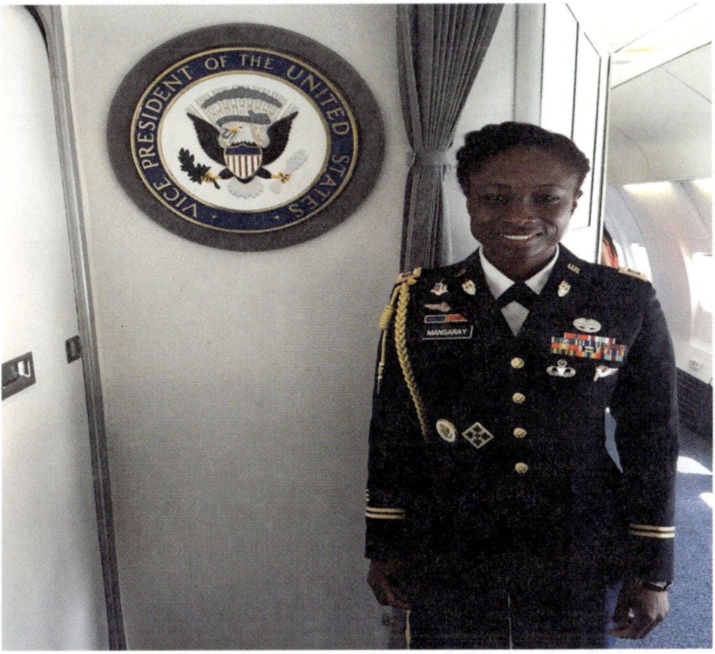

Figure 1-12. Then-Major Saibatu Mansaray-Knight during her tenure as Vice President Biden's Army military aide.
Photograph courtesy of Major (Retired) Saibatu Mansaray-Knight.

Currently, there are five PAs serving in brigade-level commands, eight in battalion-level commands, and one as a forward surgical team (FST) commander. There are two PAs who formerly served in brigade-level commands, eleven in battalion-level commands, and eight as FST commanders. In April 2019, Colonel Amy L. Jackson became the first PA to be promoted to colonel "below the zone," and on July 20, 2020, with the change of command ceremony at Keller Army Community Hospital, West Point, New York (Figure 1-14), she became the first female PA to command a level-1 military MTF.[31] "Below the zone" refers to early promotion, before the usual, expected time for consideration. These promotions "are intended to provide officers of exceptional ability an opportunity to advance quickly to more responsible positions, help retain high-quality officers, and give officers an incentive to perform at their highest potential."[32 (p19)]

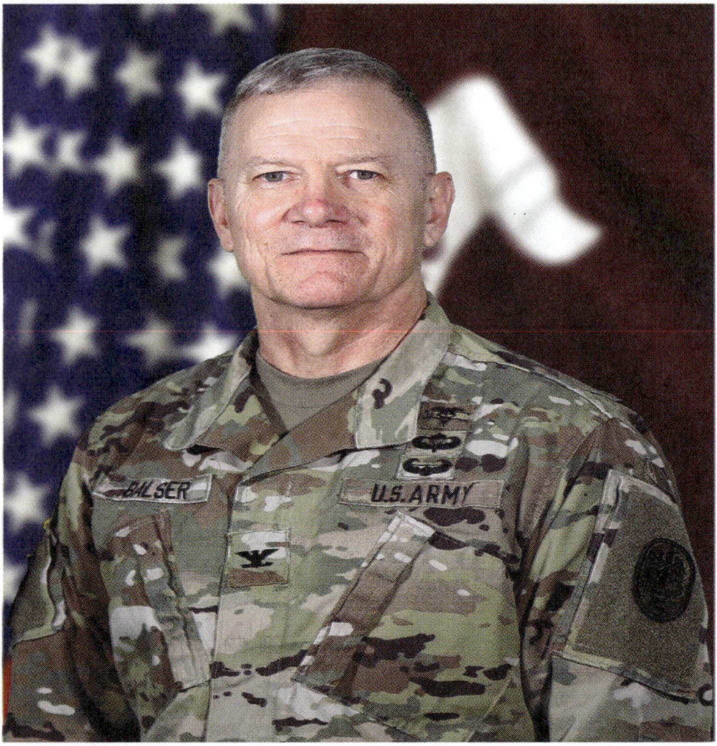

Figure 1-13. Colonel John Balser, Army Medical Specialist Corps chief. Photograph courtesy of Colonel John Balser.

On February 26, 2020, the Centers for Disease Control and Prevention reported the first case of the spread of the novel coronavirus disease (COVID-19) within the United States. The disease was first recognized in Wuhan, China, and the first US patient had recently returned from China. The ensuing global pandemic led to the activation of active and reserve military forces to support civilian authorities to battle COVID-19. Several Army PAs were instrumental in the early efforts, including Colonel David Hamilton, commander of the 9th Hospital Center, which was set up within New York City's Javits Center to take on non-COVID patients to decrease pressure on the city's health care system (Figure 1-15). Within a few days, the team began and continues

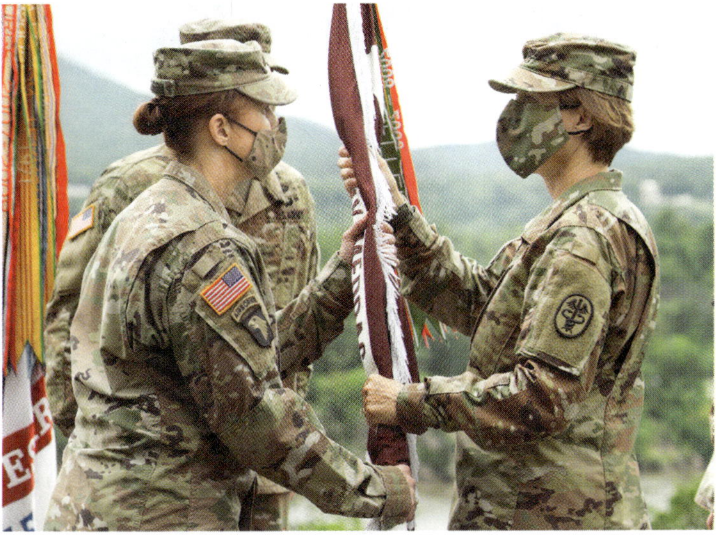

Figure 1-14. Colonel Amy L. Jackson's change of command ceremony at Keller Army Community Hospital, West Point, New York, on July 10, 2020. Brigadier General Paula C. Lodi (right), commanding general, Regional Health Command–Atlantic, passes the Medical Activity West Point flag to Colonel Amy L. Jackson, signifying the change of command from Colonel Brett H. Venable to Colonel Jackson. Photo by John Pellino/USMA PAO.
Reproduced from: Lanier RK. WPHSA, CACH welcomes new commander. *Pointer View.* Published July 23, 2020. Accessed August 4, 2020. http://www.pointerview.com/2020/07/23/wphsa-kach-welcomes-new-commander/

to take on COVID-19 patients (email from Colonel David Hamilton, April 14, 2020). As of July 30, 2020, the global number of infections was 17,067,754 cases, with 667,935 deaths. Within the United States, there were 4,431,399 infected and 150,765 deaths.[33] As the fight to contain the virus attests, military PAs have been and will continue to be at the forefront of military medicine, whether supporting combat or humanitarian missions.

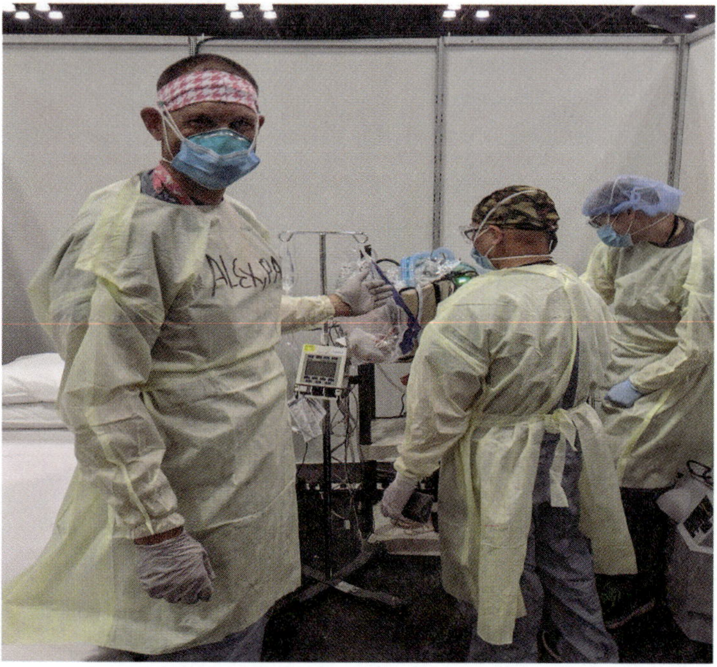

Figure 1-15. Captain Alex Merkle providing medical care to COVID-19 patients at the Javits Center, New York City.
Photograph courtesy of Lieutenant Colonel Terry "Lee" Clark.

Conclusion

Today's Army PA is not only a clinician, but also a leader. Several PAs have served in command roles, senior clinical positions, and administrative leadership roles throughout Army and military medicine. Army PAs are seasoned veterans with years of service. By drawing on their experiences, PAs can lead in both tactical and clinical settings. Today's soldiers continue to pave the way for future Army PA and AMSC leaders. The future of the Army PA is bright, and the potential is limitless. As Colonel John Balser frequently states, "PAs are the chameleons of the AMEDD, able to adjust to any mission, anywhere, at any time" (email from Colonel John E. Balser, Command Surgeon, US Army Reserve Headquarters, Fort Bragg, NC, January 20, 2016).

References

1. Carter R. Dr. Eugene A. Stead, Jr, MD. Physician Assistant History Society website. Accessed July 30, 2020. http://www.pahx.org/stead-jr-eugene
2. Hudson CL. Expansion of medical professional services with nonprofessional personnel. *JAMA*. 1961;176(10):839–841.
3. Carter R. Physician assistant history. *Physician Assistant Hist Soc*. 2001;12(2):130–132. Accessed July 30, 2020. https://pahx.org/wp-content/uploads/2016/12/Military-Ranks.pdf
4. Cawley JF, Cawthon E, Hooker RS. Origins of the physician assistant movement in the United States. *JAAPA*. 2012;25(12):36–40,42.
5. Physician Assistant History Society. Oral history interviews: Estes & Mau, 2007. Accessed July 30, 2020. http://pahx.org/oral-history-interviews-estes-mau
6. Jolly R. *Health Workforce: A Case For Physician Assistants?* Parliamentary Library (Australia); March 27, 2008. Accessed July 21, 2020. https://apo.org.au/node/1556
7. Carter RD, Strand J. Physician assistants. A young profession celebrates the 35th anniversary of its birth in North Carolina. *N C Med J*. 2000;61(5):249–256.
8. Carter RD, Clark T. Amos Johnson, MD, and Mr. Henry Lee "Buddy" Treadwell: A prototypical MD/PA practice. Physician Assistant History Society website. Accessed July 30, 2020. https://pahx.org/pdf/BuddyTreadwell.pdf
9. Ballweg R, Wick KH. MEDEX Northwest: workforce innovations, 40th anniversary issue. *J Physician Assistant Educ*. 2007;18(3):30–39.
10. Carter R. Victor H. Germino, Jr, PA-C. Physician Assistant History Society website. Accessed June 24, 2020. http://www.pahx.org/germino-victor-h

11. Carter R. Marketing the physician assistant concept to the American public: The Bold Ones TV episode and Gasoline Alley comic strip. Physician Assistant History Society website. Accessed July 30, 2020. https://pahx.org/wp-content/uploads/2016/11/Marketing-the-Physician-Assistant-Concept-to-the-American-Public.pdf

12. Morse DF Jr. *Some Considerations in the Development of a Physicians' Assistant Program in the U.S. Army*. Army War College; 1971.

13. Oral history interview with CW2 Louis R. Rocco. US Army Medical Department, Office of Medical History website. Accessed July 20, 2020. http://ameddregiment.amedd.army.mil/moh/bios/roccoInt.html

14. National Commission on Certification of Physician Assistants. About us: purpose and passion. Accessed July 21, 2020. https://www.nccpa.net?About

15. Hooker RD, Carter R, Cawley JF. The National Commission on Certification of Physician Assistants: history and role. *NCCPA Special Issue*. Accessed on July 30, 2020. https://pahx.org/wp-content/uploads/2016/12/NCCPA_History_Article.pdf

16. Potter B. SAPA history. Society of Army Physician Assistants website. Accessed July 30, 2020. http://www.sapa.org/resources/webpages/history/html

17. Colver JE, Blessing D, Hinojosa J. Military physician assistants: their background and education. *J Physician Assistant Educ.* 2007;18(3):40–45.

18. Oland DD, Hogan DW Jr. US Army Center of Military History. Department of the Army historical summary, FY 1992, chapter 7. Updated July 21, 2003. Accessed July 30, 2020. https://history.army.mil/books/DAHSUM/1992/ch07.htm

19. Rear Admiral Michael Milner. Public Health Service PA is first promoted to rear admiral. Physician Assistant History Society website. Accessed July 20, 2020. https://pahx.org/gallery/rear-admiral-michael-milner

20. Eliason MC. The saga of the Comfortless. *US Army Med Dept J.* 1992; Mar-Apr:PB 8-92-3/4.

21. Haigler TF. Operation Desert Storm—a PA's perspective. *US Army Med Dept J.* 1992;Jan-Feb;62–65. https://history.amedd.army.mil/booksdocs/AMEDDinODS/AMEDDODS1Haigler.pdf

22. Harper S. "Granny" goes to Iraq to take care of soldiers. *Fort Huachuca Scout.* October 1991.

23. Ranger Hall of Fame inductees include man from Kirkland—his heroic efforts in WWII recognized. *Seattle Times*. January 2016.

24. Interservice Physician Assistant Program. US Army Medical Center of Excellence website. Accessed July 30, 2020. http://www.cs.amedd.army.mil/ipap/

25. Best physician assistant programs, ranked in 2019. *US News and World Report*. Accessed July 30, 2020. https://www.usnews.com/best-graduate-schools/top-health-schools/physician-assistant-rankings

26. Butler FK Jr, Blackbourne LH. Battlefield trauma care then and now: A decade of Tactical Combat Casualty Care. *J Trauma Acute Care Surg*. 2012;73(6 Suppl 5):S395–402.

27. Westfall, R. Tactical Combat Medical Care Course hones combat medical readiness. Department of the *Army*. Accessed July 21, 2020. https://www.army.mil/article/220898/tactical_combat_medical_care_course_hones_combat_medical_readiness

28. Cawley JF. Doctoral degrees for PAs: What happens next? *JAAPA*. 2008;21(3):13. Accessed July 30, 2020. https://journals.lww.com/jaapa/pages/articleviewer.aspx?year=2008&issue=03000&article=00002&type=Fulltext

29. Military Times Hall of Valor. Awards and citations. Christopher B. Cordova Silver Star citation. Accessed July 20, 2020. https://valor.militarytimes.com/hero/27500

30. American Academy of Physician Assistants. Making PA history at the White House. April 10, 2015. Accessed July 30, 2020. https://www.aapa.org/news-central/2015/04/making-pa-history-at-the-white-house/

31. Physician Assistant History Society. Colonel Amy L. Jackson PA History Society Biography. Accessed July 30, 2020. https://pahx.org/assistants/jackson-amy-l/

32. Department of the Army. *Officer Promotions*. Army Regulation 600-8-29. February 25, 2005. Accessed July 30, 2020. https://armypubs.army.mil/epubs/DR_pubs/DR_a/pdf/web/r600_8_29.pdf

33. Pettersson H, Manley B, Hernandez S. Tracking coronavirus' global spread. Updated July 30, 2020. Accessed July 30, 2020. https://www.cnn.com/interactive/2020/health/coronavirus-maps-and-cases/

Chapter 2

THE COUNCIL OF JUNIOR PHYSICIAN ASSISTANTS

P. Jason E.E. Auchincloss, APA-C, MPAS, and Amelia M. Duran-Stanton, PA-C, PhD, DSc, MPAS

Introduction

The Council of Junior Physician Assistants (CJPA) originated as a team of accomplished junior Army physician assistants (PAs), eager to focus awareness on current and potential future challenges and provide relevant feedback from the field to senior leaders. This team of PAs was hand-selected by senior mentors to provide time-sensitive input regarding a host of matters affecting Army medicine. Army PAs continue to serve as the "tip of the spear" to ensure readiness and increase lethality, while also supporting Army medicine's lines of effort, ensuring that forces are ready to fight today and prepared for the challenges of tomorrow. Army PAs remain front runners in the Army's ready medical force, and serve tirelessly to promote a medically ready force. Army PAs serve throughout the military, from the battalion aid station to the corps headquarters, from the Pentagon to the White House, spanning the full spectrum of warfighting from the tactical to the strategic level. Because Army PAs often function in remote operational locations, and regularly perform duties independently, mentoring them can be a challenge. Many senior leaders provide mentorship to promote the success of the Army PA; however, sustained face-to-face interactions are infrequent due to geographical separation and autonomy.

Literature Review

There is a reported gap in mentorship between senior and junior PAs—work often gets in the way of professional guidance and mentoring, and as a result junior PAs feel they are often left to seek out mentoring opportunities on their own. Junior PAs may feel they need to "pull" knowledge from leaders, rather than having guidance routinely "pushed" from above. Recently, more emphasis has been placed on advising junior PAs to seek out a mentor and establish the mentor-mentee relationship early in their careers. Ideal mentor-mentee relationships span an extended period and require a significant time commitment by both parties.[1,2] Studies have shown that mentees initiate the most successful mentorship relationships,[3,4] and that mentorship improves the success and productivity of individuals and organizations as a whole.[5–8] The Army advocates mentorship because "mentoring develops great leaders to lead great soldiers"[9]; however, junior PAs may not know what they do not know in terms of mentorship, and how to reach out to their senior leaders.

Background

Lieutenant Colonel Amelia Duran-Stanton created the CJPA in 2017 as an informal group of junior PAs who showed initiative and drive in accomplishing projects outside the scope of their regular duties and responsibilities. The original group provided "boots on the ground" feedback on regulation updates, offered junior-level feedback to senior leaders, and processed strategic-level information and products from the Department of Defense, Department of the Army, Medical Command, Medical Specialist Corps, and civilian organizations that were then prioritized and disseminated to the PA community. The group was later formalized in 2018 with the approval of the PA consultant (then Colonel John F. Detro), and CJPA membership was extended to recipients of awards or recognitions such as the Surgeon General Physician Assistant Recognition Award (TSG-PARA), Iron Majors Week attendance, and the Junior Leadership Course attendance. Senior PA leaders identified their stellar junior PAs for inclusion. The inaugural director of the CJPA is Major P. Jason E.E. Auchincloss, the 2016 TSG-PARA.

Selection

Personnel selected informally by the PA leadership comprise the CJPA until a formal process is established. In addition to the award winners discussed above, other selectees are leaders within the organization, including brigade and division PAs, who are making great strides in the advancement of medicine within the military. Additionally, with the establishment of new 65D (Army PA) committees in 2020, the senior PA leadership in each corps (I, III, and XVIII) will identify a group of outstanding junior PAs as selectees. To date, the CJPA team has been divided among committees, as follows:

- **Senior Executive Committee**. Composed of selected colonels and their deputies, acts as the board of directors, receives and reviews the work of other committees, and coordinates strategic action.
- **Committee on Recruitment and Retention**. Includes leaders from Human Resources Command, Recruiting Command, Forces Command, Medical Center of Excellence, and corps and division leadership. Focus is on junior officer outreach and mentorship, PA recognition (awards), career and talent management, bonuses, and other recruitment and retention tools.
- **Committee on Professional Policy and Modernization**. Concentrates on regulatory policy and guidance, synergizing medical organization initiatives for modified table of organization and equipment (MTOE) changes, personnel and equipment, Defense Health Agency transformation, and privileges and credentials.
- **Committee on Combat Medicine and Medical Readiness/ Sustainment**. Applies to individual critical task lists, the postprofessional short course program, 5-year long-term health education and training plans, continuing medical education, and force generation management.

Activities

The CJPA is frequently called upon by PA senior leaders to provide timely feedback for policy revision, updates to regulations and procedures, and bottom-up input for projects that affect the medical force. Many of these tasks garner high-level visibility within the Medical Command, Medical Specialist Corps, Office of the Surgeon General, Defense Health Agency, Pentagon, and the Joint Staff. Input from the field is critical to maintaining a ready and relevant medical force, and information is also often disseminated through the CJPA to the line elements. Much of the knowledge passed to the unit medical teams is time-sensitive and carries essential policy updates and messaging. Additionally, these activities inherently provide senior leadership availability, exposure, and mentorship to CJPA members.

Roles and Responsibilities

The CJPA group is responsible for providing timely feedback based on their current location and expertise. The varied experience of each CJPA member, whether coming from their area of concentration or military occupational specialty before becoming an Army PA, or from their current duty station, must be utilized in providing diverse and comprehensive feedback and communication, both within the group and to senior leaders. CJPA members are encouraged to provide candid feedback about products and other subjects of discussions that otherwise would not have reached the PA leadership. This communication offers visibility to senior leaders working at operational and strategic levels, separated from the tactical "boots on the ground" experience. CJPA members should take personal responsibility for their careers, initiate installation-level mentorship, leverage available modern technology, seek and provide products available for continuous updates and reviews, and improve current methods of communication.

Desired Skills and Attributes

Desired skills and attributes of a PA selected for the CJPA include:

- being current in all PA skills mandated by the individual critical task lists;
- operational experience;
- the rank of captain or junior major;
- outstanding written and oral communication skills and a willingness to provide meaningful input on short notice; and
- being outspoken and eager to bring about change within the organization.

The following attributes are helpful for success:

- operational medical experience within a variety of units (eg, infantry, artillery, aviation), with a minimum of Role 1 deployment experience preferred;
- readiness experience and understanding of the tactical and operational environments;

- ability to work well with both military and civilian personnel and organizations; and
- willingness to provide honest feedback to senior Army leaders.

Training

No additional training is required for the position other than the standard credentials requirements and those expected in Department of Defense Instruction 1322.24, *Medical Readiness Training*,[10] and by the Army. However, junior PAs are encouraged to seek training availability such as Lean Six Sigma, continuing medical education, and at least one Army Training Requirements and Resource System (ATRRS) readiness course annually.

Recommended Certifications

Beyond those required for credentialing, recommended certifications include Advanced Life Support and Lean Six Sigma courses such as Lean Leader, Green Belt, Black Belt, and Master Black Belt (see Chapter 66).

Opportunities and Experiences

The CJPA provides input into medical personnel management, equipment acquisition, training, and development of a ready medical force. Through the council, opportunities exist to provide real-time modifications to regulatory guidance that affect not only the Army Medical Department but also its beneficiaries. The CJPA is keenly aware of the positive impacts it has on enabling change within the organization.

Tips for Success

Members of CJPA should:

- identify challenges within the operational environment, document these challenges, and develop ideas and ways to improve systems and processes;

- not only look for areas to improve, but also provide solutions and alternative courses of action to bring about change;
- seek self-improvement and steward the profession at every opportunity (publishing or participating in research projects are great ways to develop critical thinking and writing skills); and
- become a subject matter expert in their organization and the medical capabilities it possesses.

Conclusion

Working behind the scenes with equity holders to improve the delivery of medicine, CJPA members are groomed for further service by exposure to the experience of executive leadership. The privileges and responsibilities of elite junior PAs in the CJPA require additional work beyond daily duties; however, the rewards of influencing tomorrow's medical force, and enhancing the readiness of the military, are immeasurable to the Army readiness posture.

References

1. Hauer KE, Teherani A, Dechet A, Aagaard EM. Medical students' perceptions of mentoring: a focus-group analysis. *Med Teach.* 2005;27(8):732–734.

2. Simonton DK. Historiometric methods. In: Ericsson KA, ed. *The Cambridge Handbook of Expertise and Expert Performance.* Cambridge University Press; 2006:327.

3. Amonoo HL, Barreto EA, Stern TA, Donelan K. Residents' experiences with mentorship in academic medicine. *Acad Psychiatry.* 2019;43(1):71–75. DOI: 10.1007/s40596-018-0924-4

4. Jackson VA, Palepu A, Szalacha L, Caswell C, Carr PL, Inui T. "Having the right chemistry": a qualitative study of mentoring in academic medicine. *Acad Med.* 2003;78(3):328–334.

5. Cochran A, Paukert JL, ScalWes EM, Neumayer LA. How medical students define surgical mentors. *Am J Surg.* 2004;187(6):698–701.

6. Aagaard EM, Hauer KE. A cross-sectional descriptive study of mentoring relationships formed by medical students. *J Gen Intern Med.* 2003;18(4):298–302.

7. Sambunjak D, Straus SE, Marusic A. Mentoring in academic medicine: A systematic review. *JAMA*. 2006;296:1103–1115.

8. Straus SE, Johnson MO, Marquez C, Feldman MD. Characteristics of successful and failed mentoring relationships: a qualitative study across two academic health centers. *Acad Med.* 2013;88(1):82–89.

9. Department of the Army. *Army Medical Department Officer Professional Development and Career Management*. HQDA: September 2018. DA Pamphlet 600-4. Accessed April 7, 2020. https://armypubs.army.mil/epubs/DR_pubs/DR_a/pdf/web/ARN13783_P600_4_admin_FINAL.pdf

10. Department of Defense. *Medical Readiness Training*. March 16, 2018. DoD Instruction 1322.24. Accessed April 8, 2020. https://www.esd.whs.mil/Portals/54/Documents/DD/issuances/dodi/132224p.pdf?ver=2018-03-16-140510-410

Section 2

Training, Certification, and Career Management

Chapter 3

THE ROLE OF THE PHYSICIAN ASSISTANT AS THE SPECIALIST AND VETERINARY CORPS EDUCATION BRANCH CHIEF

Benjamin K. Kocher, PA-C, DSc, MPAS

Introduction

The education branch chief (EBC) for the Specialist (SP) and Veterinary Corps (VC) is an SP Corps immaterial officer (65X) who is assigned to the Professional Education and Training Department (PETD), US Army Medical Center of Excellence (MEDCoE), Joint Base San Antonio–Fort Sam Houston, Texas. This officer is essential to synchronizing key strategic education and training initiatives for the SP and VC. The EBC also serves as the co-chair of the SP Corps education committee. The position is essential for execution of the long-term health education and training (LTHET) programs and the post-professional short course program (PPSCP). The EBC facilitates the administrative and budgetary requirements of these programs in collaboration with the organization's resource management office and corps leadership.

Organizational Functions

PETD serves multiple roles that influence Army Medical Department (AMEDD) officers on a daily basis. The functions of the department include the following:

- Serves as the proponent and principle advisor for Army Regulation 351-3, *Professional Education and Training Programs of the Army Medical Department*; LTHET; PPSCP; and professional certification (or licensure) maintenance and supporting policies.[1]

- Coordinates AMEDD, MEDCoE, Defense Health Agency, and Department of Defense professional education initiatives with corps leadership, including the graduate education manager, area of concentration (AOC) consultants to the surgeon general, corps-specific branch proponent officers (CSBPO), and corps chiefs.
- Facilitates SP and VC corps programs—LTHET, training with industry (TWI), and PPSCP.
- Validates military training agreements and education service agreements with institutions that support LTHET and PPSCPs.

Unit Structure

The EBC is rated by the department director and senior-rated by the assistant commandant. The department was historically task-organized under the Directorate of Training and Academic Affairs. However, since the 2019 restructuring and the transition to the MEDCoE, the department is under the assistant commandant's office. The department works closely with the Office of the Surgeon General (OTSG), Army Medicine Proponency Office, AMEDD Personnel Proponent Directorate, Capability Development Integration Directorate, MEDCoE Resource Management, Department of Graduate Education (MEDCoE Graduate School), and Human Resources Command to perform its routine functions.

Program Management

Program Development and Implementation

Each program must undergo an annual multidepartment analysis. For the SP Corps, the process starts with providing a proof of concept to the education committee for review. The education committee serves as the executive body responsible for providing strategic oversight to education and training initiatives. The proof of concept must evaluate the components of doctrine, organization, training, materiel, leadership and education, personnel, facilities, and policy as follows:

- identify capability gap or requirement;
- identify training platforms capable of providing required education;
- evaluate program compliance in accordance with policies and doctrine;

- evaluate AOC and trainee, transient, holdee, and student inventory;
- identify and approve utilization tours (designated as "97" on the modified table of organization and equipment or the table of distribution and allowances);
- execute a costs and business case analysis; and
- evaluate selection processes and prerequisites for the program (eg, grade point requirements, civilian education level, military education level, and Graduate Record Examination scores).

Once reviewed, the education committee provides its recommendation to the corps chief. If approved, the packet is sent to PETD for inclusion on the board. Once a program is validated, it may be included in future boards without resubmission through the education committee. The VC has a similar process and staffs the product through executive leaders, but without a specific committee to fulfill the function.

Types of Long-Term Health Education and Training Programs

The types of programs determine the funding sources and governing policies and regulations. Three programs cover all training opportunities.

School of Choice Programs. These degree-granting programs or professional residencies matriculate at a civilian institution. PETD manages the funding requirements of these programs in conjunction with Central Training Branch. Each student has historically been authorized a $1,000 book stipend annually, and a $200 to $500 stipend with completion of a program requiring a thesis or dissertation. Temporary duty costs, candidacy fees, and board certification fees are reimbursed only if they are program and corps requirements. Board certification fees are typically reimbursed only if certification is required for the AOC designation and occurs within the contracted LTHET period. Examples include Doctor of Philosophy (PhD), Masters in Public Health (MPH), and Masters in Health Administration (MHA).

Federal Programs. A Department of Defense institution sponsors these degree-granting, professional residencies or fellowships. Typically, each program's host organization supports funding requirements in accordance with MEDCoE agreements generated by the office of Assistant Chief of Staff for Resource Management. Examples include the following:

- Laboratory Animal Medicine Programs
- Uniformed Services University of the Health Sciences
- US Army Medical Research Institute of Infectious Diseases
- Walter Reed Army Institute of Research
- DOD Veterinary Pathology Residency (DODVPR), Joint Pathology Center
- US Army–Baylor/MEDCoE Graduate School Programs
- Doctor of Science in Occupational Therapy
- Doctor of Science in Physical Therapy
- Doctor of Science in Physician Assistant Studies
- Fellowships
- Test and Evaluation Fellowship, AMEDD Board
- Point-of-Care Ultrasound Fellowship (Brooke Army Medical Center and Madigan Army Medical Center)

Training With Industry. Civilian internships, residencies, or fellowships sponsored and managed by the Department of the Army are separate from the LTHET offerings. However, they are included as part of the AMEDD LTHET validation board to fulfill Army requirements. The Department of the Army has quotas for these programs, and the corps must provide an order-of-merit list if they are requesting multiple training-with-industry positions. The sponsoring civilian organization typically funds program requirements. Offerings include:

- American Academy of Physician Assistants
- National Commission on Certification of Physician Assistants
- National Registry of Emergency Medical Technicians

Validation Process

After the SP and VC populate their program information into the annual program and position requirements worksheet (PPRW), PETD reviews the products to ensure compliance with governing policies and regulations. The Army Medicine Proponency Office then holds an electronic voting board using the automated PPRW to staff the annual

LTHET offerings for the AMEDD. Historically, the corps chief delegates the duty of voting and corps representation on the electronic board to the CSBPO. PETD summarizes the results and forwards them to the surgeon general through the MEDCoE commander for final approval. The surgeon general retains Title 10 authority over education and training of AMEDD officers under the reorganization.

Physician Assistant Planning Cycle

It is imperative that all PAs understand the validation process for LTHET and PPSCP. The process for LTHET programs occurs approximately 2 years prior to execution, whereas the PPSCP process occurs approximately 1 year prior to execution. With this in mind, PAs should coordinate emerging requirements and new courses approximately 3 years in advance to provide ample time for the required staffing and implementation. In preparation for the annual board, the graduate education manager, AOC consultant, CSBPO, and EBC work together to populate the key staff products. This primarily involves creating the PPRW for LTHET and TWI offerings, along with submitting the course administrative data sheets for the PPSCPs.

LTHET and TWI Planning Cycles

- October–November: LTHET military personnel (MILPER) message releases
- November–January: Applications submitted to, and staffed by, Human Resources Command
- January–February: Application waiver review and disposition
- February–March: PPRW input, TWI memo, and course administration datasheet generation
- April: LTHET / TWI / PPSCP validation board and selection panel
- June–July: LTHET results released
- August–September: Application and MILPER message revision

Skills and Attributes

The PETD position requires an experienced officer with a background in academia who collaborates effectively with multiple entities and senior AMEDD leaders. This officer advises and ensures that education and training requirements are incorporated into life-cycle management and integrated into all changes to doctrine, organization, training, materiel, leadership and education, personnel, facilities, and policy decisions affecting corps officers.

At PETD, a major or lieutenant colonel with the following experience historically serves as the EBC:

- knowledge of military and deployed medicine readiness requirements;
- experience in graduate professional education across multiple professions;
- prior academic leadership and program budget management;
- prior experience as a project officer for a PPSCP, functional course, or continuing education unit or continuing medical education activity;
- knowledge of national professional certification and license maintenance requirements for multiple disciplines;
- knowledge of personnel database systems such as the Force Management System website, Medical Operational Data System, and Total Officer Personnel Management Information System;
- effective verbal and written communication skills, including the ability to produce cogent staff materials designed for diverse audiences; and
- completion of Intermediate Level Education (recommended).

Duties and Responsibilities

On a daily basis, the EBC has many routine requirements, including the following:

- coordinating student tuition and associated program costs with Central Training Branch,
- validating and processing execution costs for PPSCPs,
- participating in briefing corps leadership on education and training activities, and

- analyzing AMEDD initiatives to provide input or recommendations to corps office staffing functions.

Routinely, the EBC is engaged in the following activities:

- speaking at junior officer mentorship programs (Basic Officer Leader Course, Captains Career Course, professional conferences, and graduate school programs),
- conducting SP Corps education committee (monthly),
- briefing the SP corps chief update (quarterly) and VC leadership upon request,
- submitting articles to the SP *Corps Connection* newsletter (quarterly),
- briefing the SP Corps Strategic Advisory Board (biannually) on education and training initiatives,
- co-authoring the SP corps handbook (annually),
- facilitating tuition waiver requirements (January–March),
- conducting LTHET student in-briefs (April–May),
- facilitating program validation and PPRW submission (April–May), and
- facilitating MILPER and LTHET application updates (August–September).

Lessons Learned

The EBC position may be challenging for individuals without a diverse background in academics, resource management, or the US Department of Education infrastructure. Each of the managed programs and courses have specific friction points that the EBC must be aware of to mitigate potential issues. This is complicated by managing two separate corps, because the officer requires familiarization with ten different AOCs and their associated education offerings and roles within the AMEDD. Early communication and research with AOC consultants and the CSBPO is essential to success. Familiarization with commonly used regulatory guidance is a vital step to professional success as the EBC.

Conclusion

The EBC provides a broadening opportunity for a field-grade officer to serve in a job that influences multiple disciplines of the AMEDD. The individual holding the position will gain key knowledge of AMEDD planning processes and will work collaboratively with multiple organizations and agencies throughout the Department of Defense. PAs are well suited for this position with their diverse understanding of multidisciplinary care in the deployed environment and military medical treatment facilities. The position provides officers with the potential to affect long-term AMEDD initiatives and shape multiple professions.

As of 2020, and as part of the MEDCoE reorganization, this authorization will be repurposed to the Directorate of Training and Doctrine. In this new role, the officer will be acting as the subject matter expert for the SP Corps and be working to develop education and training platforms for the MEDCoE across operational, institutional, and self-development (OISD) domains.

Reference

1. US Department of the Army. *Professional Education and Training Programs of the Army Medical Department.* DA; 2007. Army Regulation 351-3. Accessed July 29, 2020. https://armypubs.army.mil/epubs/DR_pubs/DR_a/pdf/web/AR%20351-3.pdf

Additional Sources

- US Army Medical Center of Excellence website. Professional Education and Training Department. Updated May 13, 2019. Accessed July 29, 2020. https://www.cs.amedd.army.mil/Portlet.aspx?id=4ac06b51-6b3e-4ab4-91c5-0e4120193c01
- US Army Medical Center of Excellence website. AMEDD Student Detachment. Updated July 21, 2020. Accessed July 29, 2020. https://www.cs.amedd.army.mil/portlet.aspx?id=21052884-7e41-4fc8-bfac-60adb11fd63d

Chapter 4

ACADEMIC LEADERSHIP ROLES, PROFESSIONAL EDUCATION, AND TRAINING OPPORTUNITIES FOR PHYSICIAN ASSISTANTS

Benjamin K. Kocher, PA-C, DSc, MPAS; Matthew S. Douglas, PA-C, DSc, MPAS; Amelia M. Duran-Stanton, PA-C, PhD, DSc, MPAS; Amy L. Jackson, PA-C, MPAS; Sharon Rosser, PA-C, DSc, MPAS; Luis Vidal, APA-C, MPAS; and John F. Detro, APA-C, MPAS, MSS, MEd

Introduction

As Army medicine continues to evolve to meet the needs of the warfighter, physician assistants (PAs) are more essential than ever in meeting the Army and Army Medical Department (AMEDD) mission. Army medicine's professional education programs are integral to developing future leaders and providing qualified officers to man the generating and operational force.[1] These professional education programs are also vital to the continuum of care for service members and their families by expanding access to emergent and surgical services. This chapter reviews the roles and relationships of officers involved in professional education and discusses broadening opportunities available to the military PA. The attachment at the end of the chapter provides additional operational, medical, predeployment, and leadership training resources.

Education and Training Support Structure

Professional education initiatives specific to PAs are the responsibility of the Specialist Corps (SP) Office and are primarily managed by the PA consultant. The PA consultant leverages corps and PA academic leadership to perform these duties and manage the programs on a routine basis. The following key academic leaders influence PA education: corps-specific branch proponent officer (CSBPO) and personnel proponent officer, Army Medicine Personnel Proponent Directorate (APPD); education branch chief (EBC), Professional Education and Training Department (PETD); PA capability manager, Capability Development Integration Directorate (CDID); graduate education manager (GEM), an additional duty historically assigned to a US Army Medical Center of Excellence (MEDCoE) officer; associate dean, MEDCoE Graduate School; and program chairpersons and directors of PA education. These leaders synergize PA educational initiatives through multiple working groups and committees, including the SP Strategic Advisory Board, SP Education Committee, SP Research Committee, PA Senior Executive Committee, and PA Committee on Combat Medicine and Medical Readiness/Sustainment.

All programs go through an annual validation process that includes the review and approval of the six AMEDD Corps proponent offices. Secondary to the reorganization of the MEDCoE under US Army Training and Doctrine Command (TRADOC) in 2019, training and education program service quota validation will be transitioned to the MEDCoE Training Programs Management Division of the Directorate of Training/Doctrine (DOTD), using the Army Program for Individual Training model described in Army Regulation 350-1, *Army Training and Leader Development*,[2] and the TRADOC Training Requirements Analysis System methodology, including the structure manning decision review (SMDR) and training resource arbitration panel (TRAP) processes. Services request training requirements 3 years out (reevaluated at 2 years) through the SMDR, then the TRAP determines what is supportable based on resources and priorities for the execution year.

Roles and Responsibilities of Academic Leaders

This section provides an overview on the different roles and responsibilities, command and control relationships, and support structures of the education programs for PAs. Figures 4-1 and 4-2 show the relationships of these leaders within the education structure. Figures 4-3 through 4-5 represent the annual planning cycles discussed in this section.

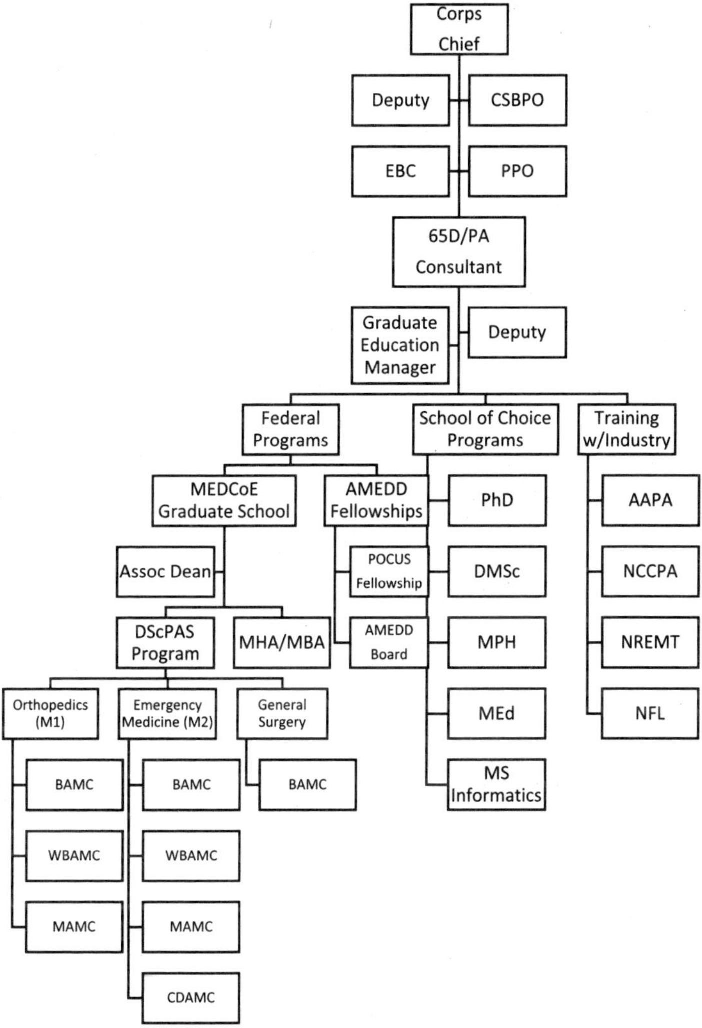

Figure 4-1. The education infrastructure for physician assistant postgraduate education programs and US Army Specialist Corps leadership.

AAPA: American Academy of Physician Assistants; AMEDD: Army Medical Department; BAMC: Brooke Army Medical Center; CDAMC: Carl R. Darnall Army Medical Center; CSBPO: corps-specific branch proponent officer; EBC: education branch chief; MAMC: Madigan Army Medical Center; MEDCoE: Medical Center of Excellence; NCCPA: National Commission on Certification of Physician Assistants; NFL: National Football League; NREMT: National Registry for Emergency Medicine Technicians; POCUS: Point-of-Care Ultrasound; PPO: personnel proponent officer; WBAMC: William Beaumont Army Medical Center

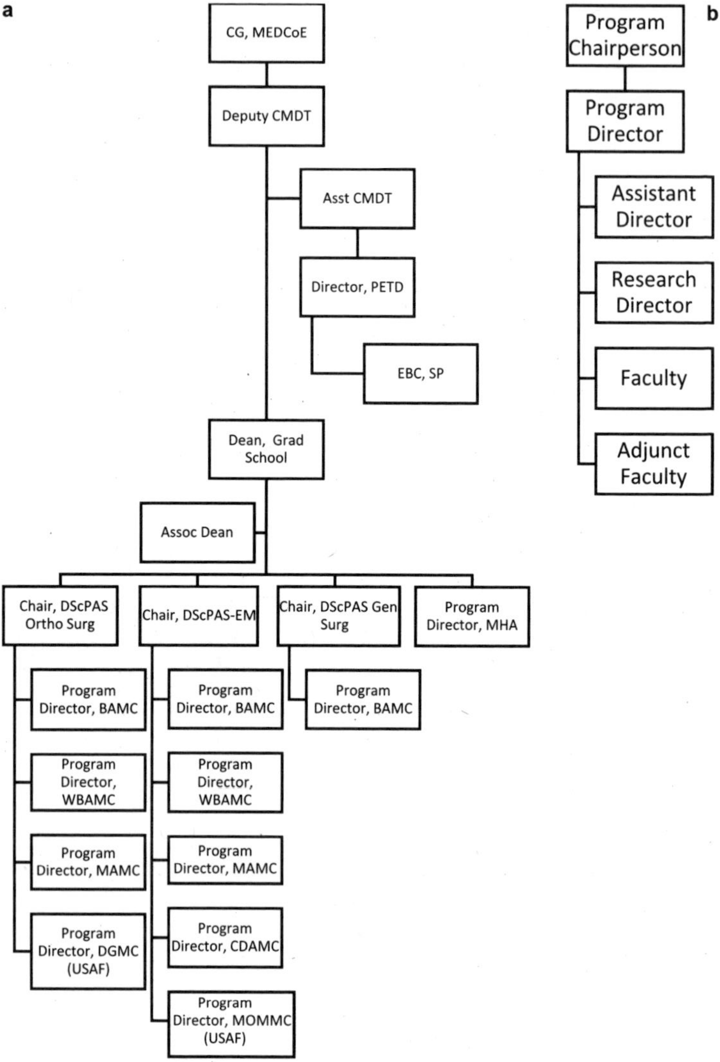

Figure 4-2. (a) The academic infrastructure for federal programs that reside under the Medical Center of Excellence Graduate School; **(b)** DScPAS program infrastructure and faculty organization.

BAMC: Brooke Army Medical Center; CG: commanding general; CDAMC: Carl R. Darnall Army Medical Center; CMDT: commandant; DGMC: David Grant Medical Center; EBC: education branch chief; EM: Emergency Medicine; MAMC: Madigan Army Medical Center; MOMMC: Mike O'Callaghan Military Medical Center; PETD: Professional Education and Training Department; Ortho: Orthopedic Surgery; Surg: General Surgery; USAF: US Air Force

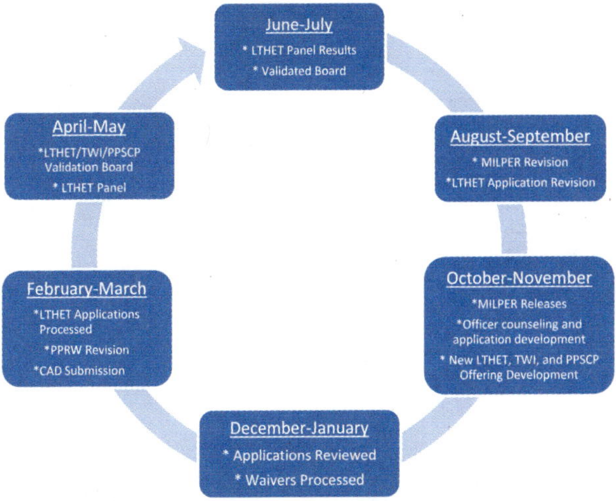

Figure 4-3. Professional Education and Training annual planning cycle.
CAD: course administrative data sheet; LTHET: long-term health education and training; MILPER: military personnel; PA: physician assistant; PPRW: program and positions requirement worksheet; PPSCP: post-professional short course program; TWI: training with industry

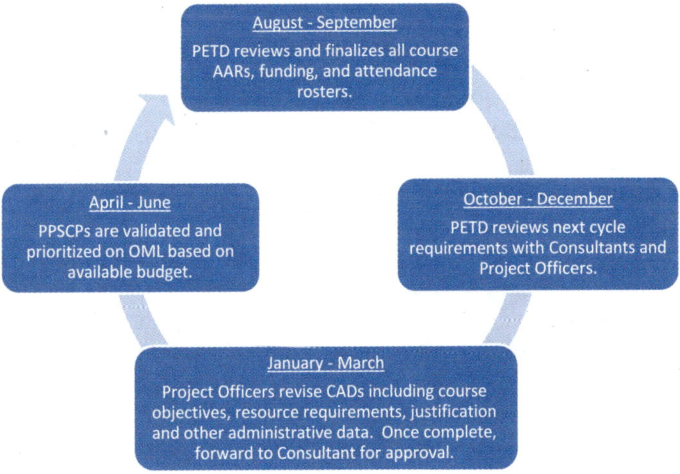

Figure 4-4. Post-professional short course program annual planning cycle.
AAR: after-action review; CAD: course administrative data sheet; LTHET: long-term health education and training; OML: order-of-merit list; PA: physician assistant; PETD: Professional Education and Training Department; PPRW: program and positions requirement worksheet; TWI: training with industry

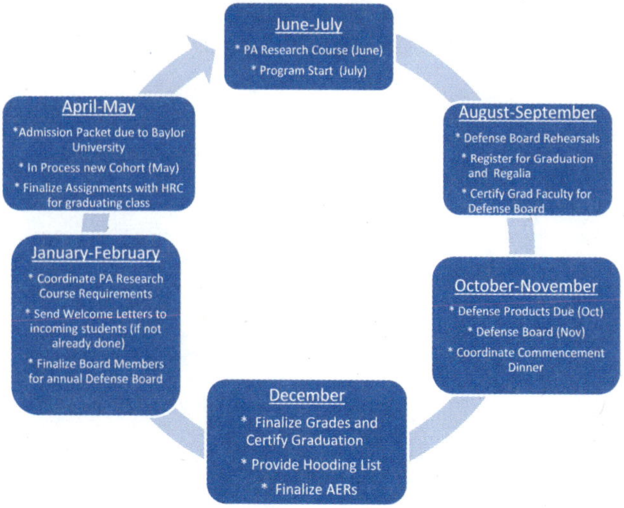

Figure 4-5. DScPAS program annual planning cycle.
AER: academic evaluation report; GEM: graduate education manager; HRC: Human Resources Command; LTHET: long-term health education and training; PA: physician assistant; PPRW: program and positions requirement worksheet

PA Consultant

The SP chief and PA consultant are ultimately responsible for coordinating, validating, and executing education for PAs. The consultant serves the following management roles in professional education:

- Coordinates and provides justification of new courses and programs, facilitated by the SP Education Committee. Each new program must undergo a multi-department analysis that identifies: capability requirement, training platform with a training agreement (PETD), and a validated utilization tour (APPD). This typically occurs during late fall and must be finalized prior to populating the program and position requirements worksheet (PPRW) and the annual validation cycle.
- Validates program and course offerings on an annual basis and provides updated program justification, narrative, and funding requirements on the PPRW.

- Provides academic oversight, validation of graduation requirements, and program accountability for officers enrolled in long-term health education and training (LTHET), training with industry (TWI), and the post-professional short course program (PPSCP).
- Reviews LTHET applications and provides consultation to the SP chief for officer waivers.

Education Branch Chief

The EBC is a 65X (branch immaterial) position responsible for coordinating all staff functions of professional education for the SP Corps. Multiple PAs have served in this role, most recently Lieutenant Colonel (Retired) Pamela Roof and Lieutenant Colonel Ben Kocher. This position has been repurposed under DOTD in 2020 with the reorganization of the AMEDD Center and School into the MEDCoE. Significant duties and responsibilities include:

- Coordinates AMEDD and DOD professional education initiatives with corps leadership including the GEM, consultants to the surgeon general, CSBPO, Human Resources Command (HRC), and SP Chief.
- Serves as vice-chair of the SP Education Committee, managing agenda and staffing products for the CSBPO (the committee chair). In conjunction with the consultant and GEM, provides updates to students enrolled in education programs such as LTHET and PPSCP. Coordinates new program requirements for presentations at board meetings.
- Assists the PA consultant and GEM in providing academic oversight to education programs through reviewing degree plans and coordinating student actions with program leadership.
- Validates graduation and funding requirements with the consultant and the GEM.
- Processes documentation that directs payment of tuition and execution fees. Also processes officer reimbursement requests with MEDCoE G8 (budget) staff.
- Facilitates staffing requirements of the annual validation process with key stakeholders. Reviews PPRWs with the CSBPO, PA consultant, GEM, APPD, and PETD director to ensure an accurate and comprehensive staffing product. Provides training to new leaders as required.

- Markets and recruits LTHET programs during junior officer leadership programs (Basic Officer Leader Course and Captains Career Course), professional conferences, and graduate school officer professional development events.

Graduation Education Manager

The GEM is the linchpin that synergizes PA education by interfacing with all key stakeholders and coordinating programmatic requirements at the direction of the PA consultant. This role is an additional duty. The GEM is appointed by the SP Corps office, with endorsement by the PA consultant, to serve as the consultant's principal advisor on PA education and training programs. It has historically been assigned to either a previous program chair or director of one of the Doctor of Science in Physician Assistant Studies (DScPAS) programs at Brooke Army Medical Center ("DSc" is used as the degree designation in signature blocks). The SP established the additional duty in 2006 due to the expansion of programs and increased requirements for student oversight. Previous officers filling this role include Colonel Rick Villarreal, Major (Retired) Paul Allen, Lieutenant Colonel Sharon Rosser, Colonel Brian Burk, Lieutenant Colonel Ben Kocher, Lieutenant Colonel James Jones, and Major Kerri Van Arnem. Significant duties and responsibilities include:

- Coordinates with CDID and APPD to project force management requirements to inform the annual validation board. Publishes the 5-year plan based on these projected requirements to synchronize program starts and utilization requirements.
- Member of the SP Education Committee, SP Research Committee, and PA Committee on Combat Medicine and Medical Readiness/ Sustainment.
- Appointed to the graduate faculty of MEDCoE graduate programs. Eligible to serve as chair or member of doctoral defense boards for the DScPAS program.
- Assists in developing the annual LTHET guidance by advising on issues such as numbers needed to train and necessary selection qualifications of PAs for postgraduate training.
- Responsible for managing the LTHET application process for PAs, including recruitment, the application process, and post-selection placement, working closely with PETD, HRC, and SP leadership throughout the application and selection process.

- Provides updates to the SP Research Committee on research efforts within the postgraduate programs; works closely with the program directors to align research efforts and track scholarly and research activities.
- Advises the PA consultant on student actions. If a student in a postgraduate program does not meet standards and requires discipline, remediation, probation, or release from the program, the GEM works closely with program leadership and the SP Education Committee to ensure the student receives due process.

Requirements for the GEM additional duty include:

- Terminal (professional or research) doctorate degree.
- Rank of lieutenant colonel (preferred).
- Intermediate Level Education graduate.
- Must meet requirements to be appointed to the graduate faculty of MEDCoE Graduate School affiliated universities.

Desired skills and attributes for the GEM additional duty include:

- Prior experience in an academic leadership position in a graduate program.
- Must be an excellent role model with the desire to mentor others.
- Comprehensive leadership, administrative, and academic skills.
- Strategic vision for future education and training requirements.

Associate Dean, Graduate School

The associate dean is a 65D (PA) position serving as the principal advisor to the dean on hospital-based training programs, which include all branch programs under the MEDCoE Graduate School. Specifically for PAs, these programs include Doctor of Science degrees and Phase 2 (hospital-based/clinical phase) of the Interservice Physician Assistant Program (IPAP). Previous officers filling this role include Lieutenant Colonel Sharon Rosser, Lieutenant Colonel Randolph "Scott" Harrison, and Lieutenant Colonel Matthew Douglas. Significant duties and responsibilities include:

- Manages accreditation requirements for programs under the Graduate School; primary liaison to the supporting institution's Office of Institutional Effectiveness.

- Responsible for providing organizational oversight and program standardization of DScPAS programs and other hospital-based training programs.
- Coordinates admissions process and other student in-processing requirements with the degree-granting university programs.
- Coordinates graduate faculty, professorial rank, and adjunct faculty appointments. Publishes the standard operating procedure for the process and ensures standardization of appointments.
- Coordinates graduate activities including student in-processing, faculty development, football events, and commencement activities.
- Manages graduation certification and filing requirements. Maintains student records in accordance with accreditation standards.
- Appointed graduate faculty for affiliated institutions. Eligible to serve as a chairperson or member of defense boards for the DScPAS program.
- Member of the SP Education Committee, SP Research Committee, and PA Committee on Combat Medicine and Medical Readiness/ Sustainment.

Requirements for the associate dean include:

- Terminal (professional or research) doctorate degree.
- Rank of lieutenant colonel.
- Intermediate Level Education graduate.
- Must meet requirements to be appointed graduate faculty of MEDCoE Graduate School affiliated universities.

Desired skills and attributes for the associate dean include:

- Prior experience in an academic leadership position in a graduate program.
- Must be an excellent role model with the desire to mentor others.
- Solid leadership, administrative, and academic skills; strategic vision for future education and training requirements.

Duty Descriptions for the Doctor of Science Programs

The positions below (program chairperson, program director, assistant program director, research director, and Specialized Interservice

Physician Assistant Program Instructor) apply to DSc programs for orthopedic surgery (see Chapter 5), emergency medicine (see Chapter 6), and general surgery (see Chapter 7), with similar roles and responsibilities. All PAs in these positions must be appointed in a professorial rank of assistant professor and above, maintain appointment to the graduate faculty of the degree-granting university, and serve as staff providers for their discipline.

Program Chairperson

Each discipline (orthopedic surgery, emergency medicine, and general surgery) has a program chairperson who is responsible for synergizing and orchestrating the training within their program across all training sites. The chairperson manages the accreditation requirements of the program and ensures standardization for the program and discipline. They are the primary liaison for the program with Army leadership, including the MEDCoE Graduate School, SP Office, PA consultant, and collaborative specialty consultants. Additionally, they serve the following functions:

- Provides academic leadership and oversight to the program directors by ensuring the entrusted professional attributes, program milestones, and procedural competencies are assessed and validated at each training site in accordance with governing policies and regulations. Ensures training is relevant to possible future capability gaps across the Department of Defense (DOD).
- Publishes and revises their program manual, policies, faculty handbook, and resident handbook to provide guidance to program faculty and matriculating students.
- Recommends faculty appointments in accordance with Graduate School policy and provides professional development and mentorship to program staff.
- Principal advisor to the specialty consultant to the Army surgeon general, the PA consultant to the Army surgeon general, and the SP chief. Responsible for identifying capability gaps within the specialty and providing recommendations on the use and placement of PAs within the profession throughout the services. Synchronizes education and research initiatives with the SP Education Committee, SP Research Committee, and other executive steering committees.

Program Directors (Site-Specific)

Each discipline assigns a program director for each training site. The directors are responsible for managing the program's accreditation requirements and ensuring compliance at their site. They are the primary liaison between the program and their site. They interface regularly with supporting Accreditation Council for Graduate Medical Education (ACGME) programs and other graduate professional education programs. Additionally, they serve the following functions:

- Serves as graduate faculty at the degree-granting university, responsible for managing all grade reporting, rotation evaluations, and doctoral defense preparation and coordination with the MEDCoE Graduate School.
- Ensures all programmatic policies are followed and objectives achieved by the matriculating officers.
- Responsible for managing the degree plan, coordinating medical-related rotations and training affiliation agreements. Also performs didactic instruction and mentors residents in clinical research.
- Coordinates academic requirements and student actions with the supporting graduate medical education committee or the institution's executive committee that governs professional education.
- Manages research initiatives and performance improvement projects for the programs, which includes performing research approved by the institutional review board (IRB), as well as assigning it to students and faculty and assisting them in completing it. Ensures that research initiatives support the SP Corps lines of research.
- Coordinates institutional support and serves as a preceptor for other graduate professional education programs such as the Uniformed Services University of the Health Sciences, IPAP, and nurse practitioner programs.

Assistant Program Director (Site-Specific)

Each site director assigns an assistant to support the residency site. The assistant directors are responsible for helping the director manage the accreditation requirements of the program and ensure compliance at their individual site. They are the alternative liaison between the program and their site. Assistant program directors interface regularly with supporting ACGME programs and other graduate professional education programs. Additionally, the assistant program director has the following functions:

- Serves as program director in their absence or when required.
- May be assigned additional administrative duties, including as research director.
- Ensures all faculty members are compliant with productivity requirements based on duty description and additional duties.
- May serve as an IPAP Phase 2 coordinator.

Program Research Director

Each program assigns a research director to coordinate research activities and synchronize efforts for the students and faculty. The assigned faculty member will align efforts with the SP research program. Additionally, the research director serves the following functions:

- Responsible for tracking and assisting ongoing research efforts including publications, podium presentations in front of an audience, and poster presentations. Coordinates with the SP Education and Research Committee and with the program chairperson to establish a collaborative research effort within the SP.
- Ensures that all IRB-approved research projects are tracked and reported to the program chairperson, directors, the GEM, and the SP Education and Research Committee.
- Maintains a list of preproposal research projects within the established lines of research and task areas and provides immediate coordination of proposal ideas to collaborators within the SP Corps.
- Ensures that each student's research question has scientific merit (is novel and relevant) and is feasible to answer during the DSc program.
- Assists students in developing their protocol (study design as well as the IRB process) and makes sure the students follow the research timeline and submit quarterly counseling comments to the program director at each residency site.
- Conducts individual written performance counseling as needed.
- Monitors the participation of staff mentors in students' research; intervenes as needed to ensure ongoing mentorship.

- Reviews or coordinates mentor review for all students' manuscripts and offers comments.
- Organizes and conducts the defense of doctoral research projects and arranges practice for the defense. Performs as the main point of contact for DSc site program research.
- Serves as a 0.50 FTE (full-time equivalent) clinical provider.
- May serve as an IPAP Phase 2 coordinator.
- May be assigned additional administrative duties.

Specialized Interservice Physician Assistant Program Instructor

The IPAP (refer to Chapter 38 in this handbook) instructors for emergency medicine, orthopedics, and general surgery serve as associate professors for the Master of Science in Physician Assistant Studies (MPAS) program and as their specialty expert for the IPAP at the MEDCoE. They also serve as guest providers in their specialty, maintaining a minimum of 40 patient care hours per year, along with additional requirements by the credentialing and privileging facility. The specialized PA (in either emergency medicine, orthopedics, or general surgery) assigned to IPAP:

- is responsible for providing over 80 hours of instruction to Department of Defense PA students in their specialty;
- provides didactic instruction on anatomy and physiology, differential diagnosis, emergent evaluation and stabilization, appropriate ancillary studies, and patient management in their specialty;
- provides clinical practicums on their specialty's procedures, point-of-care stabilization, wound care and suturing, and bedside clinical and trauma procedures in accordance with specialized guidelines;
- updates IPAP curriculum and policy as a key member of program committees;
- directly mentors Phase 1 (didactic phase) IPAP students through routine and situational counseling, master's thesis development, and professional development activities;
- performs or assists in IRB-approved research and performance improvement projects; and
- educates and trains consulting providers, PAs, nurses, and medics in the management and appropriate disposition of their specialty-care patients.

Corps-Specific Education and Training Opportunities

There are three basic types of LTHET programs for SP officers. Each type is administered and funded differently, so it is important for PAs to understand how the programs are organized. The three types are:

- **School-of-choice programs**. Degree-granting or professional residencies sponsored by a civilian institution, including any of the programs conducted at an academic institution outside of the military. These programs typically result in master's degrees in public health (MPH), education (MEd), health administration (MHA), and informatics, as well as professional doctorates (DMSc) and research doctorates (DSc and PhD). Officers in these programs are assigned to the AMEDD Student Detachment (ASD) and funded through MEDCoE.
- **Federal programs.** Degree-granting, professional residencies or fellowships sponsored by the DOD or other government institution. Officers in these programs are assigned to their respective training academic medical centers and funded through their supporting organization. Examples include:
  - US Army MEDCoE Graduate School programs
    - MHA
    - DScPAS with specializations in:
      - Orthopedics (additional skill identifier [ASI] M1)
      - Emergency medicine (ASI M2)
      - General surgery and trauma (ASI M4-pending)
  - Federal training internships and fellowships
    - Point-of-Care Ultrasound Fellowship
    - Training and Evaluation Internship (with the AMEDD Board)
- **Training with industry.** Internships, residencies, or fellowships that are detailed to a civilian organization and sponsored by the Army (unlike LTHET offerings). However, AMEDD boards these programs as part of the LTHET validation process to fulfill Army requirements. There are quotas for these programs, and the SP Corps must provide an order-of-merit list if they request multiple TWI positions. Program requirements are typically funded through the civilian organization sponsoring the collaboration. Officers in these programs are assigned to the ASD and, if not funded by the sponsoring agency, the officer

may seek financial support through MEDCoE, based on availability of funds. The following are the programs that fall under TWI:

- American Academy of Physician Assistants
- NCCPA
- National Football League
- National Registry for Emergency Medicine Technicians

Qualifications

Qualifications for LTHET applicants are published in an annual military personnel (MILPER) message and are subject to change. Currently, prospective LTHET applicants must meet the following qualifications to be considered for an offering (all waiverable unless otherwise specified):

- be active duty, in the rank of captain to lieutenant colonel;
- be a graduate of the rank-appropriate military education level;
- have 5 to 13 years of active federal commissioned service, or be prior service and have less than 17 years active federal service;
- have completed 36 months of time on station (or 24 months with an HRC waiver) for stateside assignments prior to the start of the program;
- if assigned overseas, have completed the entire overseas tour, including any extension, without curtailment prior to the start of the program;
- be eligible for promotion (must not be in a non-select status);
- have not previously attended a funded equivalent-level LTHET degree program (if the applicant has completed a different degree at the level of the requested LTHET program, they must have completed the previous active duty service obligation prior to the start of the current program);
- have 3 years of clinical experience (2 years with an HRC waiver) at the start of the course[3];
- have received a general subjects GRE score greater than 300 combined for all degree-granting programs (note: individual universities determine the qualifying GRE scores for school-of-choice programs, and essay component is university- and program-dependent); and

- have completed 40 clinical-shadowing hours in the desired specialty or DSc program-approved alternative (if a PA desires to apply to more than one DSc program, they must complete shadowing for all programs they are applying for; the shadowing form is typically included with the application).[3]

Application Information

All PAs who want to participate in LTHET must be selected by the HRC LTHET panel. The digital application is posted on the HRC LTHET portal[3] and annual application guidance is published through a MILPER message posted on the portal in October or November. An applicant checklist is also posted, containing specific directions, deadlines, and the GEM's contact information.

In addition to the documents listed above, applicants need to review and update their individual Army military human resource record and officer record brief (ORB). The final application submission deadline is given in the annual MILPER message, usually in mid-February. Once the applicant receives the application with HRC, PA consultant, and corps endorsement from the GEM, the applicant must submit the completed checklist, LTHET application, DA Form 3838, official (degree-conferring) school transcripts (if not already posted on the military human resource record), and official GRE scores to the LTHET team according to the date and directions provided in the MILPER message.

Annual Planning Cycle

Prospective applicants should review the LTHET MILPER for the previous cycle to their projected application (1 year in advance). Although there may be some changes in the future checklist, a year will provide adequate preparation time to meet any application requirements, such as the GRE and clinical shadowing. Once eligible, applicants must review the current application guidelines in the annual MILPER message, usually no later than early December. LTHET selection panel results are generally published in June or July, approximately 1 year prior to the program start dates. For example, applications received in February 2021 will have selection panel results published in June or July 2021 for programs starting in summer 2022.

Utilization Tours

Each LTHET program must have an identified use, otherwise known as utilization tours. These are dependent on the program of completion, and are predetermined as part of the validation process. Before applying for training, prospective applicants should discuss utilization tours with the current GEM, previously trained PAs in the desired specialty, and the PA consultant.

Post-Professional Short Course Program

The PPSCP was developed to address military-unique medical training requirements and certification maintenance for AMEDD officers. These training opportunities were designed to align with deployment readiness requirements and later revised to train PAs on individual critical task lists. Due to the MEDCoE reorganization and alignment with TRADOC processes, responsibility for maintaining readiness has moved from the institutional to operational domains, and these programs have lost funding. However, some courses remain relevant and will continue to be sponsored.

Annual Planning Cycle

The PPSCP annual planning cycle mirrors the LTHET planning cycle. Each PPSCP has a course administrative data (CAD) document that is used to provide administrative information, course objectives, staffing requirements, funding requirements, and other resourcing information. Similar to LTHET, all new requests for training and courses occur in the late fall (October or November) and are due at the same time as the PPRW and populated in early spring. The PA consultant is responsible for assigning a project officer (course director) to each PPSCP offering to coordinate and execute the course. The project officer is responsible for development and coordination of the course's curriculum and required resources, and should be familiar with the PPSCP planning cycle, course curriculum, continuing medical education (CME) accrediting processes, and budgetary management.

PPSCPs are evaluated by the AMEDD corps offices using force development, health care delivery, and health readiness as key factors. Based on these factors, the courses are then prioritized on a four-point scale:

- Priority (highest). A program that meets regulatory requirements, such as training required for graduate professional education, GME, or dental graduate education. Programs that meet requirements for attaining an area of concentration or ASI are also considered priority.
- High priority. Programs that are directly tied to the surgeon general's priorities and lines of effort and have AMEDD relevance. Courses that maintain certification or licensure fall in this category as well.
- Moderate priority. Officer and leader development programs or training that provides education otherwise available at civilian institutions. The most common PPSCPs in this category are the Junior Leadership Course and Iron Majors Week Course.
- Low priority. Generalized institutional courses designed for federal employees and all service members.

Once prioritized, these courses are sequenced on an order-of-merit list and resourced based on available funding for the program.

Additional Educational Opportunities

A multitude of additional professional development opportunities, in both medicine and officer professional education, are offered by centralized and decentralized programs. All education that improves an officer's fund of knowledge and increases capability from the tactical to strategic roles of the AMEDD is encouraged. With exceptions as identified by DOD instructions, Army regulations, or annual programs not aligned with AMEDD, PAs are recommended to pursue all available education that improves their ability to support soldiers and the AMEDD. The National War College education system and the Army War College (aligned with Army University) offer strategic course matter that may also improve the ability to expand into joint operational force management.

Defense Strategy Course (Army War College)

A foundational military education course from the Army War College is the Defense Strategy Course, a 4-month nonresident/distant learning course offered twice a year.[4] The course is intended to improve officers' understanding of the DOD's role in the development of the national security strategy, and the strategy's role in the international environment.[4] The course is recommended for majors and lieutenant colonels, and enrollment is limited to 50 active duty, 25 reserve, and 25 National Guard officers.[4] The course is highly competitive and strongly recommended for senior PAs for several reasons: the training helps leaders develop critical thinking skills required for strategic-level decision-making; it presents the opportunity to attend various fellowships; and it provides an ASI (6Z) per DA Pamphlet 611-21, *Personnel Selection and Classification: Military Occupational Classification and Structure*.[5]

To be eligible, applicants must have credit for military education level 4, and they must not be enrolled in or have completed a Senior Service College program. Enrollment information is as follows:

- Review the course curriculum at https://dde.carlisle.army.mil/curriculum.cfm.[4]
- Notify your assignment manager of your interest in attending the course.
- Submit a DA Form 3838 to your assignment manager.
- In the Army Training Requirements and Resources System (ATRRS), the school code is 217 and the course number is DSC.[6]

The Defense Strategy Course is divided into four sections with 13 lessons each. Each lesson requires approximately 7 to 10 hours to complete. As described on the course website, the sections are as follows:

Section 1, Introduction: introduces the student to the online format of the course and critical thinking concepts.
Section 2, Strategic and Military Theory: examines classical thinking about strategic theory, the military schools of strategic thought, the international system, strategy formulation frameworks, and states and strategy.[4]
Section 3, The Department of Defense: reviews the roles of the DOD, civil control of defense, the interagency framework, and homeland security.
Section 4, Policy Development and Security Environment: examines policy making, globalization and economic development, the current strategic environment based on both opportunities and

threats, cultural relations and dimensions, multinational operations, centers of gravity analysis, and strategy at the combatant command level.[4]

Graduates receive an Army War College certificate signed by the college's commandant. Although the course awards an ASI, recorded in the ORB under military education, it does not award a formal military education level, nor does it provide college course credits. There is no formal academic evaluation report, although PAs can apply CME (continuing medical education) category 2 credits for professional development to support their credentialing requirements (see Chapter 10, Maintaining Certification and the CME Categories, for further details). Graduates should provide the course completion certificate to their assignment officer to have the course and 6Z ASI added to their ORB.[4]

Additional Professional Military Education

Upon completion of the Defense Strategy Course, additional professional military education (PME) opportunities are available to PAs. The Defense Planners Course is a distant learning course focused on joint planning. The Army Force Management School has multiple course offerings in capability development and force management, including the "How the Army Runs" course (results in a 3R ASI). The US Navy has a robust online PME program; for example, the US Naval War College's College of Distance Education accepts applications from Army majors and above, as well as civilians in grades GS-11 and above, for some of its courses.[7] Additional offerings can be found through distance learning offered by the Air War College, the senior school in the Air Force PME system. The college's 44-week course for lieutenant colonels trains senior leaders for strategic-level employment of air, space, and cyberspace forces. The curriculum emphasizes coalition warfighting and national security, and includes seminars, simulation exercises, electives, international travel, and a national security symposium (contact the Air War College registrar directly for enrollment procedures).[8] The Joint Knowledge Online website also has multiple courses such as acute care provider modules and Military Health System course modules.[9]

Conclusion

Professional education is a key component for PAs to maintain critical wartime skills and meet the demands of future engagements. Understanding the roles of strategic academic leaders, professional education programs, and broadening training opportunities will assist PAs in managing their career and ensuring they are prepared for future deployments.

References

1. US Department of the Army. *Professional Education and Training Programs of the Army Medical Department*. DA; October 15, 2007. Army Regulation 351-3. Accessed August 14, 2020. https://armypubs.army.mil/epubs/DR_pubs/DR_a/pdf/web/AR%20351-3.pdf

2. US Department of the Army. *Army Training and Leader Development*. DA; December 10, 2017. Army Regulation 350-1. Accessed August 14, 2020. https://armypubs.army.mil/epubs/DR_pubs/DR_a/pdf/web/ARN18487_R350_1_Admin_FINAL.pdf

3. US Army Human Resources Command. Long-Term Health Education MILPER 19-369, AY2021 AMEDD-4 Long-Term Health Education and Training (LTHET) Program Selection Panel Announcement. Accessed July 28, 2020. https://www.hrc.army.mil/milper/19-369 [CAC required]

4. US Army War College. Department of Distance Education website. Accessed July 28, 2020. https://dde.carlisle.army.mil/curriculum.cfm

5. Department of the Army. *Personnel Selection and Classification: Military Occupational Classification and Structure*. DA; January 2007. DA Pamphlet 611-21. Accessed August 14, 2020. https://armypubs.army.mil/ProductMaps/PubForm/Details.aspx?PUB_ID=1004900

6. Department of the Army. Defense Strategy Course. Army Training Requirements and Resources System. Accessed July 28, 2020. https://ssl.armywarcollege.edu/dde/curriculum.cfm

7. US Naval War College. Online professional military education. Accessed August 14, 2020. https://www.usnwc.edu/Student-Information/Online-Professional-Military-Education

8. US Air Force. Air University website. Accessed April 30, 2020. https://www.airuniversity.af.edu/

9. Department of Defense. Joint Knowledge Online courseware and capabilities catalog. Published February 2020. Accessed July 28, 2020. https://jko.jten.mil/docs/JKO_CW_CL_QTR_02282020.pdf

Additional Sources

- Department of the Army. US Army War College Blackboard. Accessed August 14, 2020. https://usawc.blackboard.com/ (CAC required)
- Department of the Navy. Naval Postgraduate School Distance Learning. Accessed August 14, 2020. https://nps.edu/web/dl
- Joint Forces Staff College. Advanced Joint Professional Military Education. Accessed August 14, 2020. http://jfsc.ndu.edu/Academics/Advanced Joint Professional Military Education/AJPMEProspectiveStudent.aspx

Attachment: Long-Term Health Education and Training/Training with Industry (LTHET/TWI) Program Descriptions

This attachment lists additional courses that PAs may attend to enhance their operational readiness, prepare for upcoming positions and new duties, and gain CME credit. Follow the directions below for the Army Training and Requirements Resources System (ATTRS) and Defense Medical Readiness Training Institute (DMRTI) courses:

- ATTRS (https://www.atrrs.army.mil/): Click on "Course Catalog" at the right of the screen and insert the course number into the search engine. This will bring up the course. Double click on the course, and the dates and locations, scope, and points of contact for the course will be shown. (To enroll, apply through your operations office or directly to the course point of contact.)
- DMRTI (http://www.dmrti.army.mil/): Click on "Courses" at the top of the screen. Tabs will appear for all DMRTI courses, providing contacts, dates, CME credits, training focus, and requirements for who can attend.

Doctor of Science in Physician Assistant Studies (DScPAS) with specialization in Orthopedics

Program Length: 1.5 years **ADSO**: 3.5 years

Program Narrative

The Doctor of Science of Physician Assistant Studies in Orthopedics (DScPAS-O) is an 18-month program of subspecialty rotations, formal didactic instruction, and clinical research. This graduate program prepares physician assistants (PAs) with the knowledge and expertise to provide perioperative care to a full spectrum of musculoskeletal injuries and conditions. Students matriculate at one of four academic medical centers: San Antonio Military Medical Center, Joint Base San Antonio–Fort Sam Houston, Texas; Madigan Army Medical Center, Joint Base Lewis-McChord, Washington; William Beaumont Army Medical Center, Fort Bliss, Texas; and David Grant Medical Center, Travis Air Force Base, California. Current graduates serve in expeditionary surgical teams and combat surgical hospitals to provide stabilizing measures for battlefield injuries. This program results in a research doctorate degree and an M1 additional skill identifier.

Doctor of Science in Physician Assistant Studies (DScPAS) with specialization in Emergency Medicine

Program Length: 1.5 years **ADSO**: 3.5 years

Program Narrative

The Doctor of Science of Physician Assistant Studies in Emergency Medicine (DScPAS-EM) Residency is an 18-month program that incorporates a variety of clinical rotations, formal didactic instruction, and research. The Doctor of Science program is modeled after the 3-year Emergency Medicine Physician Residency and prepares the EMPA to perform clinical research and to evaluate, diagnose, and stabilize critically ill or injured patients. The overall mission is to produce postprofessional, emergency medicine-trained PAs who provide Military Health System (MHS) beneficiaries state-of-the-art, advanced care in emergency situations. This program provides a structured environment to facilitate learning, ensure competency, practice evidence-based medicine, and conduct clinical research to benefit the warfighter, MHS beneficiaries, the US Army Medical Department, and the PA profession.

Doctor of Science in Physician Assistant Studies (DScPAS) with specialization in General Surgery

Program Length: 1.5 years **ADSO**: 3.5 years

Program Narrative

The Doctor of Science Physician Assistant Studies in General Surgery (DScPAS-GS) is an 18-month program consisting of formal academic requirements, postprofessional research, and structured clinical and surgical training. Established to train postgraduate-level Army surgical PAs to become integral members of perioperative teams in both deployed and garrison environments. The DScPAS-GS graduate's purpose is to maximize the utilization of Army surgeons and their critical skills by safely assuming non-operative surgical responsibilities and procedures, and serve as surgical (multidisciplinary) first assistants. Also, the DScPA-GS is responsible for helping to improve health care and health care policy in battlefield trauma, trauma/critical care, and surgical research. Applicants to the program must be available for Special Operations Command DScPA-GS positions, Expeditionary Resuscitation Surgical Team (ERST) forward surgical team missions, and civilian-military partnership opportunities. Graduates will be allocated to 528th Sustainment Brigade, hospitals inside and outside the United States, and Department of Defense level I trauma centers, and serve as faculty at the Army Institute of Surgical Research.

Army Medical Department (AMEDD) Board Internship in Test and Evaluation (T&E)

Program Length: 1 year **ADSO**: 3 years

Program Narrative
The Operational T&E Intern Program provides AMEDD officers with specialized training in the T&E acquisition career field and positions them as acquisition leaders. The training enables them to provide relevant data to acquisition program managers aimed at ensuring sound programmatic decisions and properly equipping operational elements to meet the Army's contingency mission requirements. T&E is described in Army Regulation 73-1, Department of Defense Instruction 5000.66, and the Defense Acquisition Guidebook as a major element of the acquisition process that provides state-of-the art medical and medical-related devices required to accomplish contingency missions. The objective of the internship is to provide the AMEDD with a pool of officers who are fully qualified to fill AMEDD T&E assignments. During the internship, students will receive hands-on practical experience in analysis, research, plan writing, report writing, oral briefings, policy development, and T&E procedures.

Doctor of Medical Science (DMSc)

Program Length: 1 year **ADSO**: 3 years

Program Narrative
This 1-year Doctorate of Medical Science Program is a professional doctorate that directly supports readiness. Graduates of this program will support educational platforms for area of concentration (AOC) 65D and train to fill operational positions that support warfighters' readiness. Examples of these educational platforms are the Interservice Physician Assistant Program (IPAP), Tactical Combat Medical Care Course, and

Brigade Combat Team Trauma Training (BCT3). The DMSc provides the requisite degree necessary for full academic faculty appointment status at affiliated universities, and is further necessary for PAs to assume leadership positions within the 65D educational programs and higher educational jobs (dean, vice provost, commandant).

American Academy of Physician Assistant (AAPA) Fellowship (TWI)

Program Length: 1 year **ADSO**: 3 years

Program Narrative
This training with industry (TWI) experience will provide in-depth training with the AAPA, the only national professional society for PAs in the United States. AAPA experiences include PA professional advocacy, state/federal governmental relations, health care policy analysis, professional education, and constituent organizational outreach. Additionally, the officer will have exposure to organizational governance, interagency coordination and communication, multidisciplinary professional outreach, information and technology affecting health care professionals, and transformations that optimize team-based medical practice.

National Commission on Certification of Physician Assistants (NCCPA) Fellowship (TWI)

Program Length: 1 year **ADSO**: 3 years

Program Narrative
This training with industry (TWI) experience will provide in-depth training with the NCCPA, the only certifying organization for PAs in the United States. This agency will provide exposure to the ever-changing world of PA certification. NCCPA experiences would include certification process/policy, exam writing, data collection, continuing medical education, current issues/problems with certification, and being part of the solution. The knowledge and skills learned in this TWI are directly applicable and invaluable to the military IPAP as well as for the subject matter expert for Army PA certification.

National Registry for Emergency Medicine Technicians Fellowship (TWI)

Program Length: 1 year **ADSO**: 3 years

Program Narrative
This training with industry (TWI) experience will provide the PA with in-depth training with the National Registry of Emergency Medical Technicians. This organization is the only national emergency medical services (EMS) certification organization that provides a valid, uniform process to assess the knowledge and skills required for competent practice by EMS professionals throughout their careers. The PA will be involved with the development of standardized EMS training, certification, and recertification process and policy.

Executive Fellow, Corps Chiefs Office Fellowship (all AOCs, captains only)

Program Length: 1 year **ADSO**: 2 years

Program Narrative
The Office of the Chief, Army Medical Specialist Corps Fellowship Program offers Army Medical Specialist Corps (SP) officers the opportunity to actively participate in the strategic development, planning, and execution of SP-related policies, initiatives, and events. Fellows assist in formulating programs and actions that influence active and reserve component SP officers worldwide and support Army medicine strategic goals and objectives. Graduates of this broadening assignment are prepared to perform as primary staff officers within the Army Medical Command, Office of the Surgeon General, Defense Health Agency (DHA), and medical brigades.

Master in Health Administration (executive track Intermediate Level Education graduates only)

Program Length: 1 year **ADSO**: 3 years

Program Narrative
The 1-year executive MHA program is for senior officers to gain business skills in data acquisition, business metrics, and analysis to understand and solve the most complex enterprise problems arising from the clinical, administrative, or training areas of the AMEDD and

DHA. Students will simultaneously engage in didactics and residency problems that combine the knowledge and application of lessons learned in the MHA program.

Point-of-Care Ultrasound Fellowship (DScPAS graduates only)

Program Length: 1 year **ADSO**: 2 years

Program Narrative
The Point-of-Care Ultrasound Fellowship is a 1-year program designed to enhance the evaluation, assessment, and treatment skills of medical providers who care for service members with injuries that could be detected using bedside ultrasound in clinic and in combat. Graduates of the Ultrasound Fellowship receive the same training as their emergency medicine physician counterparts, including program/course development, instructing students at the novice and advanced levels, research, and administration of ultrasound programs. Graduates become approved subject matter experts and certified trainers for other physicians, PAs, and medics within the force. Graduates will fill positions at the IPAP, Tactical Combat Medical Care Course, DSc program faculty, and major Forces Command installations to bring ultrasound training to the force.

Chapter 5

THE ARMY ORTHOPEDIC PHYSICIAN ASSISTANT

Robyn L. Chalupa, PA-C, DSc, MPAS; Amelia M. Duran-Stanton, PA-C, PhD, DSc, MPAS; John E. King, APA-C, DSc, MPAS; Benjamin K. Kocher, PA-C, DSc, MPAS; and John F. Detro, APA-C, MPAS, MSS, MEd

> Orthopedic Physician Assistants are critically important providers within the musculoskeletal care team, both in garrison and downrange, ensuring the readiness of our fighting force and assisting with combat casualty care. Over 80% of combat wounds involve the extremities, and musculoskeletal injuries are by far the most common disabling conditions limiting readiness of our troops at home. Orthopedic Physician Assistants are at the tip of the spear in Army Medicine. Highly trained and highly sought after, they serve alongside surgeons in the clinic and operating room to treat injury and return Service Members to duty. With a broad range of skills ranging from fracture care to surgical first-assist, Army Orthopedic Physician Assistants have an exciting and rewarding career in the Army and in civilian practice.

—Colonel Benjamin Kyle Potter
Orthopedic Surgery Consultant to the Surgeon General

Introduction

The development of the orthopedic physician assistant (PA) profession in Army medicine began in response to Medical Corps personnel shortages in both the US Army Forces Command (FORSCOM) and Medical Command (MEDCOM) in the late 1980s. The Office of the Surgeon General approved the orthopedic PA program in 1989 and extended it to an 18-month doctoral program in 2007.[1] In FORSCOM, orthopedic PAs were specifically utilized to extend orthopedic surgeons' capabilities in combat support hospitals and forward surgical teams, increasing access to orthopedic care on the battlefield. In MEDCOM, orthopedic PAs improved access to orthopedic care in the garrison environment by increasing staffing at orthopedic surgery clinics in medical treatment facilities (MTFs), including community hospitals. This increased staffing has been imperative for ensuring continued access to care for the deployed force and maintaining medical readiness.[2]

To fill the capability gap caused by personnel shortages, and to produce a cadre of competent PAs with consistent skills, capable of providing advanced care at all levels of Army medicine and covering multiple subspecialties within orthopedic surgery, formal academic education was required. Because orthopedic PAs would need to fill multiple roles in varied environments, on-the-job training would not provide the breadth of knowledge required to operate in the full spectrum of FORSCOM and MEDCOM missions.

Mission

The mission of the Army orthopedic PA is to extend orthopedic surgical care on the battlefield and to enhance the capabilities of Army orthopedic surgeons by serving in MTFs and combat support hospitals. The orthopedic PA provides perioperative orthopedic management, surgical first-assist, and minor procedures for surgical and nonsurgical patients. Orthopedic PAs also conduct performance improvement projects and research approved by an institutional review board (IRB) in order to enhance evidence-based practice and improve care in the military health system. In 2016 orthopedic PAs began contributing to the joint Special Forces mission in the United Arab Emirates, with a dedicated position performing extensive medical planning and treatment for a wide variety of patient complaints at several separate Role 1 treatment facilities. Since 2018, orthopedic PAs have been substituting for the 61M orthopedic surgeon on expeditionary resuscitative surgical teams, sometimes as team leaders.

Duties and Responsibilities

The orthopedic PA profession in FORSCOM and MEDCOM continues to expand and adapt to the Army's requirements. Today, the orthopedic PA plays four vital roles[3]:

1. **Surgeon extenders**. Orthopedic PAs effectively extend the capacity of orthopedic surgeons in all subspecialties and at all levels of military medicine from damage-control orthopedic care

on the battlefield to augmentation of subspecialties at academic MTFs.

2. **Clinical scientists**. Orthopedic PAs advance scientific and medical knowledge by performing as clinical scientists, conducting relevant and valid research that generates evidence-based practices. This ensures that Army medical centers provide consistent and effective health care to service members and their families.

3. **Educators and mentors**. As educators and mentors, orthopedic PAs optimize the education of future clinicians in Army Medical Center of Excellence (MEDCoE) graduate programs. They also act as subject matter experts who direct continued medical education and facilitate comprehensive career-long education for medical professionals at military installations.

4. **Professional service and scholarship**. Orthopedic PAs lead the PA profession at the national level and are recognized experts in PA graduate allied health education. They hold leadership positions and participate in organizational work groups in the American Academy of Physician Assistants, National Commission for the Certification of Physician Assistants (NCCPA), Accreditation Review Commission on Education for the Physician Assistant, and Physician Assistants in Orthopaedic Surgery. They also serve as peer reviewers for numerous national and international journals, including the *Journal of the American Academy of Physician Assistants*, *Journal of Bone and Joint Surgery*, and the *Journal of Orthopaedics for Physician Assistants*.

Education and Training

The US Army orthopedic PA residency and doctoral program was created as a benchmark for postgraduate education, through the pursuit of academic and clinical excellence, of PAs working in orthopedics.[3] The program is an intense 18-month curriculum that includes completion of 36 courses (59 credit hours representing over 700 hours of classroom instruction) and 10 clinical rotations (29 credit hours representing more than 5,000 clinical training hours). Training is completed in the setting of an academic medical center at one of four graduate medical education (GME) residency programs. The curriculum is modeled after the Accreditation Council for Graduate Medical Education orthopedic surgery residency programs.[3]

Orthopedic PA residents are taught alongside junior orthopedic surgery residents, with a guided educational model, and given comparable responsibilities. This comprehensive model includes both didactic and clinical instruction, on-call responsibilities, management of both inpatient and outpatient orthopedic conditions, and formal education on conducting clinical research. Daily responsibilities include inpatient rounds; outpatient evaluation of urgent, semi-urgent, and routine patients in the cast room, clinic, and emergency department; preoperative evaluation and management; and first-assist in surgical cases of all levels of complexity.

The program is separated into individual rotations by subspecialty and evaluated with formal oral and written requirements. Testing consists of multiple-choice tests administered at periodic intervals as well as oral boards. Orthopedic PA residents complete clinical rotations in general orthopedics and the subspecialties of trauma, sports medicine, hand and wrist, pediatrics, oncology, joint reconstruction, foot and ankle, and spine.

The capstone requirement for the residency is a presentation of an IRB-approved research project to a board panel that includes faculty of the residency program and university. The orthopedic PA residents are required to submit a manuscript to a journal and produce a poster for display. Upon completion, residents are awarded a doctor of science (DSc) degree and an Army additional skill identifier as an orthopedic PA (M1). Graduates incur an active duty service obligation of 3.5 years (3 years for the first 12 months of training, 6 months for the last 6 months of training).

Duty Descriptions

The positions for the specialized PAs (orthopedics, emergency medicine, and general surgery) are outlined in Chapter 4 (Academic Leadership Roles, Professional Education, and Additional Training Opportunities for PAs) to avoid duplicated descriptions for research directors, deputy program directors, program (site) managers, and specialized Interservice Physician Assistant Program instructors. The positions covered in this chapter are orthopedic PA positions. All orthopedic PAs must maintain

National Commission on Certification of Physician Assistants (NCCPA), Basic Life Support (BLS), Pediatric Advanced Life Support (PALS), Advanced Life Support (ALS), and Advanced Trauma Life Support (ATLS) certifications as required by the credentialing and privileging facility.

Orthopedic Physician Assistant (General)

Primarily, orthopedic PAs practice under the supervision of orthopedic surgeons and assist in providing specialized care to patients with orthopedic injuries and conditions. Specifically, orthopedic PAs are responsible for physical examinations, ordering and reviewing diagnostic tests, diagnosis, and developing preliminary goal-oriented treatment plans for musculoskeletal disorders and injuries.

Orthopedic PAs also provide first-assist in surgery and manage patients perioperatively. As part of this management, orthopedic PAs perform orthopedic procedures (Figure 5-1) including administration of local and regional anesthetics, therapeutic and diagnostic joint injection, musculoskeletal ultrasound, fracture fluoroscopy, fracture reduction and management, wound closure/suturing, graft preparation, complex wound debridement, perioperative wound care, skeletal traction, hardware removal, and primary management of nonoperative orthopedic conditions.

Orthopedic Physician Assistant in an Expeditionary Resuscitative Surgical Team or Combat Support Hospital

An orthopedic PA in one of these deployed positions:

- is responsible for the rapid and thorough triage, evaluation, stabilization, and management of urgent medical, surgical, or traumatically injured orthopedic patients;
- performs invasive and noninvasive diagnostic and therapeutic procedures including life-saving procedures within individual credential guidelines and privileges delineated by the hospital;
- orders appropriate available laboratory, radiographic, and other diagnostic tests;
- interprets the total medical and surgical evidence, incorporating information into an accurate diagnosis or appraisal, and initiates proper treatment;

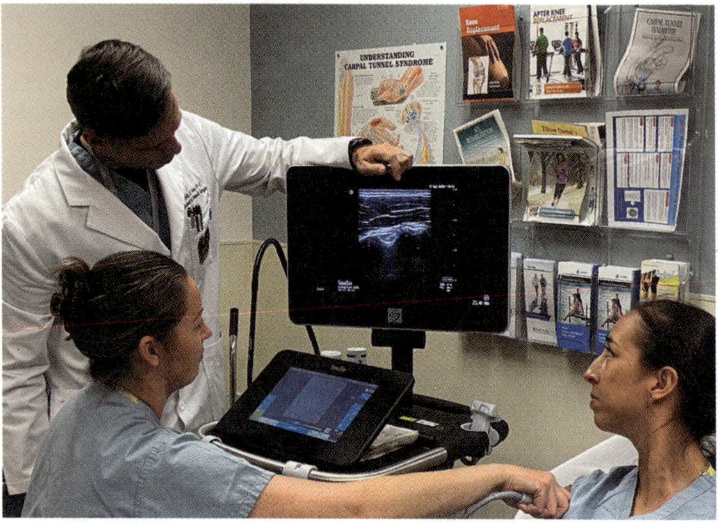

Figure 5-1. Major Timothy Pekari instructs Interservice Physician Assistant Program student officer candidates Lauren Bentley and Sherrie Jansky on ultrasound guided evaluation of the biceps tendon at Evans Army Community Hospital, Fort Carson, Colorado, in April, 2020. Photograph courtesy of Major Pekari.

- develops a patient care plan for each case appropriate to the medical assets and facilities available in the area of operations;
- facilitates patient access to continuing medical care by appropriate referrals to other health care providers and specialists, and determines necessary evacuation to higher roles of care, operating within the policies and regulations of the hospital;
- enhances medical capabilities for forward emergency and resuscitative care and expands capabilities at the tactical level by providing orthopedic stabilization at or near the point of injury; and
- augments emergency medical and orthopedic expertise in the structure of the operating forces, advising the appropriate authority on the management of orthopedic trauma patients within the area of operations.

Chief, Orthopedic Surgery Cast Clinic

The orthopedic PA assigned as chief of an orthopedic surgery cast clinic manages the daily operations for the clinic in support of the orthopedic surgical service, in a 0.75 FTE position. The orthopedic PA serving as a chief of the cast clinic:

- supervises other orthopedic PAs, the cast clinic noncommissioned officer in charge, and Army and civilian orthopedic technicians;
- ensures all faculty members are compliant with FTE and RVU productivity requirements based on duty description and additional duties;
- coordinates logistics and supplies; maintains appropriate stock level of medical and office supplies for orthopedic services;
- maintains accountability and responsibility of equipment in the clinic; and
- precepts and supervises rotational academic program students with orthopedic requirements.

Duty Locations

- Continental United States (CONUS): Fort Bragg, NC; Fort Campbell, KY; Fort Carson, CO; Fort Hood, TX; Fort Polk, LA; and Fort Stewart, GA.
- Outside CONUS: Germany, Korea, and Hawaii.
- Residency training sites: Brooke Army Medical Center, JBSA-Fort Sam Houston, TX (orthopedic PA program director, program manager, program faculty); William Beaumont Army Medical Center, Fort Bliss, TX; Madigan Army Medical Center, Joint Base Lewis-McChord, WA.

Prerequisites

- Extensive experience (including deployments) in battalion and brigade PA positions.
- Completion of long-term health education and training (LTHET) is preferred.
- Rank of major preferred.
- Intermediate Level Education (ILE) graduate preferred (or enrollment in ILE distance learning).

Skills and Attributes

- Must be an excellent role model with the desire to mentor and teach others.
- Strong leadership, administrative, and academic skills.
- Excellent oral and written communication skills.
- Solid work ethic.
- Strong organizational and time management skills.

Lessons Learned

- Orthopedic PAs should maintain their basic clinical skill sets and knowledge in primary care medicine, not only to prepare for recertification examinations, but also for routine patient management in garrison and deployments.
- Orthopedic PAs add value as clinicians and leaders in expeditionary resuscitative surgical teams.
- The vast knowledge and expertise of orthopedic PAs in medical treatment and medical planning contribute to joint Special Forces missions and Role 1 treatment facilities.

Tips for Success

- Have an excellent working relationship with the orthopedic surgeon during residency and beyond.
- Build networks early and get to know specialty staff members in physical therapy, occupational therapy, and internal medicine.
- Develop good working relationships with other members of the health care team, working as a seamless unit to best meet each individual patient's needs.
- Manage and complete documentation thoroughly. Meet with staff who can help you build templates and streamline coding for orthopedic treatment and procedures.
- Share experiences and knowledge by publishing articles.
- Individuals interested in becoming an orthopedic PA should start by shadowing one in clinic for at least a week to experience the full spectrum of assigned tasks.
- Read the annual LTHET military personnel message, which details requirements for shadowing hours and Graduate Record

Examination (GRE) scores needed to apply for the orthopedic PA doctoral program.

- Start learning about the IRB and how do conduct research at the local level by reaching out to clinicians and other researchers.
- Attend a class such as the SP Corps Mary Lipscomb Hamrick Research course before attending LTHET to learn research skills.

Conclusion

In FORSCOM, orthopedic PAs extend surgeons' capabilities in forward environments, increasing access to orthopedic care on the battlefield. In MTFs, orthopedic PAs improve access to specialty care in the garrison environment by increasing staffing in orthopedic clinics and operating rooms. Across the force, orthopedic PAs contribute to the education of general practice providers by precepting students, giving formal board review lectures, and providing patient-centered feedback. Orthopedic PAs mentor future leaders in a variety of dynamic environments, including operational medicine, clinical research, and hospital-based medicine. The orthopedic PA degree program exceeds the civilian standard of on-the-job training and certificate programs, enabling students to participate in damage-control orthopedics and contribute to evidence-based medicine. Military orthopedic PAs also serve in a number of national professional organizations, extending their sphere of influence beyond the uniform. Future orthopedic PAs will serve in a wide variety of leadership positions and further prove the value of specialty-trained PAs to supplement surgeons in far-forward units.

References

1. DeMars BJ, Chief, Army Medical Specialist Corps. *Request Approval for the Orthopedic Physician Assistant Residency Doctoral Degree (AOC/ASI: 65DM1).* Memorandum to Commander, US Army Medical Department Center and School, March 4, 2008.
2. Chief, Army Medical Specialist Corps. *Request Approval to Improve the Postgraduate Physician Assistant Residency Training Program.* Memorandum to Commander, US Army Medical Department Center and School, October 17, 2006.

3. US Army Doctor of Science Clinical Orthopedics Physician Assistant Program manual, 2018. Unpublished document available at Army Medical Center of Excellence Graduate School office.

Chapter 6

THE ARMY EMERGENCY MEDICINE PHYSICIAN ASSISTANT

Monica Casmaer, PA-C, DSc; Sharon Rosser, PA-C, DSc, MPAS; and Ryan Curtis, PA-C, DSc, RDMS

> The Army's Emergency Medicine Physician Assistant (EMPA) residency program produces the world's most highly trained Emergency PAs. Fully capable of resuscitating critically ill or injured patients, they have and are decreasing morbidity and mortality both in the Medical Treatment Facilities and on the battlefield. Highly sought after for their advanced training, EMPAs bring modern trauma resuscitation to wounded warriors, saving lives and allowing them to return home to their families.
>
> *—Colonel (Retired) Ian Wedmore*
> *Former Emergency Medicine Consultant to*
> *The Army Surgeon General*

Emergency Medicine Physician Assistant's Mission

The mission of the US Army emergency medicine physician assistant (EMPA) is threefold: (1) to be a force multiplier by providing emergency medical and trauma resuscitative care on and off the battlefield (Figure 6-1); (2) to perform as a clinical scientist to better serve Military Health System beneficiaries; and (3) to enrich the physician assistant (PA) profession with expertise in emergency medicine. This mission is met through producing EMPA residency program graduates with proficiency in clinical emergency medicine and resuscitative trauma management.

EMPAs provide rapid and thorough evaluation and management of emergent medical, surgical, neurologic, polytrauma, and critical patients (Figure 6-2). They perform emergent bedside procedures to

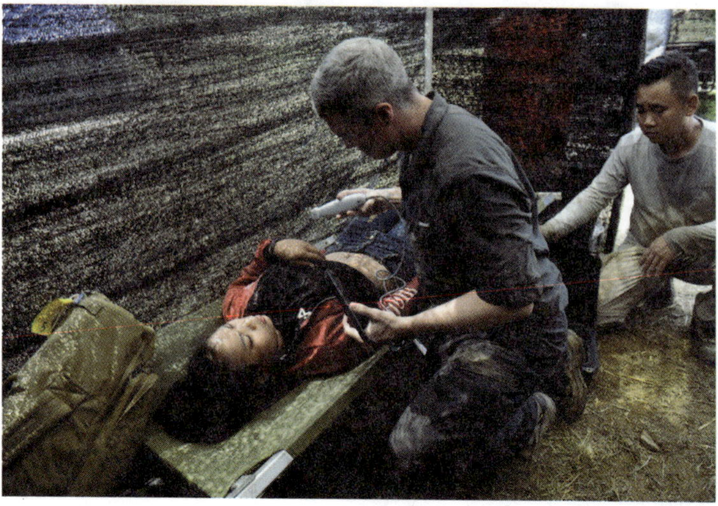

Figure 6-1. Captain Brian Ahern, an emergency physician assistant assigned to a Defense POW/MIA Accounting Agency (DPAA) recovery team, performs an ultrasound on a local worker during excavation operations in the Houaphan province, Laos, February 16, 2019. As part of the humanitarian mission, DPAA hosts a medical outreach event to treat local villagers. The team deployed in support of DPAA's mission to provide the fullest possible accounting of missing personnel to their families and the nation by searching for the remains of service members lost during the Vietnam War. Photograph by Staff Sergeant Michael O'Neal, US Army.
Reproduced from Defense Visual Information Distribution Service. https://www.dvidshub.net/image/5150551/19-2la

stabilize critical medical and traumatically wounded patients within military medical treatment facilities (MTFs). EMPAs improve access to emergency medical care in MTFs and optimize emergency department (ED) throughput and productivity, which reduces the overall health care cost burden in the current period of physician shortages.[1] EMPAs also increase medical knowledge and performance improvement (PI) by conducting research approved by the institutional review board and other PI projects related to emergency medicine.

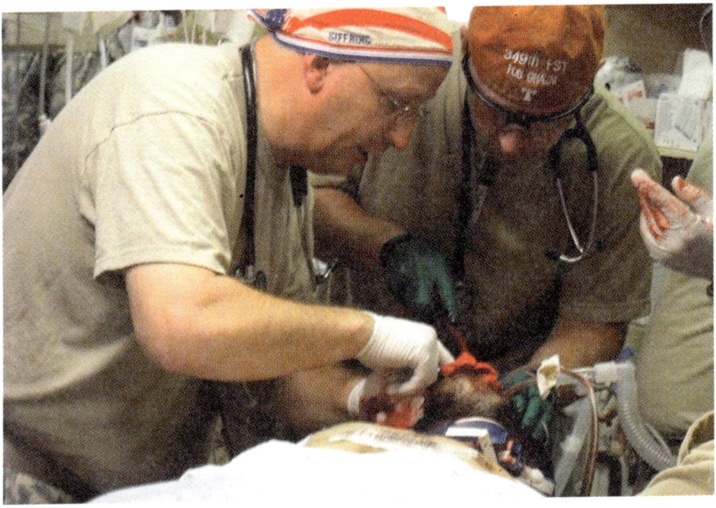

Figure 6-2. Captain Ryan Curtis, 36th Area Support Medical Company, and trauma surgeon Lieutenant Colonel Corydon Siffring, work to achieve hemostasis on a coalition partner suffering from a gunshot wound to the face. Both were assigned to the Role 2 forward surgical element at Forward Operating Base Ghazni, Afghanistan. They were deployed in support of Operation Enduring Freedom.
Photograph courtesy of Corydon Siffring, Lieutenant Colonel, Medical Corps, US Army.

Residency Program

Vision

The vision of the EMPA residency program is to create the benchmark for postgraduate EMPA education through the pursuit of academic and clinical excellence. This vision is realized by developing clinical scientists who are prepared to conduct advanced scientific research, as well as to provide quality emergency care for patients with a wide variety of illnesses and traumatic injuries in the ED and on the battlefield. These EMPA clinical scientists will develop as future leaders and mentors by establishing scholarly excellence for the PA profession.

History

In 1981, in response to an Army-wide emergency medicine physician shortage, the Army initiated training in emergency medicine for PAs. PAs were trained to augment physician staff in the perpetually busy EDs. Most assignments were to understaffed MTFs located throughout the continental United States. Selected PAs were enrolled in a training program at Darnall Army Community Hospital, Fort Hood, Texas, which already had an existing emergency medicine physician residency. The program of study was 12 months long and paralleled the second postgraduate year training for emergency physicians. However, suffering a severe PA shortage in line units and poor PA retention, the Army reduced or stopped most postgraduate training for PAs in 1986. A total of 12 EMPAs were trained during those 5 years.

In 1989, the American College of Emergency Physicians (ACEP) published a position paper in the *Annals of Emergency Medicine* on the utilization of PAs in military emergency medicine.[2] While there was some division among physicians as to the practicality of utilizing PAs in emergency medicine, the authors made the important point that training PAs in this field prepared them for the type of trauma anticipated in combat.[3] The authors maintained that EMPAs could be a valuable asset to a military ED, stressing that PAs should be used as physician extenders and not as physician substitutes. ACEP advocated that all EMPAs receive a formal course of training in either a fellowship or residency program for at least 12 months, and that the training be conducted at an approved emergency medicine physician residency program.

In 1991, the Army surgeon general approved a plan for a revised program. The first EMPA training began at Brooke Army Medical Center, Fort Sam Houston, Texas, on July 1, 1991. In 1992, a second program was established at Madigan Army Medical Center, Tacoma, Washington. A third program began in 1995 at Darnall Army Community Hospital (but closed the following year after graduating one class in 1996). All three training sites had active emergency medicine physician residency programs. Upon successful completion and graduation from EMPA training, graduates were awarded the M2 identifier to their area of concentration (65DM2).

In January 2007, ACEP issued a policy statement validating the necessity of additional training for PAs in the ED setting. The policy states that "Physician Assistants working in EDs should have or acquire specific experience or specialty training in emergency care, should participate in a supervised orientation program, and should receive appropriate training and continuing education in providing emergency care."[4] This is the first time that a non-PA organization acknowledged the necessity for advanced education of PAs.

Traditionally, entry-level training for PAs was either a bachelor's degree or, now more commonly, a master's degree program. PAs desiring doctoral degrees had to pursue the traditional academic route such as the Doctor of Philosophy (PhD), available only in nonclinical subjects. Those desiring postprofessional education emphasizing clinical skills had limited options. Most of the current programs are based on distance learning with very little faculty oversight of the clinical experience. PAs who wanted to specialize in a clinical residency training program could attend a 12-month clinical program that issued a certificate of advanced competency in the specialty upon completion.

In 2006, the US Army partnered with Baylor University to create the world's first Doctor of Science in Physician Assistant Studies specializing in Emergency Medicine (DScPAS-EM) degree. To create the new doctoral degree, the previous 12-month certificate program was extended into an 18-month clinical emergency medicine residency program with a more robust curriculum and additional clinical contact hours. The residency program was developed to provide training in emergency medical care on and off the battlefield. With emphasis on individual research, evidence-based practice, and a superior clinical curriculum, the program is unique. No other existing EMPA residency and fellowship programs can match its strengths in all areas. It has established a standard that other programs are currently attempting to emulate. With this distinction and the prestige earned by its graduates, the DScPAS-EM residency program benefits the Army by serving as a tool to recruit and retain highly qualified military graduates who wish to further their education, specialize in a highly demanding field, and provide emergency medicine capabilities to military units and MTFs (Figure 6-3).

Program Curriculum

The EMPA residency program selects residents from a pool of qualified Army PA applicants based on projected needs of the Army and per guidelines established in the annual long-term health education training

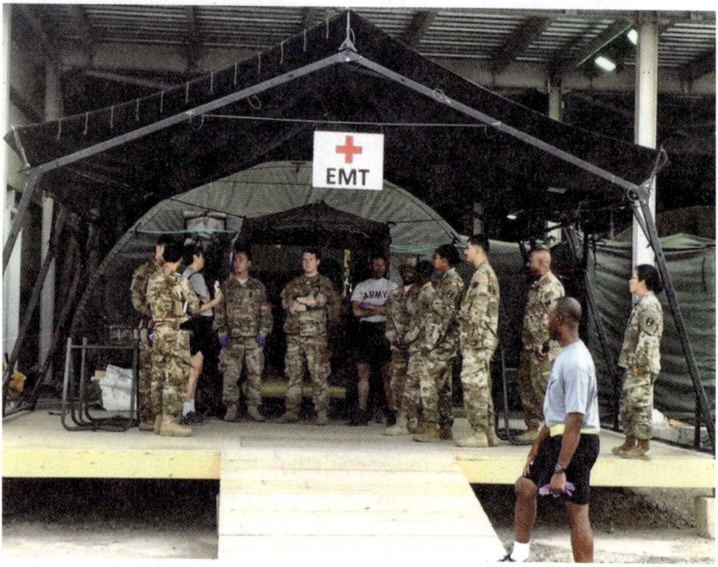

Figure 6-3. Role 3 emergency medical technician section officer in charge, Lieutenant Colonel Jason Naylor, and his team await the arrival of a patient from Baghdad International Airport. They were deployed in support of Operation Inherent Resolve in 2017.
Photograph courtesy of Jason Naylor, Lieutenant Colonel, Medical Specialist Corps, US Army.

message. New EMPA residents begin with a 2-week accelerated research course on how to design a research protocol that can be approved by an institutional review board, conduct research, collect data, analyze the research data, and complete a doctoral-level manuscript. Additionally, EMPA residents learn how to present their research in various platforms including poster presentations, scientific platform presentations, and defense of the doctoral research project.

The EMPA residents join their physician colleagues in an extensive, in-depth, 4-week introduction to critical care and emergency medicine to familiarize the PA with emergency, combat, and polytrauma medicine. During this training, the EMPA resident participates in numerous procedure labs and performs various lifesaving skills to resuscitate the sick and wounded. Next is a 4-week ultrasound training rotation that familiarizes and credentials the EMPA resident in point-of-care (bedside) ultrasonography. Procedures performed during live tissue and cadaver labs include central venous access, pericardiocentesis, arterial line placement, transvenous cardiac pacing, chest tube thoracostomy, needle thoracostomy, resuscitative thoracotomy, venous cutdown, intraosseous device placement, and lumbar puncture. Additionally, residents perform lateral canthotomy, orotracheal intubation, rapid sequence induction, cricothyroidotomy, tracheostomy, supraglottic airway device placement, and ventilator management.

The program emphasizes patient care through hands-on learning. In total, the EMPA residency consists of 16 didactic sections and 20 clinical rotations comprised of approximately 740 hours of classroom instruction and nearly 4,000 clinical hours. It includes rotations through the medical, surgical, and cardiac intensive care units, the pediatric ED, and eight separate rotations at two level 1 trauma centers with extensive trauma surgery and resuscitation exposure.

Certifications

The EMPA resident must complete the American College of Surgeons Advanced Trauma Life Support (ATLS), Advanced Life Support (ALS), Pediatric Advanced Life Support (PALS), and Basic Life Support (BLS) courses during the residency. Residents may choose to attend Advanced Burn Life Support (ABLS), Neonatal Resuscitation Program (NRP), and the Pediatric Fundamentals of Critical Care Support (PFCCS). After completion of the EMPA residency program, graduates are awarded the DScPAS-EM. Graduates from the DScPAS-EM program may apply for the 1-year ultrasound fellowship.

Ultrasound Fellowship

The ultrasound fellowship is designed to train acute care clinicians to be leaders in bedside ultrasound. It is dedicated to the principle that ultrasound is part of the clinical practice of every emergency physician and PA. The fellowship adheres to the ACEP *Emergency Ultrasound Guidelines* (2013) specifically pertaining to the site qualification requirements and fellowship criteria for graduation.[5] The program focuses on four primary competency areas: sonographer/sonologist training; ultrasound educator; scholarly activity; and administration of ultrasound continuous quality improvement programs.

The EMPA ultrasound fellow is expected to personally perform at least 1,000 ultrasound exams during the fellowship. The fellow must master the applications of diagnostic and procedural emergency ultrasound prior to graduation.[5–7]

Duty Descriptions

The positions for the specialized PAs (orthopedics, emergency medicine, and general surgery) with similar roles and responsibilities are provided in more detail in Chapter 4, Academic Leadership Roles, Professional Education, and Training Opportunities. The following are the duty descriptions specific to EMPAs.

Emergency Medicine Physician Assistant in the Emergency Department or Combat Support Hospital

- Provides direct expert patient care to patients in the ED or combat support hospital under high-stress situations. Provides care and clinical supervision for a wide range of patient presentations, ages, and conditions including emergent, urgent, and non-urgent complaints.
- Responsible for the rapid and thorough triage, evaluation, and management of the pediatric, psychiatric, obstetric, geriatric, surgical, and traumatically injured patients in the ED or combat support hospital. Performs invasive and noninvasive diagnostic and therapeutic procedures including lifesaving procedures within personal credentials and privileges delineated by the hospital.
- Responsible for utilizing considerable ingenuity in identifying symptoms of presenting patients that are often subtle or present with overlapping symptoms due to the presence of more than one condition or ailment, and that require extensive analysis and testing to determine the nature and scope of the problem.
- Orders appropriate laboratory, x-ray, and other diagnostic tests; interprets the total medical and surgical evidence, incorporating information into an accurate diagnosis or appraisal; institutes proper treatment and develops the appropriate patient care plan.
- Facilitates patient access to continuing medical care by appropriate referrals to other health care providers, operating within the policies and regulations of the hospital or MTF. Skillfully interacts with a

variety of patients and consultants in an effort to obtain desired compliance and cooperation. Maintains health and clinical records in accordance with current regulations and standards. Maintains the appropriate level of physical fitness necessary to respond to any emergency medical or trauma situation.

Emergency Medicine Physician Assistant in the Forward Deployed Surgical/Resuscitative Element, Critical Care Transport, US Disaster Response Team, Damage Control Resuscitation Team, and White House

- Responsible for the rapid and thorough triage, evaluation, stabilization, and management of urgent medical, surgical, or traumatically injured patients.
- Performs invasive and noninvasive diagnostic and therapeutic procedures including lifesaving procedures within personal credentials and privileges delineated by the hospital or MTF.
- Responsible for utilizing considerable ingenuity in identifying symptoms of presenting patients that are often subtle or present with overlapping symptoms due to the presence of more than one condition or ailment, and that require extensive analysis and testing to determine the nature and scope of the problem.
- Orders appropriate available laboratory, x-ray, and other diagnostic tests; interprets the total medical and surgical evidence, incorporating information into an accurate diagnosis or appraisal; institutes proper treatment and develops a patient care plan appropriate to the medical assets and facilities available in the area of operations.
- Facilitates patient access to continuing medical care by appropriate referrals to other health care providers and specialists and determines necessary evacuation to higher echelons of care, operating within the policies and regulations of the hospital or MTF.
- Enhances medical capabilities for forward emergency and resuscitative care and expands capabilities at the tactical level by providing specialized advanced trauma management and far-forward damage control resuscitation at or near the point of injury, to prevent deterioration and death in the urgent presurgical patient and reduce the number of deaths from potentially survivable wounds on the battlefield or in other austere conditions of operations
- Augments emergency medical expertise in the structure of the

operating forces, advising the brigade surgeon or appropriate authority on the management of trauma patients within the area of operations.

- Skillfully interacts with a variety of patients and consultants to obtain compliance and cooperation.
- Maintains health and clinical records in accordance with current regulations and standards.
- Maintains the appropriate level of physical fitness necessary to respond to any emergency medical or trauma situation.

Emergency Medicine Physician Assistant Ultrasound Fellow

- Provides education to physician residents, EMPA residents and fellows, medics, nurses, and faculty or medical students. The primary venue for teaching is scanning shifts, when the fellow will help staff hone their skills on the primary applications for emergency and critical care ultrasound, and expand their knowledge of evolving applications.
- Must be able to demonstrate 20 hours per month of hands-on teaching at the end of each 28-day rotation block.
- Runs the weekly ultrasound quality assurance review sessions, during which each bedside and training ultrasound exam is reviewed and critiqued. Exams reviewed include studies done by the fellow, residents, and students during their ultrasound electives. Responsible for educating residents and students in this forum under the supervision of the director.
- Integrally involved in the emergency medicine residency ultrasound curriculum. This involves a combination of pre-scheduled didactic and hands-on teaching sessions, ED scanning shifts, and assisting the fellowship director in leading journal review discussions.
- Presents a minimum of one grand rounds lecture during the course of the year on advanced emergency ultrasound topics.
- Assists and facilitates residents during ultrasound rotations in preparing video review clips and high-yield teaching points for grand rounds "Ultrasound Cases of the Month."
- Conducts research followed by peer-reviewed publication as a significant portion of the nonclinical workload.
- Serves as a primary investigator on one research project approved by an institutional review board and as associate investigator on a

second. Abstract publications as well as one additional publication in the form of images in clinical medicine, case report, case series, expert opinion, letter to the editor, or textbook chapter are also a requirement of the fellowship.

- Attends a national emergency medicine ultrasound section meeting during the fellowship.
- Learns how to set up, direct, and manage an ultrasound continuous quality improvement program. This entails developing a data collection instrument, a database for storing continuous quality improvement data, and a means of developing measures of quality.
- Initiates and conducts at least one interdepartmental quality assurance project to improve the use of ultrasound in the emergency medicine setting.
- Becomes familiar with national recommendations for credentialing and how they are carried out in a hospital-based emergency medicine practice.
- Attends interdepartmental and committee meetings throughout the hospital in relation to ultrasound use in the ED.
- Attends weekly emergency medicine grand rounds and departmental continuing education activities. Registered Diagnostic Medical Sonographer certification is encouraged.

Chair, Emergency Medicine Physician Assistant Program

- Identifies capability gaps the EMPA can fill. Provides recommendations on the use and placement of EMPAs throughout the Army to the emergency medicine consultant to the Army surgeon general, the PA consultant to the Army surgeon general and SP Corps chief, the PA requirements chief at the Directorate of Combat and Doctrine Development, and the Army Medical Department Personnel Proponent Directorate.
- Assists the EMPA program directors by ensuring the EMPA skill sets remain up to date and relevant to possible future capability gaps across the Department of Defense.
- Works closely with the PA graduate medical education committee and dean to ensure that the EMPA residency program is adhering to all standards and producing quality EMPAs. Provides input and recommendations to the PA graduate medical education committee and dean, PA chief, SP Corps chief, and SP Corps education

committee on recommendations for the EMPA program directors. Provides input on applicants to the EMPA residency program.

Duty Locations

- Continental United States: California (Ft Irwin); Colorado (Ft Carson); Georgia (Ft Benning, Ft Gordon, Ft Stewart); Kansas (Ft Riley); Kentucky (Ft Campbell, Ft Knox); Louisiana (Ft Polk); New York (West Point); North Carolina (Ft Bragg); Oklahoma (Ft Sill); South Carolina (Ft Jackson); Texas (Ft Hood); Virginia (Ft Belvoir); and Washington (Ft Lewis).
- Outside continental United States: Alaska, Hawaii, Germany, and Korea.
- Fort Sam Houston: Medical Center of Excellence (Interservice Physician Assistant Program instructor); Brooke Army Medical Center (EMPA program director, EMPA program faculty, and EMPA program manager).

Requirements

- Sincere desire and commitment to attain excellence in providing emergency medical care.
- Must have a Master's Degree in Physician Assistant Studies.
- Must meet Graduate Record Examination requirements for admission to Baylor University.

Desired Skills and Attributes

- Must be an excellent role model with the desire to mentor and teach others.
- Solid leadership, administrative, and academic skills.

Lessons Learned

These are important lessons learned for EMPAs:

- A 65DM2 is a subject matter expert in resuscitation.
- Resuscitation skills require honing and maintenance. This is best accomplished by working no less than 20 hours per week in an ED.

- The 65DM2 needs to be facile in integrating core emergency bedside ultrasound into the patient care flow.

Tips for Success

Along with lessons learned, the following tips for success will enable the future EMPA to succeed beyond expectations:

- If emergency medicine is truly a passion, seek a 65DM2 mentor who is fully engaged in academics and patient care.
- Truly master routine medical complaints to allow the future EMPA to focus on the finer points of emergency medical care.
- Attend the Basic Skills Course to attain a true appreciation of the DScPAS-EM Fellowship.

Conclusion

The EMPA Fellowship is an arduous training program. However, the program generates clinicians capable of handling any emergency at home or abroad. The 65DM2 will experience a career that is both challenging and extremely rewarding.

References

1. Herrera J, Gendron BP, Rice MM. Military emergency medicine physician assistants. *Mil Med.* 1994 Mar;159(3):241–242.

2. American College of Emergency Physicians. Task Force on Military Emergency Medicine. Military emergency medicine systems. *Ann Emerg Med.* 1989;18:214–221.

3. Forsberg PA. The US Army Emergency Medicine Physician Assistant Program. *Federal Pract.* 1996; March:37–42.

4. American College of Emergency Physicians. *Guidelines Regarding the Role of Physician Assistants and Advanced Practiced Registered Nurses in the Emergency Department.* ACEP Policy Statement. Approved June 2013. Accessed September 8, 2020. https://www.acep.org/globalassets/new-pdfs/policy-statements/guidelines-regarding-the-role-of-phy.-assts-and-adv-practice-registered-nurses-in-the-ed.pdf

5. American College of Emergency Physicians. *Ultrasound Guidelines: Emergency, Point-of-Care, and Clinical Ultrasound Guidelines in Medicine*. ACEP Policy Statement. Approved June 2016. Accessed September 8, 2020. https://www.acep.org/globalassets/sites/acep/media/ultrasound/pointofcareultrasound-guidelines.pdf

6. American College of Emergency Physicians Board of Directors. *Emergency Ultrasound Imaging Criteria Compendium*. ACEP Policy Statement. Approved October 2014. Accessed September 8, 2020. https://www.acep.org/globalassets/uploads/uploaded-files/acep/by-medical-focus/ultrasound/emergency-ultrasound-imaging-criteria-compendium.pdf

7. Mayo PH, Beaulieu Y, Doelken P, et al. American College of Chest Physicians/La Société de Réanimation de Langue Française statement on competence in critical care ultrasonography. *Chest*. 2009 Apr;135(4):1050–1060.

Additional Sources

- Officer of the Under Secretary of Defense for Personnel Readiness. *Joint Trauma System (JTS)*. Department of Defense; 2016 (Change 1 effective August 5, 2018). DOD Instruction 6040.47. Accessed June 15, 2020. https://www.esd.whs.mil/Portals/54/Documents/DD/issuances/dodi/604047p.pdf?ver=2018-08-06-124902-047
- US Department of Defense. *Medical Readiness Training*. DOD; 2011. DOD Instruction 1322.24.

Chapter 7

THE ARMY GENERAL SURGERY PHYSICIAN ASSISTANT

Seth Holland, PA-C, DSc, MPAS; James Huang, PA-C, DSc, MPAS; Joshua Randles, PA-C, DSc, MPAS; Jonathan Saxe, PA-C, DSc, MPAS; and Matthew S. Douglas, PA-C, DSc, MPAS

"The most important clotting factor is the surgeon."

—*Moshe Schein, MD*[1]

Mission

The mission of an Army general surgery physician assistant (GSPA) is to extend surgical and critical care far forward on the battlefield. GSPAs are force multipliers, enhancing the capabilities of Army general surgeons by extending advanced care and surgical decision-making. GSPAs serve in conventional or special operation forces to support surgical care and surgical critical care in all roles of care, including forward resuscitative surgical teams, critical care transport/emergency resuscitation teams, and deployable hospitals. In military treatment facilities, GSPAs provide perioperative, postoperative, surgical first assist, critical care, and bedside procedures to surgical patients with the goals of increasing surgical productivity, access to care, and continuity of care within the sphere of surgical practice throughout the Army. Doctorate GSPAs also conduct clinical research and performance improvement projects approved by the institutional review board (IRB) in surgery or critical care with the intent of improving care on and off the battlefield.[2]

History

In the 1960s, surgical assistants were being developed on an apprenticeship basis, although there was no formal training process. During that decade, in response to the shortage of medical providers, the PA training model was developed by Dr Eugene Stead Jr, Dr Richard

Smith, Dr Hu C. Myers, and Dr Henry K. Silver, based on World War II physician medical and nursing models.[3] The military first started training specialty PAs in the 1980s. The first military PA specialty was orthopedics, followed by emergency medicine in the 1990s.

In 1995, the idea first surfaced for developing a surgically trained PA who would serve as an extension for surgeons on forward surgical teams. A surgical PA program was developed that included clinical rotations at the University of Maryland Shock Trauma Center in Baltimore; Brooke Army Medical Center at Fort Sam Houston, Texas; and the University of Texas Health Science in San Antonio.[3] Once trained, these PAs would be able to first assist, perform triage, and provide surgical critical care, thus allowing surgeons to focus on performing operations.

In 2001, a pilot program was conducted to train a surgical Army PA. The selected trainee began a 12-month rotation through surgical services at Fort Hood, Texas. The program was a success, but further development of the program was deferred after the September 11th terrorist attacks (email communication with Major [Retired] Don Adams, January 2014).

According to the first GSPA program directors, Lieutenant Colonel David Freel and Lieutenant Colonel Patrick Sherman, the idea of the GSPA was revived in 2005. Over the next year, a curriculum was developed, and a training site was established at Brooke Army Medical Center, Fort Sam Houston, Texas (email communication with Lieutenant Colonel [Retired] David Freel, December 2013). The first class to attend the 18-month training program began in July 2009. In December 2014, the Doctor of Science in Physician Assistant Studies–General Surgery (DScPAS-GS) was awarded. The program continued to grow, incorporating Air Force PAs, and seeing its first Navy cohort in the 2018–2019 class cycle, making it a truly tri-service program. In October 2019, new operational assignments for GSPAs were added to the 528th Sustainment Brigade to provide direct surgical support to Special Forces missions.

Because of the continued surgeon shortfall, current initiatives to increase trauma surgical capability include the use of the M4 skill identifier. Through collaborative efforts of the Medical Corps and Specialist Corps via the Medical Center of Excellence Personnel Proponency Directorate, the M4 skill identifier is being proposed as a multiple branch means to collectively identify both trauma-trained surgeons and trauma-trained surgical PAs to augment Role 2 through Role 4 surgical employment.[2]

Training

The 18-month DScPAS-GS doctoral program includes general surgery clinical rotations and subspecialty (trauma/critical care, burn surgery, oncological surgery, pediatric surgery, neurosurgery, vascular surgery, plastic surgery, interventional radiology, and intensive care unit procedures) monthly clinical rotations (Figure 7-1). The following procedures are taught during the 18-month program:

- emergency and critical care ultrasound;
- endoscopy (bronchoscopy, colonoscopy, esophagogastroduodenoscopy);
- placement of central lines;
- peripheral inserted central catheter;
- pericardiocentesis;
- thoracostomy tube placement;

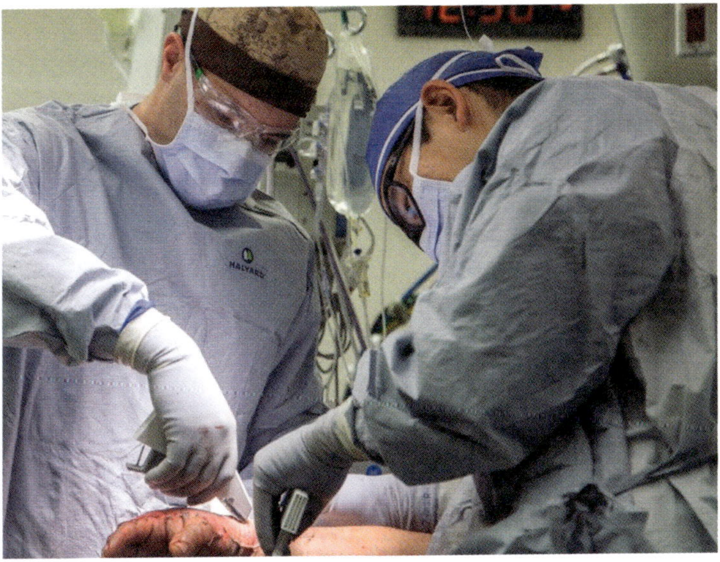

Figure 7-1. Captain Josh Randles (left) affixes an autologous split-thickness skin graft with a US Army Institute of Surgical Research staff surgeon (right); October 2019.

- lumbar puncture;
- ventriculostomy;
- surgical airways (crichothyroidotomy and tracheostomy); and
- fluoroscopic guided procedures.

Also taught are basic surgical first assist techniques for trauma, open surgical cases, and laparoscopic and robotic surgical cases. Other critical care and trauma procedures taught are airway management (intubation, crichothyroidotomy, tracheostomy); orthopedic external fixation; continuous renal replacement therapy; burn and wound care; minor procedures; thoracotomy; and ventilator management. The GSPA resident also attends training in the following certifications: Advanced Burn Life Support (ABLS); Fundamentals of Critical Care Support; Emergency War Surgery; and Advanced Trauma Life Support (ATLS).[2]

Current curricular training occurs at Brooke Army Medical Center for 17 didactic courses aligned with 16 clinical rotations and comprehensive IRB-approved doctoral research projects, culminating in a doctoral defense with the affiliated university. These programmatic events are complemented by oral examinations, simulation training/testing, case report publications, surgical presentations in morbidity/mortality and tumor board conferences, and the American Board of Surgery In-Training Examination (ABSITE).[2]

Practice and Certifications

After graduation, GSPAs have the opportunity to practice in a multitude of fields and may obtain additional certifications:

- Specialty practice
    - trauma/critical care
    - acute care surgery/emergency general surgery
    - cardiothoracic surgery
    - interventional radiology
    - neurosurgery
    - vascular surgery
    - bariatric/minimally invasive surgery
    - surgical oncology
    - colorectal surgery

- Certifications
  - Registered Diagnostic Medical Sonographer (RDMS)[4]
  - Certified Wound Care Specialist (CWS)[5]
  - Certificate of Advanced Qualification (Hospitalist)

Duty Descriptions

Chapter 4 described four positions—program director, research director, program manager, and Interservice Physician Assistant Program (IPAP) instructor—with similar roles and responsibilities in managing the DSc programs for clinical orthopedics (Chapter 5), emergency medicine (Chapter 6), and general surgery (this chapter). The following duty descriptions are specific to GSPAs:

Surgical/Critical Care Physician Assistant, Special Operations Forces

These PAs serve as surgical PAs on forward resuscitative surgical teams, providing initial trauma assessments and damage control resuscitation, assisting with damage control surgery and acute care surgery, and providing critical care. They are expected to provide operational context to the team's mission; assist with medical mission planning and training[6,7]; and advise special operations units and commanders on medical threats and permission requirements. Training for these surgical teams consists of working in civilian trauma centers and establishing overseas partnerships. These PAs must be airborne volunteers, willing to deploy at least annually, and agree to a 3-year commitment to the unit. They must be in excellent physical shape, culturally astute with good interpersonal skills, and able to think and operate at both tactical and strategic levels.

Surgical/Critical Care Physician Assistant, Conventional Forces

Positions include the White House surgical PA and PAs assigned to a forward deployed resuscitative surgical element, deployable hospital, critical care transport team, or a disaster response team in the United States. These PAs are responsible for ensuring that all assigned surgical patients receive appropriate triage, preoperative evaluation, resuscitation, and stabilization. They also provide the following care: postoperative care, surgical first assist, inpatient care, intensive care, minor procedures, ultrasound, endoscopy, and wound care. They assist with placement of external fixators (pelvic and extremity), ensure continuity of care, and perform critical care transportation as required. Additionally, they perform or assist in IRB-approved research and performance improvement projects, and educate and train consulting physicians, PAs, nurses, and medics in surgical disease processes, pathology, and treatments.

General/Trauma Surgery Physician Assistant, Fixed Facility

These GSPAs provide surgical care, under the supervision of a surgeon, for patients admitted to a military medical treatment facility. They conduct the following care: preoperative; postoperative; surgical first assist; inpatient treatment; trauma assessments; intensive care; minor clinic procedures; bedside procedures (ultrasound, central lines); endoscopy (colonoscopy, esophagogastroduodenoscopy); and wound care. These GSPAs also perform on-call duties as first call with surgeon backup, and ensure continuity of care for all patients. Additionally, they participate in morbidity and mortality conferences, cancer care conferences, and wound care conferences. These GSPAs also conduct IRB-approved research and performance improvement projects and train consulting physicians, PAs, nurses, and medics in surgical disease processes, pathology, and treatments.[2] They provide feedback and training to local Role 1 providers and medics on outcomes and possible areas for improvements.[2]

Positions and Duty Locations

- GSPA (availability contingent upon updated Defense Health Agency directives):
  - Fort Belvoir Community Hospital, Fort Belvoir, VA
  - Tripler Army Medical Center, Honolulu, HI
- Special operations surgical PA: 528th Sustainment Brigade, Fort Bragg, NC, with duty at Charlotte, NC
- IPAP general surgery instructor: US Army Medical Center of Excellence, JBSA-Fort Sam Houston, TX
- GSPA program director: Brooke Army Medical Center, JBSA Fort Sam Houston, TX

- GSPA assistant program director: Brooke Army Medical Center, JBSA-Fort Sam Houston, TX
- GSPA research director: Brooke Army Medical Center, JBSA-Fort Sam Houston, TX

Requirements

- Experience in battalion and brigade PA positions. Deployments as PA are preferred.
- Apply and be accepted to long-term health education and training (LTHET).
- Rank of captain to lieutenant colonel.
- Captains must have completed the Captains Career Course and majors and higher must have completed Intermediate Level Education prior to start of program.[2]

Desired Skills and Attributes

- Must be an excellent role model with the desire to mentor others.
- Solid leadership, administrative, and academic skills.
- Must have an interest in people.
- Must be able to encourage and assist others.
- Good spoken and written communication skills.
- Strong work ethic.
- Strong organizational and time management skills.
- Committed to working in a team environment.

Lessons Learned

- Training via LTHET is primarily an exposure to multiple practice types; the expertise in a discipline begins on becoming a staff GSPA.
- GSPAs should emphasize surgical and procedural skill maintenance as a major component of their required privileges to support surgical care in deployment.
- Open procedures and basic laparoscopic procedures (hernia, appendectomy, cholecystectomy, diagnostic laparoscopy) are the common surgical cases performed outside fixed facilities.
- Surgical care must occur along a continuum beginning with primary care, prehospital Tactical Combat Casualty Care (TCCC) initial

practice; therefore, GSPAs must be routinely familiar with primary care and TCCC practice to bridge care effectively.

- GSPAs must maintain PA-C recertification as general practitioners and must also maintain the associated knowledge and practice base.
- GSPAs are also military medical officers and must meet the milestones for professional military education and consider opportunities for broadening positions that improve the PA career field.

Tips for Success

- Exploiting a PA's career experience to bridge the knowledge gap for the surgeon from the point of injury to the surgical table and intensive care unit (ICU) bed benefits the patient and enhances shared understanding of the surgical team.
- The LTHET application process includes a good Graduate Record Examination (GRE) score, including the essay score—writing ability will have significant bearing on success in LTHET.
- Surgical research is constantly evolving; to participate, a successful GSPA must remain current in surgical and critical care research.
- Surgery is a team practice; the GSPA must carve out a role that adds value and helps the surgeon focus on their role.
- Valuable knowledge and experience can be drawn from all members of the surgical care team—operating room (OR) technicians, OR nurses, anesthesiologists, and post-anesthesia care unit (PACU) and ICU staff.
- The practice of surgery depends on understanding its judicious use in treating disease as well as appropriate nonsurgical management.
- Expertise in the OR is the result of time spent in the OR.
- More surgical care is performed outside the OR than in it.
- Thorough documentation saves lives and supports good surgical decision-making.
- A GSPA cannot rely solely on a radiologist's report; they must personally view the study ordered and know its limits (anatomy is different in 3-dimensional space).
- Elements of additional surgical disciplines (interventional radiology, neurosurgery, burn, plastics, orthopedics, vascular) should be learned in preparation for any austere surgical deployment.

- It is necessary to learn how to use equipment (loupes, headlamp, laparoscopic and other scopes, cautery, suction); GSPAs should know their intended purposes and how to compensate for their shortfalls as needed.

Conclusion

The GSPA is a well-trained and versatile specialty provider. GSPAs have a comprehensive understanding of the anatomy and pathophysiology of not only surgical disease but also traumatic injury—with the ability to manage a patient from the prehospital phase, to the trauma bay, operating room, and intensive care unit. In addition to providing treatment in all roles of care, in both conventional and unconventional forces, the GSPA can serve in force-generating roles as IPAP and LTHET faculty. They also have opportunities to conduct and publish clinical research. Those who have graduated from the training pipeline are adept and experienced health care providers. The GSPA should be a much sought-after career path.

References

1. Schein M, Rogers PN. *Schein's Common Sense Emergency Abdominal Surgery*. 2nd ed. Springer; 2005.
2. Saxe J, Holland S, Freel D, Sherman P. *US Army Doctorate of Science General Surgery Physician Assistant Program Manual*. Brooke Army Medical Center; 2013.
3. Physician Assistant History Society. Timeline: 1957 to 1970, the formative years. Accessed May 15, 2020. https://pahx.org/period02/
4. American Registry for Diagnostic Medical Sonography website. Accessed May 27, 2020. https://www.ardms.org/
5. American Board of Wound Management. CWS: why certify? Accessed May 27, 2020. http://www.abwmcertified.org/abwm-certified/cws/cws-why-certify/
6. Department of Defense. *Medical Readiness Training*. DOD; March 2018. DOD Instruction 1322.24.

7. Officer of the Under Secretary of Defense for Personnel Readiness. *Joint Trauma System (JTS)*. Department of Defense; 2016 (Change 1 effective August 5, 2018). DOD Instruction 6040.47. Accessed June 15, 2020. https://www.esd.whs.mil/Portals/54/Documents/DD/issuances/dodi/604047p.pdf?ver=2018-08-06-124902-047

Chapter 8

ATTENDING INTERMEDIATE LEVEL EDUCATION

Kane D. Morgan, APA-C, MPAS, MPH; Charlie Day, PA-C, MPAS; Margaret Kucia, PA-C, MPAS; Garrett Larson, APA-C, MPAS, MS; Johnny Wayne Paul, APA-C, DMSc, MPAS; John Joe Peña, APA-C, MPAS, MSIR; Patrick Walsh, PA-C, MPAS; Larry A. Wyatt, APA-C, MPAS; and John F. Detro, APA-C, MPAS, MSS, MEd

Introduction

Intermediate level education (ILE) broadly describes the US Army's formal education system for field-grade, mid-career Army officers preparing to serve in staff and command roles. ILE is achieved through the Command and General Staff Officer Course (CGSOC), either through resident courses, distance learning, or a combination of these programs. CGSOC programs include officers from other US military services, foreign military services, and civilian interagency leaders who intend to operate in Army, joint, interagency, and multinational environments as commanders and general staff officers.[1] CGSOC is similar to ILE programs in other services, such as Air Command and Staff College education for Air Force officers, and the US Navy College of Naval Command and Staff. Pathways to complete ILE through the US Army include:

- 10-month resident CGSOC at Fort Leavenworth, Kansas.
- 14-week resident courses at satellite locations.
- 18-month distance learning course through independent study, the Total Army School System (TASS) reserve schools option, or a combination of both.

Resident Staff College

Resident CGSOC lasts 44 weeks across three curricular components: (1) the CGSOC Common Core (16 weeks), (2) the Advanced Operations Course (16 weeks), and (3) electives (12 weeks).[2] The Common Core curriculum aims to broaden the perspective of junior majors from the tactical level to an operational level and includes seven blocks, culminating in oral and written exams:

- Foundations
- Strategic Studies
- Operational Studies
- Army Operations
- Managing Army Change
- Rise of the Western Way of War
- Leadership: Forging Success in Uncertain Times[3]

The Advanced Operations Course prepares officers to build and lead operational and tactical formations in unified land operations and covers the following subject areas:

- Today's Operational Environment
- Full Spectrum Operations
- Theory of War and Doctrine
- Conduct of War
- Commandership[3]

The elective curriculum provides students the opportunity to enhance their learning while conducting advanced studies in focus areas, across 192 class hours.[2] Students complete courses in an experiential learning environment that yields adaptive, self-aware, field-grade leaders of character and competence who are capable of shaping the joint operational environment.[1] The instruction is designed to develop students' critical and creative thinking skills, decision-making ability, character, self-awareness, leadership skills, and teamwork approaches to solving complex problems from a systems perspective.[1]

Supervision

Participants are assigned to the CGSOC US Student Detachment (USSD) at Fort Leavenworth, in student status, and placed into one of approximately 64 staff groups, each with 16 students under a group advisor.[2] A staff group consists of officers from multiple branches and various services or governmental agencies, with one or two representatives from multinational partners. Only one Army Medical Department (AMEDD) officer is in each staff group.

Roles and Duties

While assigned to the USSD, each officer participates in a leadership position within the student chain of command. These positions range from small group leader to class president, and all are designed to assist with the daily management of the staff group. Additionally, there are multiple opportunities to serve in various other volunteer positions, some of which result in elective credits toward graduation. Some of these positions include:

- class historian,
- yearbook editor,
- triathlon director,
- adjutant officer,
- international student sponsor, and
- sports and recreation director.[2]

Desired Skills and Attributes

Applicants compete for attendance under the Army special branches ILE selection board, based on the following requirements and desired attributes:

- rank of major or captain promotable;
- Captain Career Course graduate;
- extensive experience as a physician assistant (PA) and AMEDD officer, with working knowledge of the military decision-making process;
- robust oral and written communication skills;

- strong work ethic and ability to work both independently and in a group, and
- desire to think critically about the military's strategic issues.

Training and Coursework

The Fort Leavenworth ILE experience challenges AMEDD students with daily intellectual exercises, rigorous academic assignments, complex problem-solving, impassioned peer-to-peer interactions, and broad exposure to joint, interagency, and multinational perspectives. AMEDD students will be asked not only to represent the AMEDD, but also to operate well outside the normal boundaries of a medical officer within the structure and framework of an Army staff. ILE faculty members intend to produce the field-grade officers soldiers deserve: tactically proficient, professionally competent, intellectually grounded, organizationally skilled, ethically sound, and readily able to exercise disciplined initiative in a brigade, division, corps, or joint headquarters.[2]

The first 7 months of ILE residency are particularly demanding and typically require 8 in-class hours per day and 3 to 5 additional hours of reading and homework. During this time, students participate in the Common Core and Advanced Operations Course curricula, which culminate in a joint exercise with international exchange students who travel to the United States to participate.

After completion of the Common Core and Advanced Operations Course, students proceed to the 8-course elective portion. They choose elective programs or courses of study based on personal interest and professional stewardship, such as:

- Graduate degree program focus, culminating in the Master of Military Art and Science (MMAS) degree or other graduate degrees through Kansas State University, the University of Kansas, or another partnering university.[2]
- Homeland security studies focus, offering students the opportunity to develop expertise in the area of homeland security.[2,4]
- Certificate in Overseas Contingency Operations–Planning, providing students the opportunity to develop expertise critical to the execution of stability operations and reconstruction and stabilization missions.[2,4]

- Foreign language program, providing formal language instruction in a language of the student's choice, or based on projected postgraduation assignments.[2,4]
- International exchange and fellowship programs with the Australian, French, German, or United Kingdom staff colleges in conjunction with the completion of a regional studies certificate.[2,4]
- Defense Support to Civil Authorities (awarding additional skill identifier [ASI] 7A), which trains officers to navigate the challenges of multidisciplinary and interagency roles in global humanitarian assistance/disaster response, emergency operations, and interoperating with National Guard and reserve components.[2,4]
- Joint planner (ASI 3H), which trains students in the Joint Operation Planning and Execution System (JOPES) and supporting information technologies.[2,4]
- Space activities (ASI 3Y), which trains the student on the capabilities, functions, and organizations performing military space missions.[2,4]
- Air operations officer (ASI 5U), which develops the skills for becoming an air operation officer through the joint firepower course.[2,4]
- Historian (ASI 5X), which educates students on the unique skills to serve in positions as Army historians, instructors, and history detachment members.[2,4]
- Strategic studies graduate (ASI 6Z), which prepares officers for future assignments dealing with national security and military strategy.[2,4]
- Red teaming (ASI 7J or 7G), which trains the student on the ability to enhance mission accomplishment by looking at problems from the perspective of the adversary, multinational partners, or alternative strategies.[2,4]

Additional Resident Information

- The resident ILE website is https://usacac.army.mil/organizations/cace/cgsc/cgss#.
- Attendance requires a permanent change of station (PCS) to Fort Leavenworth (see information for inbound students at https://usacac.army.mil/organizations/cace/cgsc/inbound).[4]
- Attendance incurs a 2-year service obligation upon completion. Graduates are normally placed in an operational utilization tour of duty using the skills and knowledge developed during training.[4]

- AMEDD students may be credentialed at Munson Army Health Center at Fort Leavenworth, with participation in half-day clinics (preferably two to four times a month).
- Upon notification of selection to the resident ILE course, applicants have 30 days to accept or decline the assignment.[4]
- Applicants should consider moving their family to Fort Leavenworth; the post is very family-friendly, and many students who do not bring their families regret it. On-post housing for unaccompanied officers is also available. If planning to live on post, call the housing office at Fort Leavenworth as early as possible.
- Complete the required online preparatory courses, which include online tests, writing samples, and significant required doctrinal readings.
- Prior to the start of the Common Core, AMEDD officers additionally complete a 2-week on-site prep course review of tactics, symbology, operations planning, and introduction to Army warfighting challenges.[2]
- Consider whether to pursue an MMAS or master's degree from a civilian university. This work is in addition to ILE coursework.[2]

Common Core Satellite Campuses

The CGSOC satellite campuses are located at Fort Belvoir and Fort Lee, Virginia; Fort Gordon, Georgia; and Redstone Arsenal, Alabama (Figure 8-1).[5] Officers from operations support, information operations, and institutional support career fields join AMEDD officers who attend with board-selected reserve component, National Guard, and special branch officers such as judge advocate generals and chaplains. In total, 12 satellite cohorts per year receive the identical 3.5-month CGSOC Common Core curriculum. AMEDD typically receives 108 satellite campus seats annually.[5]

Satellite Course Administration

Selected students attend in either temporary duty (TDY) or TDY en-route status and stay in centrally funded lodging. All TDY students are directed to use dining facilities, and are entitled to daily meals and incidental expenses.[6] TDY student personnel actions, including leave and finance, are managed by their home unit.[5,6] Limited TDY en-route

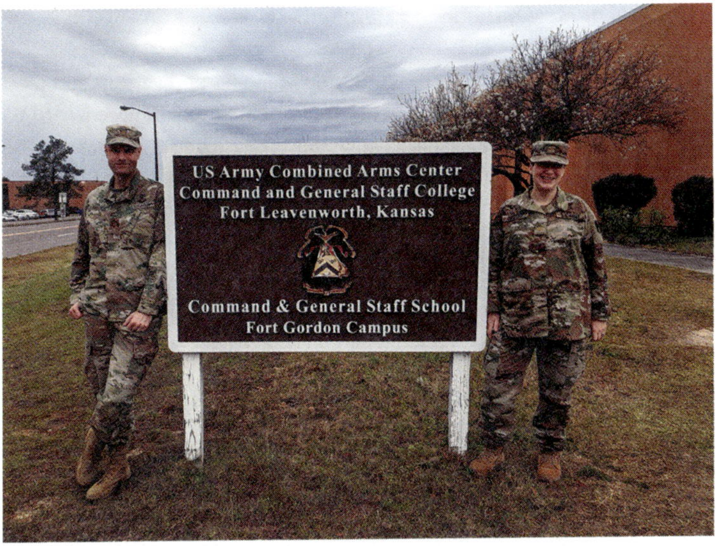

Figure 8-1. Major Garrett Larson, APA-C, and Major Lydia Zellers, PA-C, completed Intermediate Level Education through the satellite resident program at Fort Belvoir, Virginia, in March 2020.
Photograph courtesy of Major Larson.

student actions can be forwarded through the satellite campus to Fort Leavenworth for processing. Non-emergency leave during the course is not approved, except during holidays or weekends. Throughout satellite course attendance, students should not perform work activities related to their home or gaining unit. Personal or professional TDY during ILE (eg, conference or change of command ceremony attendance) is not approved unless general/flag officer requests are sent to the Combined Arms Center commander. Students attending in TDY status from duty stations outside the continental United States will not have tours curtailed or extended.[6]

Students are not eligible to attend CGSOC if currently flagged for failure to pass a record physical fitness test, or are noncompliant with Army body fat standards.[2] Temporary profiles are not authorized for incoming students unless due to pregnancy.

Satellite Course Training and Coursework

Four groups of 16 students, from multiple branches and various services, comprise each satellite course. There are typically two or three AMEDD officers in each group. A faculty group adviser leads each group, and the senior ranking student is the student group leader. The following additional duties are available:

- personnel officer
- supply officer
- technology officer
- safety officer
- after-action review officer
- homework officer
- social coordinator
- physical training coordinator
- photography coordinator

The typical satellite course training day is 0800 to 1500 hours, with plenty of free time provided for reading and reflection.[2] Organized small group physical fitness training is mandatory. Self-development undertakings such as journal article publication, scholarly projects, and physical fitness events are highly encouraged and rewarded.[2] The Common Core curriculum at satellite campuses, which differs from the structure at Fort Leavenworth, includes the following nine blocks of facilitated experiential learning instruction[2]:

1. CGSOC Foundations
2. Political and Strategic Environment
3. Joint Operations and Unified Action
4. US Army Doctrine
5. Joint Planning
6. Force Management
7. History
8. Leadership
9. Exams: a computer-based final exam and a rigorous oral board exam

Common Core Distance Learning

The Common Core distance learning (CC-DL) course is completed through independent study. Students are given access to the three phases and the same nine Common Core blocks. Distance learners use non-facilitated instruction to work independently on the Blackboard Learning Management System. Each phase represents a separate "course" in the Army Training Requirements and Resources System (ATRRS), to be completed sequentially. Students are assigned faculty advisors who monitor and support their progress through the course. Army Regulation 350-1 authorizes students 18 months to complete the course, although completion time varies by student, and depends largely on time invested by students.[7]

Total Army School System Common Core Option

Students may also enroll in the US Army Reserve TASS course option, called Command and General Staff Officer Course–Common Core (CGSOC-CC).[5] This option provides US Army Reserve students with a resident-like CGSOC experience. The TASS option is also a three-phase course. The DL and TASS phases of instruction are nearly identical, allowing students to move between either online or TASS instruction. Students enroll in the TASS version of the Common Core course in the same manner they would CC-DL, by applying for the TASS option through ATRRS.[5] TASS organizations include CGSOC-certified instructors to teach the course. For the most up-to-date information, refer to the ATRRS course catalog, www.atrrs.army.mil/atrrscc/, course number 701-1-250-ILE-CC.

Phases 1 and 3 are conducted in two ways:

1. Two-week resident courses at Fort Dix, New Jersey; Camp Parks, California; Fort McCoy, Wisconsin; Hawaii; and Germany.
2. Distance learning.

Phase 2 is conducted in two ways:

1. "2 × 8": 2 days a month for 8 months, October through May, at approximately 45 locations are across the United States, including Puerto Rico.

2. TASS accelerated "4 × 4": 4 days a month for 4 months, at seven locations across the United States, beginning the second quarter of the fiscal year.[5]

Awards

Resident

- George C. Marshall Award (distinguished graduate)
- Arter-Doniphan Award (highest grade point average)
- CGSOC Iron Major Award (physical fitness course)
- Grierson Award for Excellence in Strategic Studies (top strategist)
- MacArthur Military Leadership Writing Award
- Arter-Darby Military History Writing Award (tactical)
- Simons Center Interagency Writing Award
- Outstanding MMAS Thesis
- Excellence in Joint Command, Control, Communications, Computer and Intelligence (JC4I) Writing
- Homeland Security Studies Award
- Father Donald J. Smythe Award (military history)
- Master Tactician
- Master Logistician
- Harris Leadership Award (instructor nomination)
- Excellence in Joint Service Warfare Award

Satellite course

- General John J. Pershing Award (top graduate in each CGSOC satellite course)[2,8]

The Western Hemisphere Institute for Security Cooperation

The Western Hemisphere Institute for Security Cooperation (WHINSEC) is a tenant unit on Fort Benning, Georgia, located in the community of Columbus, Georgia.[9] WHINSEC was established in 2001 and codified in Title 10 USC, §343, as a Department of Defense training and education institution.[9,10] WHINSEC advances democratic principles and promotes interoperability, human rights, and US customs and traditions. These goals are achieved by providing security and defense training to partner nations through partnerships with academic institutions, and by fostering relationships with senior officials from the Americas and the Caribbean.[10] Of the several courses held at WHINSEC, the School of Professional Military Education delivers a 10-month in-residence CGSOC. Similar to the in-residence CGSOC offered at Fort Leavenworth, CGSOC at WHINSEC is conducted once every academic year.[2,9,10] Students completing CGSOC at WHINSEC achieve the professional military education ILE requirements for intermediate-level officers.[2]

Facilities and Class Structure

Generally, the 64 students attending CGSOC at WHINSEC are a combination of US and international officers in the rank of major (O-4) or lieutenant colonel (O-5), as well as interagency and intergovernmental civilian equivalents. Students are divided into four groups of 15 or 16 officers led by a faculty group advisor. Each group has approximately an even distribution of US and international students, with only one AMEDD officer in each group. The CGSOC at WHINSEC provides state-of-the-art classrooms in Bradley Hall that are nearly identical to those in Fort Leavenworth. Students have access to support facilities and reference facilities at the Maneuver Center of Excellence.[9,10] For most US students, this is their initial exposure to a joint, interagency, intergovernmental, and multinational environment.

Training and Education

CGSOC students receive the same training and education as those attending CGSOC at Fort Leavenworth. However, CGSOC at WHINSEC does have some differences; most notably, the course is taught entirely in Spanish, and students are fully immersed in the Spanish language (although English-language study materials are provided).[9] Therefore, US students selected to attend CGSOC at WHINSEC are required to demonstrate Spanish language proficiency with a rating of at least "2" in both listening and reading, annotated in Section V, Foreign Language, on the officer record brief. Eligible US military students earning a Spanish language proficiency rating of "1" or higher in both listening and reading may receive up to $400 in foreign language proficiency pay throughout their academic year.[11,12] A DA Form 4187, Personnel Action, is generally required to schedule the Defense Language Proficiency Test 5 at a nearby military installation education or testing office.[11,12] CGSOC at WHINSEC also includes additional classes on human rights, the rule of law, due process, civilian control of the military, and the role of the military in a democratic society.[9]

Faculty and Staff

The faculty and staff that make up the instructors for CGSOC at WHINSEC include military personnel from the different US services, military personnel from the Americas and Caribbean, and a foreign service officer from the Department of State. Guest lecturers include representatives and senior officials from Immigration and Customs Enforcement, the Department of Homeland Security, Department of Justice, Drug Enforcement Administration, United Nations, and various US universities.[9]

Additional Opportunities

Students may pursue the following additional educational opportunities while attending CGSOC at WHINSEC:

- **MMAS**. Enrolled CGSOC students may apply for admission into the MMAS program, which requires a choice of electives and an independent research project approved at the department director level. Students are also eligible to compete for CGSOC resident student awards upon submission of their MMAS thesis.[9] The MMAS may only be pursued while enrolled in the resident CGSOC.[9] Additionally, students attending CGSOC at WHINSEC have a unique opportunity to apply up to 18 hours of their CGSOC coursework to simultaneously earn a Master of International Relations in partnership with Troy University.[13]
- **School of Advanced Military Studies.** Graduates of CGSOC are eligible to apply to the School of Advanced Military Studies Program and earn a Master of Art in Military Operations.[2,9]

Attending CGSOC at WHINSEC allows for building camaraderie, establishing relationships, and further fostering the relationship between the United States and partner-nations of the Americas and Caribbean.[9] Nearly twice a month, and sometimes more often, events called "bocadillos" are held. Translated as "luncheons," bocadillos are an opportunity for partner-nation students to introduce regional cultures and customs through sharing popular food and drinks from their country. WHINSEC offers an excellent opportunity for PAs to operate outside of their comfort zone, through exposure to a joint, interagency, intergovernmental, multinational environment. WHINSEC also offers the Army ASI 3H, Joint Planner, which trains students in the JOPES and its supporting information technologies.[9]

Lessons Learned and Tips for Success

- Prior to beginning formal ILE coursework, consider themes or challenges from the AMEDD or broader military context to serve as a focal point for study and research.
- Review doctrinal publications, ranging from tactics and leadership to the Army operating concept.
- Maintain a portfolio of written work and resources throughout ILE to aid future professional development.
- Review a personal learning skills inventory to identify the manner in which learning best occurs prior to starting coursework.
- ILE courses include well-established lecture series, allowing students to learn directly from and interact with general officers, leaders, and policy makers in the Department of Defense and legislative and executive branches of government.
- Expect to study hard, develop new relationships, and interoperate with peers from diverse branches, services, functional areas, and nations.

Conclusion

ILE provides a way for AMEDD officers and PAs to expand their roles in strategic- and operational-level planning and leadership contexts. ILE represents a capstone educational experience for developing skills and addressing shared challenges in a diverse peer group, whether in person or online. While ILE centers on the personal and professional development of staff officers, this unique opportunity crucially supports and underwrites the role of PAs throughout the joint and multinational operating environment, today and in the future.

References

1. US Army Combined Arms Center. Command and General Staff School. Accessed May 28, 2020. https://usacac.army.mil/organizations/cace/cgsc/cgss

2. US Army Combined Arms Center. *US Army Command and General Staff College Catalog, Academic Year 2018–2019*. CGSS; 2018: chap 7. CGSS Circular 350-1. Accessed May 28, 2020. https://usacac.army.mil/sites/default/files/documents/cace/CGSC/CGSC_Circular_350-1_College_Catalog_%28AY2018-2019%29.pdf

3. US Army Combined Arms Center. Command and General Staff Officer's Course summary. Accessed May 28, 2020. https://usacac.army.mil/organizations/cace/cgsc/courses

4. US Army Combined Arms Center. *Student Handbook*. CGSS; 2014: appendix C. Circular 350-5. Accessed May 28, 2020. https://usacac.army.mil/sites/default/files/documents/cace/12-1/12-1_AppC_Electives.pdf

5. US Army Human Resources Command. Senior Service College–Intermediate Level Education. Accessed May 28, 2020. https://www.hrc.army.mil/content/Senior%20Service%20College-Intermediate%20Level%20Education%20AHRC-OPH-LS

6. US Department of the Army, G-3/5/7. *Institutional Training-Directed Lodging and Meal (ITDLM) Policy Handbook*. HQDA; April 1, 2016.

7. US Department of the Army. *Training and Leader Development*. DA; 2014. Army Regulation 350-1.

8. Command and General Staff College Foundation. CGSC Graduation Awards. Accessed May 28, 2020. http://www.cgscfoundation.org/newsroom/cgsc-graduation-awards/

9. US Army Fort Benning, Maneuver Center of Excellence. Western Hemisphere Institute for Security Cooperation (WHINSEC) academics. Accessed May 28, 2020. https://www.benning.army.mil/tenant/whinsec/academics.html

10. US Army Fort Benning, Maneuver Center of Excellence. Western Hemisphere Institute for Security Cooperation (WHINSEC) mission. Accessed May 28, 2020. https://www.benning.army.mil/tenant/whinsec/Mission.html

11. US Department of the Army. *Army Foreign Language.* HQDA; 2016. Army Regulation 11-6. Accessed March 5, 2020. https://armypubs.army.mil/epubs/DR_pubs/DR_a/pdf/web/r11_6.pdf

12. US Department of the Army. *Army Foreign Language Program Handbook.* HQDA; 2016. Department of the Army Pamphlet 11-8. Accessed May 28, 2020. https://armypubs.army.mil/epubs/DR_pubs/DR_a/pdf/web/p11_8.pdf

13. Troy University. College of Arts and Sciences 2019–2020 catalog. Accessed May 28, 2020. https://www.troy.edu/_assets/catalogs/_documents/2019-20/graduate/3g-arts-sciences-19-20.pdf

Chapter 9

LICENSURE, CREDENTIALING, AND GRANTING OF CLINICAL PRIVILEGES

Amelia M. Duran-Stanton, PA-C, PhD, DSc, MPAS; Terry Lee Clark Jr, PA-C, MPAS; Mary J. Coy, PA-C, MPAS, MSHS, MBA; Robyn L. Mason, APA-C, MS; and Joanna G. Sanford, PA-C, MPAS

Introduction

US Army physician assistants (PAs) are required to meet established standards of education, professional licensure, certification, and clinical competency. To maintain the highest quality of military health care, a process is in place to ensure every provider meets these standards. Credentialing and privileging can be a seemingly arduous and lengthy process; however, a basic understanding of procedures and requirements and knowing what to expect can streamline the process. Additionally, Army PAs need to know specific information depending on their component—active duty, Army National Guard (ARNG), or US Army Reserve (USAR). After defining terms, this chapter is structured to describe the overall clinical privileging process for all Army PAs, followed by specific information for the ARNG and USAR (Figure 9-1).

Definitions

Army Medical Department (AMEDD) Professional Management Command (APMC). The APMC was stood up in 2005 with the formation of the Army Reserve Medical Command (AR-MEDCOM). APMC supports USAR commanders by providing personnel, training, finance, and assignment management for medical personnel when there are critical wartime shortages. APMC also provides centralized management of medical professionals to improve readiness, including credentialing and privileging of USAR providers. APMC is a direct

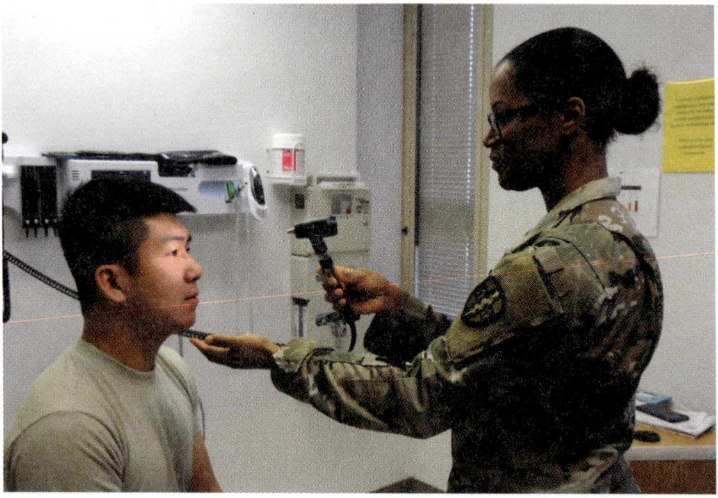

Figure 9-1. Then-Captain Erika Walker, a US Army Reserve physician assistant, conducts a periodic health assessment for Specialist Shuya Yang, an Army Reserve soldier assigned to 7226th Medical Support Unit, based out of Fort Jackson, South Carolina, in December 2017. Operation Reserve Care was an initiative run by Army Reserve Medical Command's 7458th Medical Backfill Battalion performed at Womack Army Medical Center, at Fort Bragg, North Carolina. Photo by Lieutenant Colonel Angela Wallace.
Reproduced from: https://www.dvidshub.net/image/4045101/initial-medical-screening-operation-reserve-care

reporting unit to AR-MEDCOM and derives authority from the US Army Reserve Command (USARC), with guidance from the USARC Surgeon's Office and US Army MEDCOM Quality Assurance Office, in accordance with (IAW) Defense Health Agency Procedures Manual (DHA PM) 6025.13 and Army Regulations (ARs) 40-68 and 40-66.

Health care credentialing. Refers to the process of verifying education, training, and proven skills of health care providers. Steps taken during the credentialing process include verifying licenses, completion of medical education, and completion of training such as fellowships and other certifications.

Privileging. Refers to the granting of permission to provide patient care in an institution within the framework of defined clinical practice.

Interfacility credentials transfer brief (ICTB). The ICTB is a summary of the contents kept in the practitioner credentialed file (PCF), used for all privileged providers when applying for privileges at a temporary duty (TDY) or temporary change of station (TCS) location.

Joint Centralized Credentials Quality Assurance System (JCCQAS). The JCCQAS (https://ccqas.csd.disa.mil/Account/Splash?ReturnUrl=%2f) is a military and civilian medical workforce management and privileging system designed to maintain historical and current medical provider qualifications, certifications, and privileges. All Department of Defense (DOD) applicants possessing a common access card (CAC) must use the JCCQAS to apply for clinical privileges.

Primary source verification (PSV). Refers to verification of a provider's credentials by going to the "primary source"—the entity that provided the education, license, or other credential to ensure the accuracy of the information given by the health care provider.

Practitioner's credentials file (PCF). The PCF is a comprehensive, permanent file containing documentation relevant to an individual's education, experience, licensure/certification, training, and professional history.

Physician Assistant Credentialing Requirements

Education. Army PAs must meet certain educational criteria for commissioning as a 65D (the Army PA area of concentration). According to Army Regulation (AR) 135-101,[1] all PAs must be graduates of a PA training program accredited by the Accreditation Review Commission on Education for the Physician Assistant.

Certification. All PAs (active duty, ARNG, USAR, and civilian) are required to possess current certification by the National Commission on Certification of Physician Assistants (NCCPA) before regular clinical privileges are granted or renewed. PAs who received their training from the Interservice Physician Assistant Program (IPAP) must take the Physician Assistant National Certifying Examination (PANCE) at the first available testing period following Phase 2 of IPAP training, and must receive a passing score within 12 months.[2]

Recertification. The PA National Recertification Examination is required every 10 years.[3] PAs who are unsuccessful in passing this examination after two attempts will have their privileges revoked and are prohibited from practicing in their area of concentration. PAs with an existing active duty service obligation (ADSO) for training will be processed for involuntary branch transfer, IAW AR 614-100.[4] Individuals with no ADSO may be eliminated from service, IAW AR 600-8-24.[5]

Licensure. 10 US Code § 1098 requires individual practicing health care professionals in the military health system to be licensed. For PAs, the DOD accepts the successful passage of the PANCE as the appropriate authorizing document. State PA licensure requirements are currently waived for active duty PAs due to variations among state regulations (although state licensure is required for off-duty employment).[6–8] The American Academy of Physician Assistants (AAPA) provides open source tools and resources for state licensure at https://www.aapa.org/advocacy-central/state-advocacy/state-licensing/. This site lists all 50 state license requirements and their licensing boards; statutory and regulatory requirements for initial licensure and license renewal; and state laws and regulations. The AAPA also provides licensing tips for members.

National Practitioner Data Bank. A web-based repository of reports regarding medical malpractice payments and adverse actions related to providers.[9]

Clinical Privileging Process

The following is a general overview of the credentialing and privileging process, which may vary slightly from one facility to another.

Initial Application for Clinical Privileges

The new provider (recent IPAP graduate or direct commissioned PA) must establish contact with the credentials office at the gaining military medical treatment facility (MTF) to request privileges and initiate a JCCQAS application. Once contact is established, the gaining credentials office will send a welcome letter listing the required documentation needed to begin the privileging process (outlined below). The MTF credentials staff will use these documents to create a PCF for the new provider in JCCQAS.[2] The provider will then receive two emails from the JCCQAS system. The first will be a notification that there are tasks to complete in JCCQAS, and the second email will contain a JCCQAS username and password. The following are documents required for initial application for clinical privileges:

- consent form,
- copy of government-issued photo identification,
- official military orders,
- diploma from accredited institution,
- NCCPA certificate,
- national provider identification (apply online at https://nppes.cms.hhs.gov),
- updated curriculum vitae (signed and dated),
- current Basic Life Support (BLS) certification,
- performance assessment completed and signed by the IPAP Phase 2 clinical coordinator or civilian equivalent for direct accession, and
- two peer review questionnaires (current within the last 24 months).

Once these documents are in hand, the credentials staff completes the following: (1) the PSV to ensure accuracy of the education, training, and licensure of the health care providers; and (2) a query to the National Practitioner Database (NPDB), a web-based repository of reports on medical malpractice payments and adverse actions related to health care providers[8] ; to ensure the applicant has no adverse actions against them. The application is then reviewed by the appropriate department chief. If everything is in order, the department chief will forward application to the credentials committee, which is presided over by the deputy commander of clinical services (DCCS). The committee reviews the application. If approval is recommended, it is forwarded to the MTF commander for final approval.

Periodic Reappraisal and Renewal

Clinical privileges are in effect for a period not to exceed 24 months from the date granted. It is the responsibility of each provider to request the renewal of their clinical privileges every 2 years. Requirements for renewal (accomplished in JCCQAS) are the following:

- JCCQAS application for renewal of clinical privileges,

- performance assessment report completed by supervising physician,
- current BLS certification,
- current NCCPA certification, and
- documentation of continuing medical education (100 credits must be earned every 2 years).[3]

The completed application for renewal of credentials goes through the same approval process as an initial application.

Renewal of Privileges Following Permanent Change of Station or Transfer to Another Medical Treatment Facility

Upon notification of an impending PCS or transfer to a new facility, the provider must notify the losing MTF credentials office, which will then initiate transfer of electronic and hard copies of the application and performance assessment report. The transfer of privileges goes through the same approval process as an initial application or renewal of credentials.

Credentialing and Privileges for Temporary Change of Station or Temporary Duty

Military providers who perform temporary duty (TCS or TDY) require an ICTB to render patient care at another location. Requirements (accomplished in JCCQAS) include the following:

- Notify local credentials staff of upcoming TCS/TDY.
- The credentials staff at the parent (sending) MTF initiates the ICTB.
- An email notification is automatically sent to the provider alerting them that there are tasks to complete in JCCQAS.
- The provider logs into JCCQAS and completes a new application for clinical privileges for the gaining MTF.

From this point, the PSV and review processes are similar to those for the original application, with a few important exceptions:

- All provider licenses, certifications, and registrations, as well as those credentials that need to be verified but were not previously verified, must undergo the PSV process. Professional education and other static credentials that generally are not updated over time do not have to undergo PSV if they have already gone through PSV verification in JCCQAS.

- A new NPDB query is also required.

The privileging authority is the gaining MTF commander. Once the application is approved, the system will import the new privileges into the "Privileges" section of the provider's ICTB record. The system will also automatically calculate new privilege expiration and staff appointment expiration dates for the provider, based upon the end date for the ICTB duty.

Modification of Privileges at Request of the Provider

Modification of privileges requested by the provider can be accomplished at any time, including during a periodic renewal. Requirements (performed in JCCQAS) include:

- a new JCCQAS application with requested modifications, and
- documentation of training or certification and appropriate experience.

From this point, the PSV and review processes are similar to those of the original application upon which the modification is based, with a few exceptions. For a modification of approved privileges, only the provider's licenses, certifications, or registrations and those credentials that require verification but were not previously verified need to undergo the PSV process. A new NPDB query must also be performed. Once the modification application has been reviewed and approved by the privileging authority, the credentials manager will issue the appropriate notifications and complete the application process.

Physician Assistant Scope of Practice and Basic Core Privileges

PAs are awarded privileges commensurate with their education, experience, competence, and the operational needs of the unit they are assigned to. The scope of privileges for a PA includes the evaluation, diagnosis, and treatment of patients of all ages with any symptom, illness, injury, or condition. PAs provide medical services within the scope of practice of the collaborating physicians,

Table 9-1. Basic core privileges for US Army physician assistants.

Diagnosis and management

- Prescribe all medications, controlled substances (including Schedule II through V), and therapy regimens including orthotics and prosthetics required within the scope of practice.
- Recommend temporary limited duty profiles in accordance with service policy.
- Perform occupational and medical surveillance program physical exam.
- Perform examinations in accordance with the Occupational Safety and Health Administration (OSHA) and service policy.
- Provide evaluations of nuclear and chemical surety activities in accordance with applicable law and regulation.
- Place patients on quarters in accordance with service policy.
- Perform electrocardiogram preliminary interpretation.
- Prescribe all medications, controlled substances (including Schedule II through V), and therapy regimens including orthotics and prosthetics required within the scope of practice.

Procedures

- Laceration repair, minor (one layer).
- Excision of superficial cysts and skin lesions.
- Irrigation of the eye, ear, and wounds.
- Indirect laryngoscopy.
- Fluorescein staining.
- Splinting and stabilizing of spine or extremity injuries.
- Casting of extremities.
- Tonometry and tonography.
- Color vision testing.
- Laceration repair requiring more than one layer of closure.
- Aspiration and injection of joints and musculo-tendonous units.
- Complete or partial nail removal with or without destruction of nail matrix.
- Incision and drainage of cysts and minor abscesses.
- Cryosurgical removal of skin lesions.
- Arthrocentesis.
- Reduction of simple closed fractures and dislocations.
- Thrombosed hemorrhoid incision and drainage.
- Needle thoracostomy.
- Emergency cricothyroidotomy.
- Wound debridement.

Anesthesia

- Topical and local infiltration anesthesia.
- Peripheral nerve block anesthesia.

Skin biopsies

- Punch biopsy.
- Shave biopsy.

including routine primary and preventive care of children and adults. PAs may refer patients to specialty clinics, and assess, stabilize, and determine disposition of patients with emergent conditions. However, privileges to treat certain age groups may vary depending on facility and mission requirements. Deviation from core privileges requires documentation of training and experience and approval by the privileging authority. The basic core privileges of the US Army PA are listed in Table 9-1.

PAs with advanced education, training, and experience, and the appropriate privileges, may serve in specialty practice settings such as aviation medicine, cardiovascular perfusion, emergency medicine,

Table 9-2. Advanced privileges for US Army physician assistants (additional training required).

Advanced privileges

- Intrauterine device (IUD) insertion.
- IUD removal.
- Diaphragm fitting.
- Flexible sigmoidoscopy with and without biopsy.
- Subcutaneous contraceptive rod insertion and removal.
- Paracentesis.
- Thoracentesis.
- Tube thoracostomy.
- Lumbar puncture.
- Management of fingertip amputation.
- Direct laryngoscopy.
- Placement of posterior nasal packs or balloons.
- Vasectomy.
- Ultrasonography exam and interpretation for trauma.
- Moderate sedation.
- Regional nerve block anesthesia.

Additional advanced privileges (may depend on specialty)

- Prescribe all medications, controlled substances (including Schedule II through V) and therapy regimens including orthotics and prosthetics required within the scope of practice.
- Recommend temporary limited duty profiles in accordance with service policy.
- Perform occupational and medical surveillance program physical exam.
- Perform examinations in accordance with the Occupational Safety and Health Administration (OSHA) and service policy.
- Provide evaluations of nuclear and chemical surety activities.

occupational health, and orthopedics. Additions and deletions of PA specialties are approved by the Army surgeon general. Advanced privileges that require additional training are listed in Table 9-2.

Army National Guard and Army Reserve Physician Assistants

Most of the information in this chapter applies to all Army PAs; however, a few important differences exist in the credentialing and privileging processes for the ARNG and USAR PAs. These different processes are described below.

Army National Guard Physician Assistants

The Credentials Certification and Privileging Preparation (C2P2) Board credentials ARNG PAs and state surgeons award state privileges. The C2P2 Board holds the authority to approve state-level credentials but does not have the authority to award privileges. The C2P2 Board operates under authority from the ARNG Office of the Chief Surgeon, with guidance from the ARNG Medical Advisory Group and the MEDCOM Quality Assurance Office, IAW DHA PM 6025.13,[6] AR 40-68,[7] and AR 40-66[10] (everything in this chapter applies to the ARNG based on these regulations unless otherwise indicated). AR 40-68 is used for PAs in Title 32 status, and the DHA PM for PAs in Title 10 status. State licensure is required for all ARNG PAs, including Title 32 Active Guard Reserve (AGR) PAs; however, Title 10 AGR PAs can waive the state licensure requirement per DHA PM 6025.13.[6] Title 10 AGR PAs function in the same capacity as the active Army PA, so all regulatory guidance for active Army PAs applies to the Title 10 AGR.

ARNG PAs must contact their state credential coordinator to request privileges. The coordinator then initiates the credentialing process and coordinates with an ARNG credentialing contracted vendor and Office of the Chief Surgeon to prepare the PA's file for the C2P2 Board. The board reviews the file and recommends and approves the PA's credentialing (and additional skill identifier, if applicable). The approved credentials are then sent to the appropriate state surgeon. The state surgeon, an ARNG officer, is the delegated authority to award state privileges for delivering health care to eligible beneficiaries. ARNG

PAs who are mobilized for annual training and for missions outside of the United States require verification of credentials and privileges through the mobilizing MTF.

Army Reserve Physician Assistants

Like the ARNG, USAR PA credentialing and privileging are distinct processes. Credentialing and privileging for the USAR is a two-step process beginning with the APMC and completed by an active component MTF IAW DHA PM 6025.13 and AR 40-68. Providers often think the process is complete after ICTB submission via APMC, but the process is not complete until a designated MTF grants privileges and the provider accepts the approved privileges in JCCQAS. Credentials are managed and maintained by APMC. Privileges are granted by a designated active duty facility. Everything discussed in this chapter applies to the USAR based on these regulations.

APMC verifies credentials every 2 years, and all providers are required to maintain currency at all times. Current, verified credentials are mandatory for a PA to perform readiness evaluations outside an MTF during weekend battle assembly or annual training. USAR military providers who work in an MTF during battle assembly or annual training and are mobilized to a US location, or are deployed outside of the United States, require verification of credentials by APMC, and the generation of an ICTB to the privileging MTF in order to start the privileging process.

Privileges are required to perform any type of clinical duty in an MTF during weekend battle assembly or annual training, or in conjunction with a mobilization or deployment. As stated above, privileging is location dependent and granted by the MTF; APMC does not privilege providers. The privileging facility for USAR and ARNG PAs is determined by deployment location. For example, providers mobilizing out of Fort Bliss, Texas, or Fort Hood, Texas, are privileged through those respective MTFs; Landstuhl Regional Medical Center in Germany is responsible for Europe, Qatar, Jordan, and Kuwait; and MEDDAC (Medical Activity) Bavaria in Germany is responsible for all of Africa.

The process is as follows:

- Upon receipt of the request, APMC will re-verify credentials and request any missing documentation from the soldier.

- Once credentialing is complete, APMC generates the ICTB and sends it to the appropriate MTF.
- The provider logs into JCCQAS and completes a new application for clinical privileges for the gaining MTF.
- Once submitted, the request is reviewed by the gaining MTF privileging committee for approval.
- Once the gaining MTF approves the request, privileges need to be accepted and signed by the provider.
- Access to a CAC-enabled computer and military email is essential for completing the privileging phase. Providers will not deploy from continental US replacement centers without approved privileges.

Additional Information

See the US Army Medical Department Office of Quality Management website (https://www.qmo.amedd.army.mil/credentialing/cp.htm) for the latest information and updates about credentials and privileges.[11] The most current Army PA (65D) credentialing forms are also on the website (https://www.qmo.amedd.army.mil/credentialing/FY19/Physician_Assistant_AOC_65D.pdf).[11]

Conclusion

Licensure, credentialing, and privileging affect readiness. A PA who is not able to see and treat patients hinders the Army's ability to be a medically ready force. PAs must take personal responsibility for these requirements. Additionally, licensure and credentialing are important if the PA will be working in the civilian sector. PAs should always remain aware of their privileges and practice at the highest level of their licenses and credentials, depending on their current training, education, and experience.

References

1. Department of the Army. *Appointment of Reserve Commissioned Officers for Assignment to Army Medical Department Branches*. HQDA; February 15, 1984. Army Regulation 135-101.

2. Department of the Army. *The Interservice Physician Assistant Training Program*. HQDA; August 17, 2009. Army Regulation 601-20.
3. National Commission on Certification of Physician Assistants website. Accessed April 20, 2020. http://www.nccpa.net
4. Department of the Army. *Officer Assignments, Policies, Details and Transfers*. HQDA; January 10, 2006. Army Regulation 614-100.
5. Department of the Army. *Officer Transfers and Discharges*. HQDA; September 13, 2011. Army Regulation 600-8-24.
6. Defense Health Agency. *Clinical Quality Management in the Military Health System, Volume 4: Credentialing and Privileging*. August 29, 2019. Defense Health Agency Procedures Manual 6025.13. Accessed August 17, 2020. https://www.health.mil/Reference-Center/Policies/2019/09/01/DHA-PM-6025-13-Implementation-Guidance-Volume-4
7. Department of the Army. *Clinical Quality Management*. HQDA; February 26, 2004. Army Regulation 40-68.
8. Assistant Secretary of Defense. *Waiver of Licensure Requirements for Physician Assistants*. DOD; January 15, 2004. Health Affairs Policy Memorandum 04-002.
9. US Department of Health of Health & Human Services. National Practitioner Data Bank. *About Us*. Accessed August 14, 2020. https://www.npdb.hrsa.gov/topNavigation/aboutUs.jsp
10. Department of the Army. *Medical Record Administration and Healthcare Documentation*. HQDA; June 17, 2008; Rapid Action Revision January 4, 2010. Army Regulation 40-66.
11. US Army Medical Department Office of Quality Management website. Physician Assistant AOC 65D. Accessed August 17, 2020. https://www.qmo.amedd.army.mil/credentialing/FY19/Physician_Assistant_AOC_65D.pdf

Chapter 10

MAINTAINING CERTIFICATION AND THE CONTINUING MEDICAL EDUCATION CATEGORIES

Lucas Allmon, PA-C, MPAS; R. Scott Harrison, PA-C, MPAS; James J. Jones, PA-C, PhD, MPAS; and Amelia M. Duran-Stanton, PA-C, PhD, DSc, MPAS

Introduction

Every Army physician assistant (PA) must maintain both military PA requirements and civilian-equivalent requirements for certification to practice. This certification is the reason for the "C" on PA credentials (PA-C). In the military, certification is vitally important to obtaining military treatment facility credentials, receive bonuses, and ensure educational proficiency as PAs.

Maintaining Certification

Maintaining the "C" (certification) in "PA-C" is required in accordance with Army Regulation 40-68, *Clinical Quality Management,*[1] and Health Affairs Policy 04-002, *Waivers of Licensure Requirement for Qualified Military Physician Assistants*.[2] According to the National Committee on Certification of Physician Assistants (NCCPA), maintenance of the 10-year certification includes five 2-year cycles. The PA must log 100 continuing medical education (CME) credits online during each cycle. The CME logging window begins May 1 in the PA's certification issuance year and continues through December 31 of the certification expiration year.[3]

At the end of the 10-year cycle, PAs are required to take the Physician Assistant National Recertifying Exam (PANRE). They must also submit a certification fee by December 31 of their certification expiration year.[3]

Continuing Medical Education

CME "consists of clinical and professional education activities that maintain, develop or increase the knowledge, skills, and professional performance and relationships that a PA uses to provide services for patients, the public and the profession."[4] After PAs pass the Physician Assistant National Certifying Exam (PANCE), they maintain certification by completing the required number of credits from two categories of CME options.

Category 1 Continuing Medical Education

There are four types of category 1 CME: (1) regular, (2) certification programs, (3) process improvement [PI-CME], and (4) self-assessment.[5] Fifty credits in each 2-year cycle are required to be from category 1 CME. Category 1 CME includes certification and recertification courses preapproved and classified by the American Academy of Physician Assistants (AAPA), such as seminars, journal post-tests, conferences, and online resources. The following sponsors offer Category 1 CME[5]:

- AAPA
- American Medical Association, with providers accredited by the Accreditation Council for Continuing Medical Education
- American Academy of Family Physicians
- American Osteopathic Association
- Royal College of Physicians and Surgeons of Canada
- College of Family Physicians of Canada
- Physician Assistant Certification Council of Canada

Regular Continuing Medical Education. Programs or certificate-producing courses preapproved by one of the previously mentioned sponsors comprise regular CME. An example is the AAPA annual conference.

Certificate Program Continuing Medical Education. Certificate programs are preapproved by the AAPA for category 1 CME regardless of the program or location. Examples are Basic Life Support and Advanced Trauma Life Support courses.[6]

Performance Improvement Continuing Medical Education. PI-CME activities compare the PA's clinical practice to clinical practice guidelines and other established metrics. PAs apply what they have learned in these activities to improve their practice. PI-CME is conducted alone or in partnership with a physician or others in the practice. Each clinician working on these CME projects can receive credit for PI-CME. Each PI-CME activity follows a three-stage model[7]:

Stage I—performance measurement. Compare your practice to an established evidence-based metric or standard.

Stage II—intervention and improvement plan. Develop and implement a plan to improve your practice based on the standards.

Stage III—remeasurement. Evaluate the impact of the improvement plan on your practice. For example, a PA chooses a PI-CME activity focused on asthma. For stage I, the PA records key data such as disease duration, exacerbations, levels of control, current medication, and other information for current asthma patients. The PA then measures their current practice against the current standard of medical care. In this case, the PA compares patient data to the National Asthma Education and Prevention Program's *Expert Panel Report 3: Guidelines for the Diagnosis and Management of Asthma,*[8] using a tool that quantifies asthma severity and treatment response.[9] In stage II, the PA corrects the existing clinical practice, based on the current standard of care. Stage III allows the PA to evaluate the improvements based on the adjustments. This final step completes the PI-CME activity, and the PA receives category 1 CME credit for the module.

Self-Assessment Continuing Medical Education. Self-assessment activities provide a systematic way to review each PA's performance, knowledge base, and skill set. In these CME activities, students typically choose a topic, take a pretest, review current evidence-based material, and take a written or multiple-choice test to assess learning.[5]

In this example, a PA chooses exercise-induced asthma (EIA) as a self-assessment CME subject. The module begins with a quiz on the PA's current understanding of the disease process and treatment. Second, the PA receives evidence-based medical information about EIA.

After reading the information, the PA must pass a multiple-choice test. This final step completes the self-assessment CME activity and the PA receives a category 1 CME credit for the module.

As with all category 1 CME, PI-CME and self-assessment CME activities must be preapproved by AAPA to meet requirements. Since August 2016, NCCPA awards 50% additional credit for SA-CME and PI-CME.[10] Therefore, an SI-CME course worth 10 credits is converted to 15 credits. Additionally, the first 20 PI-CME credits logged during each cycle are doubled.[10]

Category 2 Continuing Medical Education

Category 2 CME consists of any medical-related activity that enhances the role of the PA.[5] This type of CME includes activities such as journal reading, studying for the PANRE, medical writing, and attending medical lectures.[4] Quantification for credit is based on an honor system of how many hours the PA spends. For example, if the PA spent an hour studying for the PANRE, they would log 1 credit hour for category 2 CME.

Logging Credit

In addition to earning CME credit, it is important to log credits earned through the NCCPA website.[3] For national certification maintenance, the PA must provide the following information[3,11]:

- program title,
- provider (the organization that administered the program),
- number of CME credits earned, and
- sponsor (the organization that designated CME credit to the program).

Certification

New Certification Holders

When PA students graduate, their first CME cycle may vary depending on the time of year they graduate and when they successfully pass the PANCE.[12] For example, a PA student may graduate on January 24, 2020; take the PANCE 8 days later; and receive the PANCE score February 15, 2 weeks after the examination. This PA's CME earning cycle will begin on February 15, 2020, and last through December 31, 2022.

Ten-Year Certification Cycle

Before 2014, the PA certification cycle was 6 years. Now, PAs who pass the PANCE or PANRE enter a 10-year certification period. This cycle consists of five 2-year certification maintenance cycles. Table 10-1 shows an example of the 10-year certification cycle.

Lost Certification

If a PA fails to log the appropriate 100 hours of CME and pay the maintenance fee by the due date at the end of the 2-year maintenance period, they must take PANCE or PANRE to regain certification.[13]

Administrative Certification Extension

If a PA does not earn or log all requirements by 2359 hours (Pacific Time) on December 31 of their certification expiration year, they are granted a 1-month administrative certificate extension to complete requirements.[3] If requirements are not met by January 31, current NCCPA policies

Table 10-1. Example of the 10-year certification cycle.

CME Cycle Window	SA-CME (Cat 1)	PI-CME (Cat 1)	Regular Cat 1 CME	Cat 2 CME	Total CME
1 May 2020–31 Dec 2022	20	0	30	50	100
1 May 2022–31 Dec 2024	0	20	50	30	100
1 May 2024–31 Dec 2026	5	15	80	0	100
1 May 2026–31 Dec 2028	15	5	30	50	100
Total Goal: 40 of each SA/PI in first 4 cycles	*40*	*40*			
1 May 2028–31 Dec 2030	0	0	100	0	100

Cat: category; CME: continuing medical education; PI-CME: performance improvement CME; SA-CME: self-assessment CME determine options and procedures for regaining certification. Appeals for an additional extension are allowed only for extraordinary extenuating circumstance with appropriate documentation.[3]

Lost Certification Due to Disciplinary Proceedings

Under current NCCPA policies, PAs who have lost certification may regain it by completing CME requirements and passing the PANRE. However, PAs who have lost eligibility for certification based on NCCPA disciplinary proceedings must first apply to reestablish eligibility.[3]

Audits

PAs must keep their category 1 CME documentation for the current and previous CME cycles. For example, if a PA is currently on a 2020–2022 cycle, they should keep that documentation and the 2018–2020 CME cycle documentation.

For quality control purposes, the NCCPA randomly conducts audits of category 1 CME after the completion of the previous year's cycle. PAs selected to participate in the audits have 6 weeks from receipt of the written notification to provide NCCPA with completion certificates for all category 1 CME performed during the audit timeframe. If an audited PA cannot provide this documentation, they retain certification but will be re-audited the following certification period and must pay a re-audit fee of $100. The PA must also complete any additional unsubstantiated category 1 CME from the previous audit timeframe. These PAs may face additional random audits over the next three certification maintenance cycles. Failure to comply adequately within 6 weeks of notification in these additional audits results in immediate loss of certification. NCCPA does not audit category 2 CME.[14]

Summary

Understanding the PA certification process, including CME requirements, is vital to avoid losing certification. Obtaining and logging CME is a regulatory requirement for maintaining certification. It is the PA's responsibility to maintain certification as a matter of principle and accountability.

References

1. US Department of the Army. *Clinical Quality Management*. DA; 2004 (rapid action revision issue date: May 22, 2009). Army Regulation 40-68, Chap 4–16. Accessed May 26, 2020. https://armypubs.army.mil/epubs/DR_pubs/DR_a/pdf/web/r40_68.pdf
2. Assistant Secretary of Defense (Health Affairs). *Waivers of Licensure Requirement for Qualified Military Physician Assistants*. DOD; January 15, 2004. Health Affairs Policy 04-002.
3. National Commission on Certification of Physician Assistants website. Maintaining certification. Accessed May 26, 2020. https://www.nccpa.net/CertificationProcess
4. Accreditation Council for Continuing Medical Education website. CME Content: Definition and Examples. Accessed May 26, 2020. https://www.accme.org/accreditation-rules/policies/cme-content-definition-and-examples
5. National Commission on Certification of Physician Assistants website. Category 1 and 2 CME. Accessed May 26, 2020. http://www.nccpa.net/ CMECategoryTypes
6. National Commission on Certification of Physician Assistants website. Preapproved Certification Programs. Accessed May 26, 2020. https://www.nccpa.net/cme-preapproved
7. American Academy of Physician Assistants website. Category 1 CME for performance improvement (PI). Accessed May 26, 2020. https://www.aapa.org/cme-central/aapa-cme-accreditation/category-1-cme-for-performance-improvement-pi/
8. US Department of Health and Human Services, National Asthma Education and Prevention Program. *Asthma Care Quick Reference, Diagnosing and Managing Asthma*. DHHS; 2012. NIH Publication 12-5075. Accessed May 26, 2020. https://www.nhlbi.nih.gov/sites/default/files/media/docs/12-5075.pdf

9. American Academy of Allergy, Asthma & Immunology website. A new tool for quantification of asthma severity and treatment response. October 8, 2019. Accessed May 26, 2020. https://www.aaaai.org/global/latest-research-summaries/Current-JACI-Research/quantification

10. National Commission on Certification of Physician Assistants website. Finding self-assessment and performance improvement category 1 CME. Accessed May 26, 2020. https://www.nccpa.net/finding-sa-and-pi-cme

11. American Academy of Physician Assistants website. Logging CME. Accessed May 26, 2020. https://www.aapa.org/cme-central/cme-faqs/#tabs-3-logging-cme

12. National Commission on Certification of Physician Assistants website. About CME requirements. Accessed May 26, 2020. http://www.nccpa.net/continuingmedicaleducation

13. National Commission on Certification of Physician Assistants website. Lost Certification? Accessed May 20, 2020. https://www.nccpa.net/LostC

14. National Commission on Certification of Physician Assistants website. CME audit policy. Accessed May 26, 2020. http://www.nccpa.net/CMEAudit

Chapter 11

CAREER MANAGEMENT

Luis Vidal, APA-C, MPAS; Amelia M. Duran-Stanton, PA-C, PhD, DSc, MPAS; and Amy L. Jackson, PA-C, MPAS

Introduction

Career management for an Army physician assistant (PA) is multifaceted and requires thoughtful consideration. The first question to answer is, "What do I want to accomplish while I'm wearing the uniform?" The answer will differ from one individual to the next. Personal and professional aspirations are intertwined, and together form the foundation of the path that ultimately shapes a military journey.

A PA's career options will vary depending on timing, the flexibility of the individual's plan, and current and emerging Army requirements. Army PAs should develop a plan focused on factors that are important for their professional experience while balancing their personal and family objectives. This chapter will assist the PA in understanding the key factors to consider in developing a prospective plan to carry them through their military career. It will show how the PA can be proactive in preparing and managing their career in the military and beyond. Included is information on regulations, planning tools, resource documents, lessons learned, and tips for success. The chapter will cover career planning, the domains of leader development, mentorship, the officer record brief (ORB), and computer systems used in these processes. At the end of the chapter are several links and references with additional helpful information on PA career management.

Charting the Path

Army PAs will choose from a variety of challenging and rewarding paths or tracks as they begin their military career. Usually, PAs start their career in an operational assignment with a company, battalion, or brigade. Thereafter, positions are available in different tracks—clinical; research; broadening assignments, such as recruiter, inspector general, or aide-de-camp; education, such as long-term health education training (LTHET) or teaching in the Interservice Physician Assistant Program (IPAP); and leadership or other nonclinical roles such as a commander or executive staff member. Each Army PA career is unique, and it is important for all PAs to be aware they have the ability and responsibility to manage their own career.

For a junior PA who just finished PA school or a direct-accession PA who still has much to learn about the Army, a 5-year career timeline may seem unfathomable or even untenable given their limited knowledge. However, it is important to start planning early and establish long-term, mid-term, and short-term goals and objectives. An excellent starting point is to "begin with the end in mind," and find a mentor to assist in charting a career path toward that goal. For example, if a PA desires to be assigned to the 82d Airborne Division, an airborne physical must be obtained, and the PA must be willing and able to participate in airborne operations.

A career map is a living document that is developed, maintained, and validated as a PA moves through the ranks. Within this career timeline, the Army PA can incrementally plot a 5-year plan as a starting point that optimally projects several courses of action for the next two jobs, including educational pursuits, while reflecting on personal interests (Figure 11-1). The plan should be revisited as frequently as necessary to manage expectations and reflect changes in goals, priorities, and opportunities. Plans must also consider the needs of the Army; availability of positions will vary from time to time, and desired duty locations may not have a position that matches the PA's rank or skill set. For example, the PA position in the 3rd Infantry Division (the Old Guard), at Fort Myer, Virginia, is a two-deep position designed for a captain that opens about every 3 years.

In revisiting the plan, the Army PA should consult with mentors, Human Resources Command (HRC) career managers, and family members, taking into consideration personal and professional goals and realistic objectives. Various personal issues such as family dynamics (a new child, children in high school, new marriage, divorce, aging parents, unexpected illness or disease) can affect the PA's flexibility for certain assignments. The PA may start their career on a certain track (typically

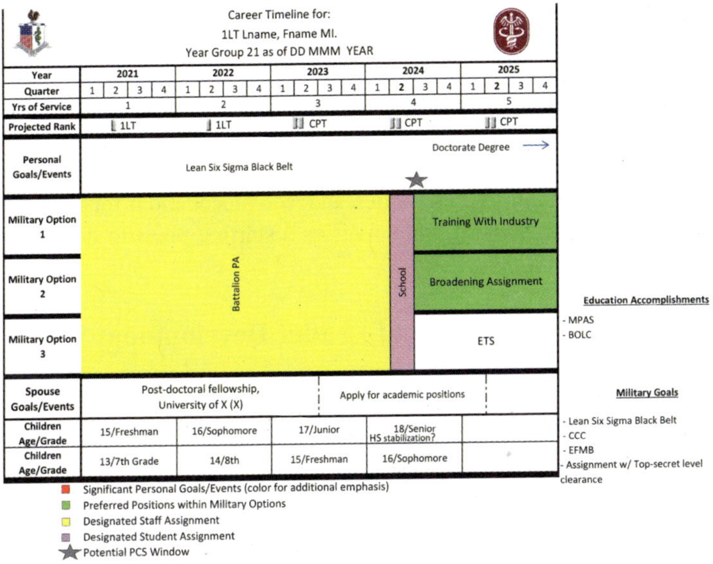

Figure 11-1. Example of a 5-year plan.

operational) and decide to pursue clinical positions, further education or research, perhaps even command, recruiting, and leadership.

Staying in the Army until retirement may be a viable option, and it is important to understand the factors that will affect retirement benefits and options. Some of these factors are retiring as an officer versus a noncommissioned officer for those who are prior enlisted, and accumulating 30 years of active federal commissioned service time versus reaching the mandatory retirement age of 62. The key to success in execution of a proposed career timeline is establishing achievable objectives and milestones along a path toward an individual's personal definition of success. Additionally, PAs must be flexible and recognize opportunities along the way.

Additionally, PAs must recognize and be familiar with the regulations that govern the process of career management. Army competitive category (ACC) officers in the Army derive their guidance from Army Regulation 600-3, *The Army Personnel Development System*.[1] The Army provides guidance to the Army Medical Department (AMEDD) and the

Army Medical Specialist Corps (SP) in Department of the Army (DA) Pamphlet (PAM) 600-4, *Army Medical Department Officer Professional Development and Career Management,* specifically chapters 3 and 4.[2] This pamphlet provides information about expectations for career progression, promotions, positions, and educational opportunities, as well as a lifecycle map. The lifecycle map lays out military educational requirements, training opportunities, and recommendations for positions to be held for each rank, and serves as a starting point to develop a 5- to 10-year plan.

Three Domains of Leader Development

The career plan must take into account the three domains of leader development: institutional training, operational assignments, and self-development.[2] Professional military education is structured to correspond with ranks and promotions, as discussed below. A variety of assignments and positions are necessary to become a well-rounded leader and officer. Self-development includes individual study, research activities, professional reading and writing, completion of certifications and degrees, and continual self-assessment. The Army has developed the Army Career Tracker as a tool to aid officers with professional development, planning, and structured mentorship.[3]

Institutional Training

Professional Military Education. It is important for all officers to attend the appropriate military schools to attain the level of military education and development commensurate to their rank and remain competitive with their peers for promotion. Professional military education focuses on core competencies and leader development to produce competent and technically and tactically proficient officers. It begins with initial military training at the Basic Officer Leader Course (BOLC).

Once an officer is a first lieutenant (promotable), they may request enrollment in the Captains Career Course (CCC) by submitting a DA Form 3838 to their commander (a lieutenant colonel/O-5 or above) for approval by the HRC career manager, or enroll directly in coordination with a permanent change of station (PCS) reassignment with temporary duty en route. Four 9-week CCC resident courses are offered annually. Additionally, a 20-week pilot CCC for AMEDD officers began in

January 2020 (refer to Chapter 56, CCC). The CCC carries a 1-year active duty service obligation (ADSO). The course should be completed prior to the major promotion board and is a prerequisite to taking a command assignment or starting LTHET. Intermediate Level Education (ILE) is the Army's training for field-grade officers. (Chapter 8, Attending ILE, provides in-depth information. Other education that enhances professional development is covered in Chapter 4, Academic Leadership Roles, Education, and Additional Training for PAs.)

Civilian Education. All PAs are required to have civilian education to at least a bachelor's degree level,[4] although the profession is currently based primarily on master's degree-level education. The IPAP awards a bachelor's degree after completing phase 1 and a master's upon graduation. Army PAs can also come from other accredited civilian PA programs. Beyond the entry-level degree requirement, several opportunities for further education are available, such as the LTHET program, in which PAs can earn additional master's or doctorate-level degrees. One of these opportunities is the Doctor of Science degree in emergency medicine, orthopedics, or general surgery (see chapters 5 through 7 for information on these specialties). The Army PA may also attend a civilian school of their choice through the LTHET, and every year there may be different education opportunities. The Army PA incurs ADSO for LTHET; however, they can elect to complete a graduate degree via distance learning, such as a DSc, DMSc, or PhD without incurring an ADSO.

Operational Assignments

PAs can achieve diversity through a balance of operational, clinical, research, educational, SP, and AMEDD developmental and immaterial (can be held regardless of an individual's area of concentration) positions (refer to Section 3 of this handbook for various roles of PAs). SP immaterial positions (designated 65X) include recruiter, recruiting battalion executive officer, corps-specific branch proponency officer, HRC branch chief, SP branch executive officer and fellow, and AMEDD Personnel Proponent Directorate staff officer. AMEDD immaterial positions (designated 05A) include warrior transition unit deputy commanding officer, aide-de-camp, executive assistant, and several strategic staff officer positions at both the Defense Health Agency and the Army Medical Command. At the rank of major (promotable) and lieutenant colonel, opportunities exist to compete for command select list (CSL) command (for further information about CSL, use the search engine on the HRC website[5] and enter "command management branch").

Key components of a career timeline are the positions, and the experience provided by each one, that are fundamental to becoming a well-rounded officer. At this time, the AMEDD has no positions coded as key and developmental, but there are many duty assignments that serve a similar purpose in PA career development. Examples of potential key developmental jobs are senior brigade combat team PA, division PA, corps PA, Forces Command PA, IPAP phase II coordinator, IPAP program director, IPAP program manager, IPAP instructor and other medical training instructors, and Department of Combat Doctrine and Development staff officer.

Self-Development

Self-development begins with discipline and organization. One tactic is to implement a battle rhythm that orchestrates reading, writing, research, studying, and skill set improvement. For example, one could read a medical journal article once a month, read the news daily, monitor S1Net (https://www.milsuite.mil/s1net)[6] for Army human resources (HR) updates, attend online courses, or obtain new credentials to meet an identified need that will benefit a patient population. The important thing is to have a plan for self-development and tailor it to meet professional needs—as a soldier, leader, clinician, and individual.

Meeting with Mentors

It is important for Army PAs to seek mentorship early and often. The mentor-mentee relationship is bilateral; each person benefits from the other during the course of the mentorship. Mentors should review the mentees' ORB, curriculum vitae (CV), and officer evaluation reports (OERs) before providing guidance, and the mentees should assemble these documents to prepare for meetings.

Officer Record Briefs

The ORB is a military resume, a snapshot of a career, credentials, and accomplishments. Commanders may use the ORB to determine which position inbound officers are best suited for and what they need for career progression. In addition to the courses listed above, any Army-sponsored school or program recognized by the Army Training and Requirements Resources System (ATRRS) that lasts more than 40 hours can be recorded in the ORB's military education section.

The ORB must be updated on a regular basis, preferably annually, perhaps as a birth month audit. Additionally, updates are recommended when being considered for a new position, moving to a new unit, receiving a new award or rank, going before any board, or returning from a deployment. Job titles on the ORB should describe what duty or position was held, such as deputy, chief, director, assistant chief, or officer in charge.

It is important that the designations "known losses" or "surplus soldier" do not appear in the ORB's assignment information when it is sent before any board, whether for a promotion, education, or other selection processes. These phrases demonstrate lack of attention to detail and could be negative factors in the boards' decisions. The Army photo, once an important element of promotion selection boards, was suspended from use effective August 1, 2020.[7]

Curriculum Vitae

Along with the ORB, a professional CV that provides a snapshot of accomplishments is a good document to maintain and is required by most military medical treatment facilities as part of a credentialing packet. Often, HRC will announce opportunities that require nominees to submit a packet including the ORB, a CV, and the last five OERs. The CV should highlight current and past experiences; civilian and military education; certification and affiliations; projects, publications, and presentations; features and recognitions; awards and decorations; special skills; and references. (Note that the CV is different from the Assignment Interactive Module 2.0 [AIM.2] resume that will be discussed later in this chapter.)

Officer Evaluation Reports

OERs, used to assess an officer's performance during a rating period, are an additional communication tool for promotion boards and mentors. An OER provides a concise representation of the officer's performance as evaluated by their rater and senior rater. Several products available on the HRC and MilSuite websites provide tips for officers and their

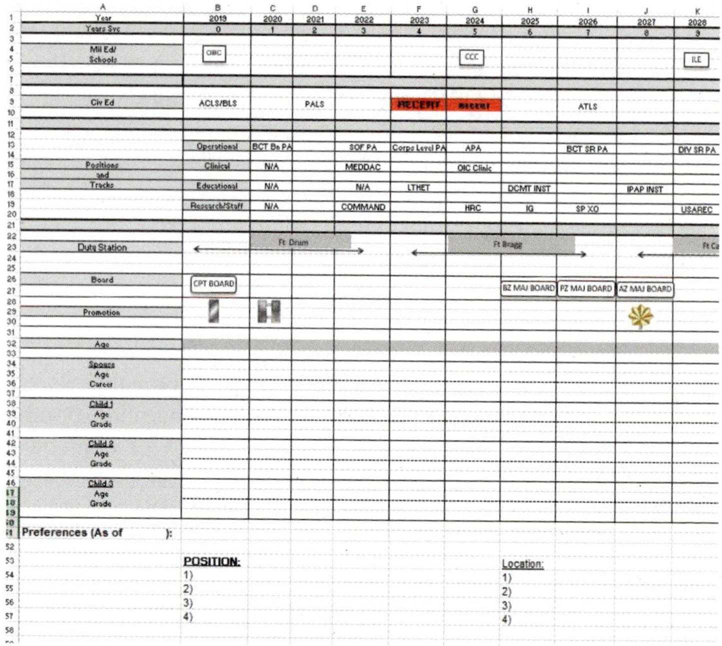

A	B	C	D	E	F	G	H	I	J	K
Year	2019	2020	2021	2022	2023	2024	2025	2026	2027	2028
Years Svc	0	1	2	3	4	5	6	7	8	9
Mil Ed/ Schools	OBC					CCC				ILE
Civ Ed	ACLS/BLS		PALS		RECERT	RECERT		ATLS		
Positions and Tracks	Operational	BCT Bn PA		SOF PA	Corps Level PA	APA		BCT SR PA		DIV SR PA
	Clinical	N/A		MEDDAC		OIC Clinic				
	Educational	N/A		N/A	LTHET		DCMT INST		IPAP INST	
	Research/Staff	N/A		COMMAND		HRC	IG	SP XO		USAREC
Duty Station		Ft Drum				Ft Bragg				Ft Ca
Board	CPT BOARD						BZ MAJ BOARD	PZ MAJ BOARD	AZ MAJ BOARD	
Promotion										
Age										
Spouse Age Career										
Child 1 Age Grade										
Child 2 Age Grade										
Child 3 Age Grade										

Preferences (As of):

POSITION:
1)
2)
3)
4)

Location:
1)
2)
3)
4)

Figure 11-2. Example of a career timeline map.

raters on maximizing the OER as an opportunity to reflect the officer's performance and potential. For more information on ORBs, see DA PAM 600-8-104, Chapter 5.[8]

Creating a Career Plan

Once the foundations of a career plan and mentorship have been established, the Army PA can put pen to paper and draft a timeline. There are several examples of career plans, such as Figure 11-2, that can be modified based on individual preference. The timeline should include date, age, years of service, military education, civilian education, deployments, assignments, duty station locations, promotions, spouse's career milestones, and children's milestones. Leave space under the timeline to note future assignment preferences based on location and

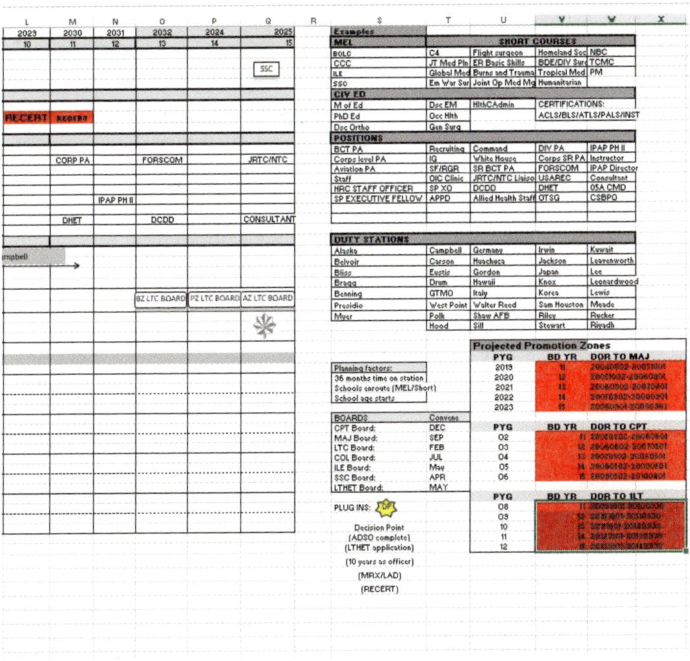

position. These preferences should be considered during timeline reviews and meetings with mentors.

Promotions and Boards

The Army PA must track possible promotions and prepare for them. The HRC website is a great tool to help plan the career timeline in coordination with when promotions may occur, depending on the Army PA's year group. For example, a PA in year group 2012 can expect their primary zone for promotion to major in the year 2020, and if selected, promotion in 2021. Officers may view their projected timeline based on their cohort year group in the AIM.2 website under branch pages. A recommendation is to plot the "below the zone" board, the primary or "in the zone" board and if desired, "above the zone" board. Other boards to follow are LTHET boards (if applying, one must start planning 2 years prior to the board to meet qualifications and appropriately prepare and also plan to be PCS-eligible during the application process), ILE and senior service education selection boards, and CSL command boards. One board no PA will likely forget is the recertification board for national certification. Plotting the first and second year of eligibility to take the test will promote preparedness for this key event. Once all the boards are plotted, it may be a good time to input assignments and positions; this is best accomplished after a discussion with mentors, career managers, and family members.

Assignment and Position Opportunities

The first time a PA has the opportunity to use the "marketplace" to find positions and compete with others in the same permanent change of station cycle, they should pay attention to available options of interest and their locations. One method is to first determine the desired position, and be open to several locations where the position can be held. Knowing that most assignments are at a duty location for approximately 3 years (with some exceptions), a plan to diversify or garner additional experiences at that location should be considered. If a desired position at a senior rank requires certain skills and education, the junior PA should pursue the requirements to be competitive when they achieve that rank. Additionally, they should reach out to officers who have held or currently hold the role to seek additional guidance on how to prepare. Deployment plotting is key as well; certain tasks must be done before or after deployments, such as sitting for certification boards, attending in-person training or certification, and updating board files with documentation that is not available during deployment.

Family Members

Family members are an important part of any Army PA's career planning; for example, individuals may need to care for their parents, or have spouses with their own careers. Children's milestones must also be considered; for example, high school "stabilization" allows parents to remain in one area so a child can stay in one high school.

Assignment Interactive Module Career Management Platform

AIM.2 is a web-based information system designed to enhance the effectiveness and efficiency of the officer management process, and facilitate communication among soldiers, units, commanders, and the HRC Officer Personnel Management Directorate.[9] AIM.2 was developed to improve officer management by integrating multiple aspects of career management that were previously processed through separate mechanisms. The system links many aspects of officer records to ensure they are factored into career management efficiently. AIM.2 uses data in a regulated market system to match officer talent with unit requirements, providing an opportunity for each to learn about each other, and influence both of their preferences.

AIM.2 does more than assist with reassignment actions; it also serves as a communication portal to advertise opportunities, branch information, volunteer assignments, and strategic billets. It allows communication between officers and their career managers, links officers to other electronic records, allows viewing of Army photographs, and processes special actions such as high school stabilizations, Exceptional Family Member Program stabilization, compassionate reassignment requests, and Security Force Assistance Brigade (SFAB) volunteering (see Chapter 13, SFAB, for more details).

An essential element of successful participation in AIM.2 is to prepare and maintain a resume in the system. Officers can build and review their resume on their AIM branch webpage at https://aim.hrc.army.mil/ (select "My Resume").[9] Unit leaders are able to view your resume as a participant in a PCS movement cycle. The resume has two main pages, the ORB (previously discussed), and the officer self-professed talents section. In the self-professed talents section, an officer can advertise more information about themselves beyond what is in their ORB, sharing more information about their knowledge, skills, and attributes, to show they are the best fit for desired assignments. The section has eight parts: summary, education, civilian, assignments, cultural, travel, language, and references. PAs should use this section to add greater depth in these areas, such as education not entered in the ORB, specifics on language skills they possess, and more detail on travel experiences. An officer's communication via the resume can help leaders decide who their preference will be in the market process.

There is no current mandatory way for officers to complete their resume, though they should be written as thoroughly as possible. Officers may be interested in consideration for assignment opportunities at any time, and having an AIM resume ready enhances their opportunities for selection. Like the ORB, the resume should be regularly updated for accuracy. The AIM.2 system is meant to bridge active duty officer talent management during the transition to the Integrated Personnel and Pay System–Army (IPPS–A).

Integrated Personnel and Pay System–Army

The IPPS-A is a web-based HR system that provides integrated personnel and pay capabilities and a comprehensive HR record for all soldiers in each component. Once IPPS-A is fully deployed, the system will enable HR transactions to automatically trigger soldier pay. IPPS-A's ability to combine personnel and pay functions (eg, a promotion or call to active duty) will address current inefficiencies caused by complex interfaces among more than 40 "stove-piped" HR systems. As a result, IPPS-A will leave fewer opportunities for error and will become the authoritative and comprehensive source of Army personnel and pay information.[10] In addition, soldiers will have common access card (CAC) access to their own personal information 24 hours a day via the self-service web portal.

This system will be used by all soldiers across all components of service, active duty, Army National Guard, and Army Reserve, as well as by the HR professionals who support them. It will be launched incrementally in phases. Training is planned for all users based on their roles and phase of integration. A mobile application is available for current service members with access to IPPS-A, and will be available as the system is activated for their components during fielding to the rest of the Army.[10] The program is currently active in the Army National Guard, and at the time of this writing was successful in Pennsylvania and in the process of implementation across the remainder of the National Guard through 2020. The next release is projected to begin integration of active duty and the Army Reserve. For more information on IPPS-A, see https://ipps-a.army.mil/.[10]

Lessons Learned

- PAs should attend and participate in 65D (PA) and SP Corps forums, which are open discussions led by experts and leaders over audio or video media. Often the latest and most relevant information is communicated in these forums.
- PAs should seek advice and mentorship from health service and ACC mentors.
- PAs must develop a strategy to achieve military career goals before leaving the Army. However, they must also remain flexible enough to adjust because their goals may change over time.

Tips for Success

- Review the career timeline at least quarterly with family members, mentors, and leaders.
- Meet with the chain of command in the beginning of each evaluation period, at least quarterly, and again at least a month prior to an OER deadline.
- Let the chain of command know that the Army PA field-grade promotions are not "fully qualified" boards, they are "best qualified" boards (not everyone who is qualified will get promoted).
- Attend at least one military course a year.
- Attend a centrally funded course en route to every PCS.
- Review the ORB and always make an effort to improve at least one aspect of the OER, whether that be military education, civilian education, weight, or a new language.
- Be well read and well rounded; read at least one professional and one personal book a month, and routinely try new skills.
- Be aware of assignment considerations terms for career planning (see the attachment to this chapter provided by Colonel John Detro and Major Drew Kennedy at HRC).

Conclusion

Career management is an individual responsibility. It requires careful thought and the ability to maximize the use of existing tools and resources, while remaining flexible and available when rare opportunities arise. To make the most informed planning decisions, Army PAs must reach out to mentors and leaders for career guidance. They also have a responsibility to lead and mentor others, guiding junior officers and peers to be as successful as possible while maintaining the role of the AMEDD in ensuring the US Army remains the premier and most talented fighting force in the world.

References

1. US Department of the Army. *The Army Personnel Development System*. HQDA; September 16, 2019. Army Regulation 600-3.
2. US Department of the Army. *Army Medical Department Officer Professional Development and Career Management*. HQDA; March 30, 2020. DA Pamphlet 600-4.
3. US Department of the Army. The Army Career Tracker website. Accessed May 13, 2020. https://act-now.army.mil
4. US Department of the Army. *Military Occupational Classification and Structure*. HQDA; July 19, 2018: DA Pamphlet 611-21. Accessed May 13, 2020. https://armypubs.army.mil/epubs/DR_pubs/DR_a/pdf/web/ARN8940_P611_21_FINAL.pdf
5. US Army Human Resources Command website. AMEDD Command Management. Accessed May 13, 2020. https://www.hrc.army.mil/content/AMEDD%20Command%20Management
6. US Department of Defense. MilSuite S1Net website. Accessed May 13, 2020. https://www.milsuite.mil/s1net
7. McConville JC, McCarthy RD. *Elimination of Department of Army (DA) Photos, and Race, Ethnicity and Gender Identification Data for Officer, Warrant Officer, and Enlisted Selection Boards (Updated)*. DA; June 26, 2020. Accessed July 28, 2020. https://www.milsuite.mil/book/docs/DOC-831018
8. US Department of the Army. *Army Human Military Resource Record Management*. HQDA; February 12, 2019. DA Pamphlet 600-8-104. Accessed May 13, 2020. https://armypubs.army.mil/epubs/DR_pubs/DR_a/pdf/web/p600_8_104.pdf

9. US Army Human Resources Command. Assignment Interactive Module 2.0 (AIM.2). Accessed May 8, 2020. https://www.hrc.army.mil/site/assets/directorate/OPMD/What%20is%20AIM%202.pdf

10. US Department of the Army. Integrated Personnel and Pay System–Army website. Accessed May 13, 2020. https://ipps-a.army.mil/

Attachment: Assignment Considerations Terms

High School Stabilization (HSS). Intended to provide stability to officers with family members in their senior year of high school and avoid disruption of the school schedule. HSS packets are submitted through AIM.2, after March 1 of the student's sophomore year and before September 30 of the junior year. Assignments officers can provide instructions and sample packets on request.

Married Army Couples Program (MACP). To the maximum extent possible and consistent with valid Army vacancies, married officers enrolled in MACP are assigned to a location where they can establish a joint domicile within a 50-mile radius or 1-hour driving time of their spouse's assignment. Army requirements and readiness goals are paramount, and married Army couples must be prepared to meet military obligations regardless of assignment. Initial enrollment is conducted through the officer's S1. Enlisted IPAP students must re-submit MACP applications upon commissioning and should inform their assignments officer of their MACP status when requesting initial assignments.

Compassionate Reassignment. Officers with serious family problems that can only be alleviated by an assignment to a particular geographical area may request reassignment, deletion, or deferment. The request must involve the health and welfare of a family member. Compassionate reassignments are generally for 12 months only.

Consecutive Overseas Tours (COTs) and In-Place Consecutive Overseas Tours (IPCOTs). A COT requires the officer to PCS between OCONUS duty stations and complete both prescribed tours. An IPCOT requires the officer to complete the first prescribed tour and remain at the current duty station for a second full prescribed tour. Officers must serve the prescribed tour lengths for both tours. Officers applying for COT/IPCOT are eligible for leave with paid travel and transportation expenses to the home of record for the officer and command-sponsored dependents.

Exceptional Family Member Program (EFMP). Officers enrolled in the EFMP receive consideration of their exceptional family member's special needs during the assignment selection process. Enrollment in the EFMP is mandatory for officers with family members with special medical and/or educational needs. Assignment officers will submit requests to ensure the gaining installation can appropriately manage the family member. Officers must pay close attention to their EFMP expiration date; they will not be placed on accompanied orders if EFMP is not approved. Officers cannot waive EFMP for an accompanied tour but may elect to serve an unaccompanied (12-month) tour at a location outside the United States.

Section 3

Physician Assistant Positions and Roles

Chapter 12

ROLE OF THE BATTALION AND SQUADRON PHYSICIAN ASSISTANT

Robert Gipson, PA-C, MPAS; Colt Crutchfield, PA-C, MPAS; Craig J. Edwards, PA-C, MPAS; Darron Fritz, PA-C, MPAS; Amy L. Jackson, PA-C, MPAS; Scott A. Kavan, PA-C, MPAS; Jay M. Lloyd Sr, PA-C, MPAS; Manish Rawat, PA-C, MPAS; Bradley Tibbetts, PA-C, MPAS; Jeremiah Tyler, PA-C, MPAS; and Amelia M. Duran-Stanton, PA-C, PhD, DSc, MPAS

Introduction

Being a battalion (BN) or squadron (SQN) physician assistant (PA) is arguably the most significant assignment PAs hold in the Army. These are the first and most forward levels of care during deployments. Working at this level, the PA must be prepared to provide a wide variety of medical services to soldiers under potentially adverse conditions. The PA's primary function is to maintain the health, readiness, and welfare of the service members in their unit. This includes more than just providing direct health care to individual soldiers; PAs must also ensure the soldiers of their unit are medically ready for worldwide deployment to austere environments. Non-deployable service members must receive dispositions promptly through the appropriate systems. Fighting and winning the nation's wars is why the US Army exists, and unit PAs must direct their efforts toward that end. The PA must prepare to provide care in austere and constrained environments with limited logistical resources. Additionally, in the conditions of current operations, the unit PA must prepare to provide medical care to host country nationals and other coalition force service members.

Requirements

To serve in this position, a PA must:

- graduate from an accredited PA program, pass the Physician Assistant National Certifying Examination, and maintain certification with the Physician Assistant National Recertifying Exam through the National Commission on Certification of Physician Assistants;
- hold the rank of first lieutenant or captain;
- graduate from the Basic Officer Leader Course;
- pass the Army fitness test and comply with height/weight standards of Army Regulation (AR) 600-9, *The Army Body Composition Program*[1];
- meet the readiness requirements listed in the 65D (PA) individual critical task list[2];
- be credentialed at the local military medical treatment facility (MTF); and
- be knowledgeable about AR 40-501, *Standards of Medical Fitness*[3]; AR 40-502, *Medical Readiness*[4]; and Department of the Army (DA) Pamphlet (PAM) 40-502, *Medical Readiness Procedures*.[5]

Desired Skills and Attributes

BN/SQN PAs should:

- be able to operate in clinical, deployed, and field settings;
- be able to communicate effectively with command teams at the company/battery/troop (C/B/T) and BN/SQN levels, fellow health care providers and specialists, NCOs, soldiers, and patients;
- have deployment experience or the ability to deploy in support of worldwide operations in accordance with AR 40-501[3];
- be able to operate independently even when not collocated with direct physician supervision (unit PAs are often separated from their supervising physician, making communication and direct oversight a challenge during deployments or field training exercises);
- be a lifelong learner and have an interest in keeping up to date on the latest research and best practices in clinical and prehospital medicine;
- have solid written and oral communication skills;
- have or develop a high level of knowledge and expertise in Tactical Combat Casualty Care (TCCC)[6];

- have the knowledge and ability to train and supervise combat medics (military occupational specialty [MOS] 68W), combat lifesavers, and other allied and ancillary health specialists in Tactical Combat Casualty Care (TCCC)[6,7]; and
- complete unit-specific schools such as airborne and air assault.

Job Duties and Responsibilities

The primary role of the Army PA at the BN/SQN level is to provide world-class health care to soldiers. The unit PA is responsible for organization and supervision of medical care at the Role 1 MTF, at the unit aid station, during field training, and in deployed environments, including prehospital resuscitation, stabilization, and evacuation. In the garrison environment, the PA operates as the primary care manager for the soldiers assigned to their unit. Daily responsibilities include:

- acute care during sick call operations;
- managing routine and chronic conditions in a clinical setting;
- ordering and interpreting laboratory and imaging studies;
- providing treatment and medication to patients;
- coordinating specialty care needs;
- consulting with the supervising physician; and
- communicating matters of medical health and readiness with the BN/SQN executive officer or commander.[8]

As the principal advisor to the commander and their staff, the PA is responsible for:

- maintaining unit medical readiness for deployment by overseeing preventive health measures such as:
  - routine and special-purpose immunizations,
  - periodic health assessments,
  - audiometry,
  - dental exams,
  - up-to-date laboratory test screening, and
  - management of chronic conditions[3];
- when appropriate (as soldiers reach the medical retention decision point), initiating permanent profiles in coordination with the physician approving authority, and referring soldiers to MOS

administrative retention review (MAR2) or enrolling them in the Integrated Disability Evaluation System (IDES);
- planning, supervising, and overseeing the medical training and employment of 68W combat medics within the medical platoon or section (Figure 12-1); and
- overall supervision of the unit's combat lifesaver (CLS) program.[9]

Professionalism

The BN/SQN PA is responsible for cultivating a sense of professionalism and unit confidence in the BN/SQN medical team, whether in garrison or deployed. The team's functionality and appearance, competence, and innate ability to accommodate any requirement are set by the PA. The PA should serve as a mentor to increase the technical and professional capabilities of all team members. The PA guides soldiers interested in becoming a PA and provides opportunities for shadowing (following the PA in performing their daily activities). BN/SQN PAs are also mentees, seeking guidance from the brigade (BDE) or unit surgeon and senior BDE combat team PA.

Collaboration is essential throughout the BDE to ensure its units are successful in their individual missions. This includes collaboration and camaraderie within the PA community for clinical success and professional development. PAs should participate in clinical and officer professional development opportunities within both the unit and the MTF. The local MTF usually has grand rounds or continuing medical education sessions already established for credentialed providers. These events provide networking opportunities and are vital to building relationships within the unit and MTF. The unit PA must demonstrate their leadership role by being visible to unit and MTF leaders. A presence at command and staff meetings, face-to-face counseling, and unit or MTF social events is essential to building relationships with the chain of command, staff peers, other providers, and specialists (such as physical therapy, behavioral health, and dental). It is also crucial the PA get to know non-medical personnel such as the chaplain, sexual assault response coordinator, and victim advocates.

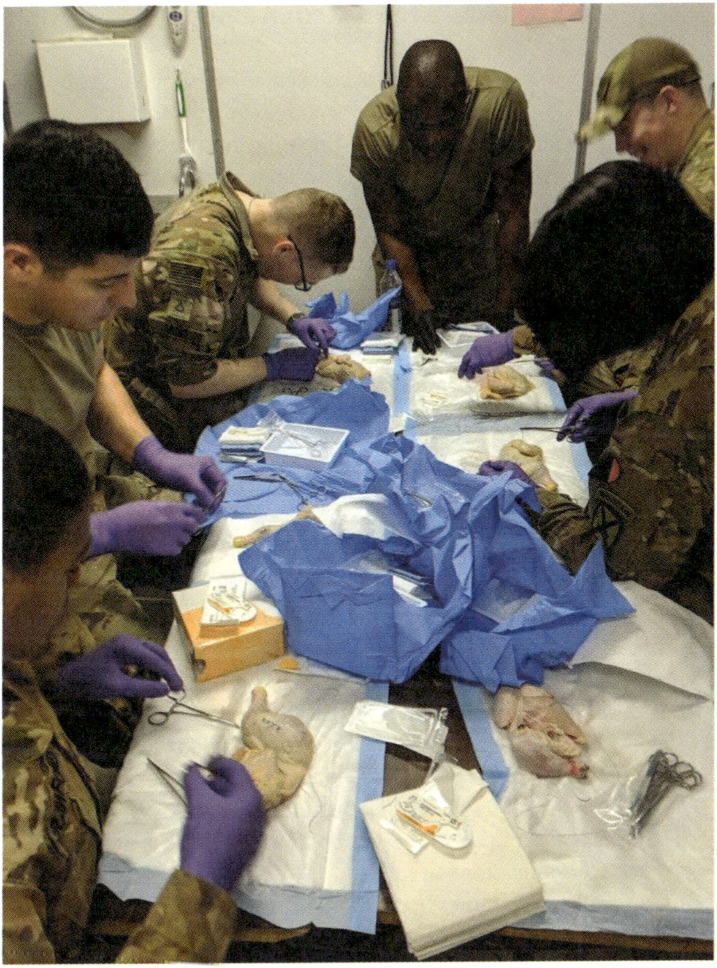

Figure 12-1. Captain Tetevi Torsoo (back end of table), 2nd Battalion, 87th Infantry Regiment, 2nd Brigade, 10th Mountain Division (Light), teaches suturing techniques to medics in Camp Dwyer, Afghanistan, April 13, 2019. Photograph courtesy of Staff Sergeant Andres Rodriguez.

Systems Access Requirements

Numerous software applications have been adopted by the Army and military MTFs for reviewing, documenting, and updating patient care and soldier readiness information. Ensuring proper systems access and being well versed in their use is an important aspect of the PA's duties. A security clearance and current Health Insurance Portability and Accountability Act (HIPAA) training certificate are required to gain access to the secure systems used by the PA. These systems are used to manage and organize vast amounts of information; as with any software application, they are subject to frequent updates and changes that the PA must keep up with. The systems listed below are intended as an outline and are not all that may be required by a PA.

- **Electronic health records** (EHRs), including the Military Health System's Genesis program and its predecessor, the Armed Forces Health Longitudinal Technology Application (AHLTA), which is being phased out, are integral to the daily routine of military PAs.[10] EHRs are used by medical professionals to order medications, request laboratory tests, and document progress notes for the 9.4 million Department of Defense beneficiaries.[10] The EHR system provides for continuity of care and sharing of information across the global military health care network and the Department of Veterans Affairs.[10] The BN/SQN PA must understand appropriate documentation and coding procedures utilizing the current EHR system employed by their MTF and clinic.
- The **Medical Operational Data System** (MODS) is an integrated system of applications used by the Army Medical Department to track medical readiness, education, manpower, and logistics.[11] Data may be exchanged among MODS applications and with Army personnel systems to expand visibility of unit readiness status.[11] The four systems below are applications within MODS, but each requires separate permission for access.
    - The **Medical Protection System** (MEDPROS) is a website that displays a comprehensive review of the medical readiness data for all medical and dental readiness requirements in accordance with AR-600-8-101, *Personnel Processing*.[12] MEDPROS (https://medpros.mods.army.mil/MEDPROSNew/) allows viewing and analysis of readiness information for individuals,

units, and custom task forces. Unit medical personnel usually use MEDPROS, while commanders use the Medical Readiness Portal's Commander Portal.

- The **Medical Readiness Portal** provides a more up-to-date version of MEDPROS with varying functionality dependent on a user's access. Within the Medical Readiness Portal, users can request access to the Healthcare Portal, Commander Portal, Senior Commander Portal, and Admin Portal.[13]
  - The **Healthcare Portal** serves as a single location for integration of medical readiness.[5,14] It provides an updated electronic profile (e-Profile) system to manage soldiers' temporary and permanent medical conditions with specific duty limitations.[15] Medical readiness information such as the Individual Medical Readiness report, PULHES data (discussed below), and immunizations are also viewable here.
  - The **Commander Portal** is a website that assists unit commanders by providing a single interface to view the medical readiness of their organization. It eliminates the need for commanders to log into multiple systems. Through this portal, commanders can view readiness deficiencies and deployment-limiting (DL) profiles, and make deployability determinations that automatically feed into the unit status report. Unit providers can access the Commander Portal and Senior Commander Portal by requesting the "BN Staff" role via MODS. Although PAs may not frequently use the Commander Portal, it is important for their situational awareness and to understand what commanders can view.[16,17]
  - The **Admin Portal** provides "reports that will pull data from all of the readiness systems."[5] Access to this portal is generally limited to users at echelons above BDE. PAs should request access to allow for ease of profile tracking.[18]
- **MEDPROS Web Data Entry** (MWDE) is the module in which the PA can update individual soldiers' medical readiness data for MEDPROS.[19]
- The **Medical Health Assessment** (MHA) is a module used to update periodic health assessments as well as predeployment and postdeployment health assessments. The completion of these requirements is automatically uploaded into MEDPROS.[20]

- The **Transportation Command Regulating and Command & Control Evacuation System** (TRAC²ES) is a significant part of a deployed medical professional's toolkit, used to coordinate and monitor patient movement between MTFs during peacetime, contingency, and wartime operations.[21]

Administrative Duties

The PA must be proficient in various administrative functions. Unit leadership will often seek information from the PA about the availability, limitations, expectations, and courses of recovery for soldiers within the unit. Proficiency in the functions listed below promote a clear understanding between medical and command teams, as well as cultivating a sense of trust within the organization.

Profiles

Physical profiling of a soldier is a medical recommendation intended to inform unit commanders of any limiting condition, provide clear guidance on the functions an individual can and cannot perform, and outline recovery expectations. PAs utilize the Physical Profile, DA Form 3349, on the Healthcare Portal to specify duty and functional limitations. When a medical condition causes a soldier to be non-deployable, the Medical Readiness Portal assigns them one of seven deployment-limiting (DL) codes in MEDPROS. It is vital to educate commanders that they must use the Commander Portal to review each physically limiting profile no more than 14 days after creation (30 days for reservists).[5] During their review, commanders can improve their units deployability by designating soldiers with DL codes 1 and 2 as deployable. Clear and concise communication on a soldier's physical limitations is imperative to allow for a correct deployability determination. Section 5 of DA Form 3349, Medical Instructions to Unit Commander, affords providers an avenue for such communication. It is helpful to organize profiles into the categories below to formulate accurate unit medical readiness data. The Unit Medical Readiness (UMR) report within MEDPROS provides PAs an easy way to view and sort soldiers with temporary and permanent profiles.[22]

- **Temporary and non-deployable**: the soldier has a temporary limitation and is NOT capable of deploying. This classification is defined by those on profiles greater than 30 days (DL 1), those who are dental readiness class 3 (DL 2), and pregnant soldiers (DL 3). PAs must communicate clearly and knowledgeably with the chain of command about the status of these soldiers. Information commanders need to know includes the total number of days on profile, the soldier's duty limitations, the required steps to recovery, and the amount of time needed to return the soldier to duty (or qualify for entry into IDES).

- **Permanent and non-deployable**: the soldier has a permanent condition and is undergoing a MAR2 (DL 4), medical evaluation board (MEB) or physical evaluation board (PEB) (DL 5), or non-duty PEB (DL 6) for not meeting the standards in AR 40-501, chapter 3. This category also includes soldiers awaiting denotation of physical category codes F, V, X, or Y (DL 7) on DA Form 3349.[3] Once listed, soldiers with code F or V remain non-deployable, while those with X or Y are deployable. Code meanings are as follows:
  - F. No assignment or deployment to areas outside the continental United States (where definitive medical care for the soldier's medical condition is not available).
  - V. Identifies a soldier with restrictions on deployment to certain areas.
  - X. Continuation on active duty or active reserve. Denotes soldiers with a disease, injury, or medical defect that is below medical retention standards, but they are granted a waiver to continue on active status.
  - Y. Fit for duty. Soldiers determined to be fit for duty after a review of a physical disability.[4]
  - Once DL codes 3 through 7 are written on DA Form 3349, commanders are unable to override them and the soldier will remain on permanent profile until their board is complete.[4] Table 12-1 provides an example of non-deployable soldier tracking.
- **Temporary and deployable**: the soldier has a temporary limitation but is available to deploy to an austere environment. For example, a soldier with routine knee pain with a "run at own pace and distance" profile with no limitations in section 4 (Functional Activities) of the DA Form 3349. This group includes those with DL code 1 or 2 who the commander designates as deployable in the Commander Portal.
- **Permanent and deployable**: the soldier has a permanent condition without a non-deployable code (F or V) on their DA Form 3349

Table 12-1. Tracking non-deployable soldiers.

Name	Rank/MOS	Days on Profile	Illness/Injury	Way Ahead
Doe, John	SPC/11B	60	Leg fracture/ surgery 9/03/20	Anticipate RTD 11/10/20
Doe, Jane	PFC/42A	98	Pregnancy, EDD: 2/15/2021	Anticipate RTD 5/15/21

EDD: estimated delivery date; MOS: military occupational specialty; PFC: private first class; RTD: return to duty; SPC: specialist

and can perform duties of their MOS. Examples include a soldier with a permanent shaving profile (facial hair allowed due to pseudofolliculitis barbae), or a 92Y (supply specialist) who meets all physical requirements of their MOS, but has a permanent L2 (lower extremity, minimal limitation) profile and performs an alternative Army fitness test event.

The Army has standardized its profile templates to facilitate physical training, recovery, and performance optimization. To assist the master fitness trainer of a unit, PAs should use the reconditioning physical readiness training (PRT) profiling program in Field Manual (FM) 7-22, *Army Physical Readiness Training*,[23] and the associated Medical Readiness Portal PRT standard templates. Commanders are familiar with references such as FM 7-22, and the PA must be able to provide profiling recommendations to commanders based on these references. To appropriately manage profiles, the PA must also understand what the Army expects of soldiers based on their MOS. The Smartbook version of DA PAM 611-21, *Military Occupational Classification and Structure*, lists physical expectations by MOS.[24] AR 40-501, chapters 3 and 7, contain information on the numerical identification of permanent profiles (1, 2, 3, 4) and the anatomical determination of performance abilities according to the acronym "PULHES": P (physical), U (upper), L (lower), H (hearing), E (eyes), S (psychiatric).[3]

Of note, BN/SQN PAs are unable to extend profiles beyond 180 days without a physician's review, except in cases of profiling pregnant soldiers. They are also limited to writing profiles for 90 days in duration at one time. Once an initial profile is written, it may be extended thereafter. For all profiles, the unit PA must specify when a soldier is eligible for a record physical fitness test. This date may be twice the length of the profile but cannot exceed 90 days. Additionally, all permanent profiles require co-signature from a physician.

Integrated Disability Evaluation System

The IDES is commonly referred to as an MEB by command teams, but it is actually a multistage process that includes the MEB—an evaluation to determine if a medical condition renders a soldier non-retainable in the military—as well as the PEB, which determines the degree of compensation, if warranted. The BDE senior PA, clinical nurse case manager, MEB Physician, and the installation Disability Evaluations Chief are typically IDES subject matter experts and can provide guidance. PAs must be familiar with their local IDES process as it varies among installations (see Chapter 30 in this handbook for a detailed overview of the IDES).

Military Occupational Specialty Administrative Retention Review

The MAR2's purpose is to retain quality service members who can no longer meet the physical requirements of their MOS in accordance with DA PAM 611-21.[24,25] Ideally, the process is completed in less than 6 weeks, and the soldier is assigned a new MOS within the limits of the permanent profile. The MAR2 is a tool to keep good soldiers in service and should not be used to move substandard performers to another MOS or unit. The BDE or division career counselor is responsible for maintaining the MAR2 program. The PA is responsible for working with command teams to identify potential candidates and, with the unit career counselor, ensure their profiles meet MAR2 criteria. Once a MAR2 is submitted, soldiers must speak to their career counselor to determine which MOS they qualify for. The career counselor will then submit the required MAR2 documents to Human Resource Command for review.[24] To ensure timely completion of the MAR2 it is good practice for the PA to notify the retention NCO when a MAR2 profile is written and signed.

High-Risk Tracking

The PA is often required to track soldiers in the unit considered "high risk" (Figure 12-2). Soldiers are regarded as high risk due to various concerns, including legal, marital, occupational, behavioral

Race:	WHITE
Gender:	MALE
Age:	20
Position:	Infantryman
Time in Service:	21 months
Time in Unit:	18 months
# of Deployments:	0
# of Dependents:	0
Marital Status:	single
Flag/Bar:	NONE
Battle Buddy:	SPC Brown
Roommate:	SPC Green
Supervisor:	SGT Grey
Risk to self/others:	YES

PFC Doe, John (Company, Battalion, Brigade)

6 DOMAINS OF FUNCTIONING (Score 1-5, 1 is healthy, 5 is unhealthy)		RISK FACTORS	Y	N	RESOURCES			
		Alcohol/Drug Abuse	●	○	Mentor / Battle Buddy	A	BH (Group)	I
Physical	4	Suicide Ideation	○	●	Chaplain	I	BH (HRCM)	I
Emotional/Behavioral	5	BH Treatment	●	○	FAP (ACS)	I	ASAP	A
Occupational	2	Work Issues	●	○	Financial (ACS)	S	SWS	N/A
Social/Interpersonal	3	Relational Issues	●	○	Legal Services	A	MFLC	N/A
Financial	2	Financial Issues	○	●	BH (Individual)	A	Community Involvement	N/A
Legal/Disciplinary	5	Legal Issues	○	●	Informed, no action		Scheduled	Attending

TOTAL SCORE:	CDR Risk Assessment:	Reason on HR Tracker	Months on HR Tracker:
21	MODERATE RISK	Alcohol Abuse/DV	3

PROFESSIONAL INPUT:	EVENTS/INCIDENTS OF SIGNIFICANCE:
BCT SURGEON:	
BH PROVIDERS:	CURRENT UPDATE:
BCT JAG:	
COMMANDER ASSESSMENT:	UNIT PLAN OF ACTION:

UNCLASSIFIED v.3 (May 2020)

Figure 12-2. Example of a tracking card for high-risk soldiers.

health, polypharmacy, and physical issues.[26] The US Army Soldier Leader Risk Reduction Tool assists commanders in identifying these soldiers and is a useful reference for what behaviors or circumstances constitute "high risk."[26] The PA should be aware of soldiers involved with polypharmacy medications, controlled substances, and substance abuse, as well as the impact that soldiers' physical illness or injury can have on their ability to function. The PA must routinely assess their soldiers for these high-risk behaviors. For example, there is often a correlation between recent legal troubles and increased use of sick call. Establishing a two-way dialogue with the command teams and the BDE behavioral health officer is the fastest way to identify and maintain visibility of these soldiers. It does not matter who identifies the soldier (command, behavioral health officer, or PA); what matters is that all three are in agreement regarding the soldier's status, monitoring, treatment, and projected disposition. Appropriate awareness may allow the PA to identify and address underlying issues on behalf of the soldier. These stressors should be identified and discussed between the PA, behavioral health officer, and leadership. The sole provider medication program is available to PAs wishing to restrict medication access to high-risk soldiers. This program prevents soldiers from receiving specific medications from providers other than those the PA designates. It is useful for soldiers on controlled medications or those with a high likelihood or past history of abuse. PAs should speak to their MTF's clinical pharmacist for the program specifics and enrollment paperwork.

Enlisted Separation for Certain Physical or Mental Conditions

AR 635-200, *Active Duty Enlisted Administrative Separations,*[27] describes ways in which enlisted soldiers can be separated (discharged) from the Army. PAs must clearly understand AR 635-200's paragraph 5-17, which states that a commander may separate a soldier "on the basis of other physical or mental conditions not amounting to disability . . . that potentially interfere with assignment to or performance of duty."[27] The type of separation described in this paragraph is almost exclusively utilized for behavioral health conditions, and it contains numerous guidelines and exclusionary terms. In particular, the section is a tool to determine if soldiers may not be fit for military service due to the inability to cope with stressors. However, this form of separation should not be used instead of an MEB for known medical conditions that make a soldier unfit for service, per AR 40-501, chapter 3.[3] The BDE behavioral health officer should be consulted for any consideration of a paragraph 5-17 separation.

Operating an Aid Station

Established for 24-hour operations, the aid station often serves as the point of entry into the medical system during field training exercises and deployments. It typically exists as a multifunctional center that can serve as a medical command post, treatment facility, classroom, counseling area, living quarters, or mass casualty (MASCAL) anchor, based on various mission requirements. It can provide "tailgate" medicine (giving care based on what is readily available in a vehicle) until care can be provided at a more established site, such as a tent or other facility in the area of operation. The unit PA is responsible for establishing the aid station based on mission requirements.

The aid station has capabilities to perform sick call, advanced trauma management, basic laboratory procedures, patient administration, and medication supply management, and it must be able to move or relocate at a moment's notice. The aid station is assigned evacuation resources such as field litter ambulances and nonstandard vehicles such as utility vehicles, but the availability of the nonstandard vehicles is based on local resources, space, and local standard operating procedures (SOPs) and MASCAL procedures. When establishing the aid station, the BN/SQN PA must also designate an easily accessible landing zone to facilitate rapid aeromedical evacuation.[28]

In a deployed environment, requests for medical care are often made by individuals who are not authorized to receive it from military assets. The task force commander decides on the medical rules of engagement, which determine when and to whom military health care providers are allowed to provide medical care (eg, to save life, limb, or eyesight, or stabilize and evacuate patients to a local national medical facility). The needs of the mission, available resources, and capability of the host nation's medical system will significantly affect these decisions. Planning for these situations is imperative. Before the start of the operation, all medical personnel must understand the commander's expectations.

The aid station provides the organizational structure that comprises the medical support system for the unit and its area of responsibility. A thorough understanding of aid station operations is found in Army Techniques Publication (ATP) 4-02.3, *Army Health Systems Support to Maneuver Forces*.[29] Situational training exercises are an opportunity for the medical team to set up its aid station, establish protocols and procedures, and integrate the aid station with unit operations.

Mass Casualty Operations

A MASCAL event is defined as a situation in which "the number of casualties exceeds the available medical capability to rapidly treat and evacuate them."[30] Various options exist for managing a MASCAL event. A holistic or flexible approach can allow for individuals to move among multiple roles as the operation develops and needs are identified; however, a predetermined plan consisting of specific assignments for each individual team member can provide clear understanding within the entire unit. The critical success factor in handling a MASCAL situation is the preparation and tone set by the BN/SQN PA. This section will focus on the BDE medical team in a deployed MASCAL setting. Appendix A of ATP 4-02.3 is an excellent resource and strongly recommended for review before developing a MASCAL plan.[29] Chapter 4 of ATP 4-25.13, *Casualty Evacuation*,[30] also provides valuable information when developing a MASCAL evacuation plan.

Planning

It is critical for the PA to have input in the development and implementation of a MASCAL plan at the earliest opportunity in both the deployed and field settings. The PA must coordinate with the medical operations officer to determine and implement a feasible MASCAL plan. MASCAL plans should be as simple as possible; personnel should not need to make complicated decisions during a MASCAL situation. Personnel responding to a MASCAL situation may be new to the organization, unfamiliar with traumatic events, or simply overwhelmed by the current conditions. A simple plan will be remembered under stress and is often the most successful plan.

Plans should be based on the unit's capabilities; for example, a combat arms (infantry, armor, or field artillery) NCO can serve as a traffic control officer or organize litter teams. The plan must account for ongoing combat operations and limited personnel and resources. Litter bearers who are not medical personnel must be identified so that medical assets are reserved for providing medical care. In MASCAL situations, medical care may be competing with other priorities; for example, a firefight may be ongoing or evacuation assets may be unavailable due to operational requirements or weather constraints. The PA must utilize NCO leadership (medical and non-medical) in both planning and execution. These leaders are the backbone of any operation and will give it structure throughout the process.

The plan must include knowing "the way out": how the unit will get the casualties to where they need to go. The PA is responsible for planning care for all patients in the unit's geographic area of responsibility, which entails the preparation of mobile trauma sets, designation of alternative treatment locations, evaluation of remote locations for storing medical supplies, and plans for moving casualties to and from remote locations. Questions to ask include the following: What is the next level of care? What assets are available at that facility? What modes of transportation are available to move patients? What capabilities does the aid station have to provide care en-route? This line of decision-making prior to an incident will instill confidence that the plan has a legitimate solution in place. In a deployed setting, the medical regulating officer (MRO) can help answer these questions.[31] MROs work in every Role 3 hospital and medical mission command headquarters.[32] They are responsible for regulating and supporting patient movement and in-transit visibility requirements under the guidance of the division surgeon or subordinate MTF.[29]

Once a MASCAL plan has been formalized and approved, it must be rehearsed until done correctly and repeated periodically to maintain readiness; the PA should strive to create "muscle memory" within the organization. Moreover, rehearsals do not have to be a formal exercise. The PA should quiz personnel on MASCAL procedures at various opportunities (eg, waiting in line at a dining facility or following a routine sick call encounter). It is likely the unit already has a MASCAL plan which is formalized in their Tactical SOP. Upon arriving to a new unit PAs should speak to their BN's operations officer and obtain a copy for review. The PA can then discuss MASCAL procedures with medical personnel and the BN's leadership to determine where a need for improvement or revision exists.

Triage and Evacuation

Triage is the assignment of degrees of urgency to illnesses or wounds in order to decide the priority of treatment for a large number of casualties. It is based on medical supplies and assets available, regardless of the number of patients or casualties.[29] The best way to triage is to use the "DIME" acronym (delayed, immediate, minimal, and expectant) to categorize the severity of casualties' injuries. Triage categories prioritize the casualties for treatment, and evacuation categories (urgent, priority, and routine) prioritize them for evacuation. Patients must be periodically reevaluated to check whether their status has changed. Changes in the patient's condition should immediately prompt a change in the assigned triage or evacuation category. A nine-line medevac (medical evacuation) request is used when calling for evacuation of patients from designated units by ground or air. Information on the request includes the patient's evacuation category, if the patient is litter or ambulatory, and any special equipment (eg, ventilator or hoist) needed.[31]

Accountability

During the MASCAL event, there must be accountability of assigned weapons and equipment as well as controlled medications. A unit's S-4 officer (logistician) typically manages supply and property accountability. Controlled medications must be accounted for inside and outside the aid station. There are several options for accounting for medications outside the aid station, and procedures should be matched with mission requirements. One option is to store a portion of the aid station narcotics in "ready-bags," such as a plastic sandwich bag with two autoinjectors of morphine and one vial of intravenous diazepam; an RSI (rapid sequence intubation) ready-bag; or the small Pelican 1030 (Pelican Products Inc) medication cases (national stock number: 8145-01-573-2533) included in medical sets (these are a more expensive option). The PA should be familiar with and adhere to the process for signing out and storing narcotics in accordance with AR 190-51, *Security of Unclassified Army Resources (Sensitive and Nonsensitive)*, chapter 4.[33]

Patient Tracking

Patient tracking and documentation are often the most overlooked aspects of casualty operations. Commanders are entitled to know the location and status of their soldiers, and the PA is responsible for having a plan in place for recording medical encounters. Medics must

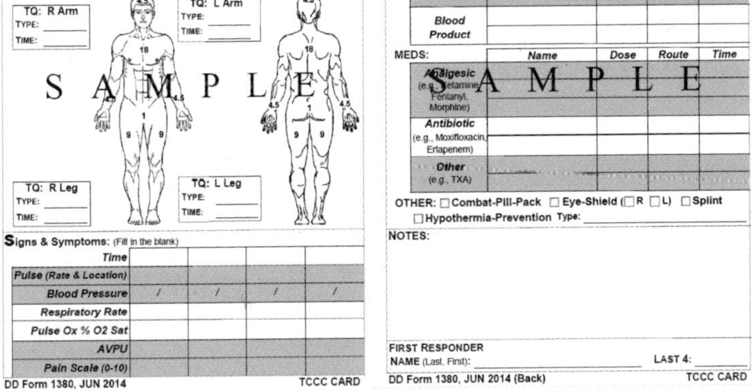

TACTICAL COMBAT CASUALTY CARE (TCCC) CARD
BATTLE ROSTER #: ________
EVAC: ☐ Urgent ☐ Priority ☐ Routine
NAME (Last, First): ________ LAST 4: ________
GENDER: ☐ M ☐ F DATE (DD-MMM-YY): ________ TIME: ________
SERVICE: ________ UNIT: ________ ALLERGIES: ________
Mechanism of Injury: (X all that apply)
☐ Artillery ☐ Blunt ☐ Burn ☐ Fall ☐ Grenade ☐ GSW ☐ IED ☐ Landmine ☐ MVC ☐ RPG ☐ Other: ________
Injury: (Mark injuries with an X)
TQ: R Arm TYPE: ____ TIME: ____
TQ: L Arm TYPE: ____ TIME: ____
TQ: R Leg TYPE: ____ TIME: ____
TQ: L Leg TYPE: ____ TIME: ____
SAMPLE

Signs & Symptoms: (Fill in the blank)

Time				
Pulse (Rate & Location)				
Blood Pressure	/	/	/	/
Respiratory Rate				
Pulse Ox % O2 Sat				
AVPU				
Pain Scale (0-10)				

DD Form 1380, JUN 2014 TCCC CARD

BATTLE ROSTER #: ________
EVAC: ☐ Urgent ☐ Priority ☐ Routine
Treatments: (X all that apply, and fill in the blank) Type
C: TQ- ☐ Extremity ☐ Junctional ☐ Truncal ________
Dressing- ☐ Hemostatic ☐ Pressure ☐ Other ________
A: ☐ Intact ☐ NPA ☐ CRIC ☐ ET-Tube ☐ SGA ________
B: ☐ O2 ☐ Needle-D ☐ Chest-Tube ☐ Chest-Seal ________

C:	Name	Volume	Route	Time
Fluid				
Blood Product				

MEDS:	Name	Dose	Route	Time
Analgesic (e.g., Ketamine, Fentanyl, Morphine)				
Antibiotic (e.g., Moxifloxacin, Ertapenem)				
Other (e.g., TXA)				

SAMPLE
OTHER: ☐ Combat-Pill-Pack ☐ Eye-Shield (☐ R ☐ L) ☐ Splint ☐ Hypothermia-Prevention Type: ________
NOTES:

FIRST RESPONDER
NAME (Last, First): ________ LAST 4: ________
DD Form 1380, JUN 2014 (Back) TCCC CARD

Figure 12-3. DD Form 1380 (Tactical Combat Casualty Care Card) example.

recognize the importance of maintaining accountability for those treated, including their name, injury, and location if evacuated. Necessary medical information is rapidly captured on DD Form 1380, the TCCC card (Figure 12-3). A simple white board in the aid station should also be used to provide redundancy and prevent information loss. When time allows, conversion of analog documentation into EHRs must occur. The Medical Communications for Combat Casualty Care (MC4) computer is used to accomplish this task.

It is imperative that every casualty is accurately accounted for throughout the process. Patient tracking starts with the S-1 (officer in charge of personnel accountability), who uses the TCCC cards attached to the patients as they are evacuated to ensure pertinent information is captured. The BN/SQN PA should contact the unit liaison (either intra- or inter-theater, depending on unit preference) for the commander to gather timely patient tracking status. PAs should provide patient location and disposition to commanders every 24 hours. The Joint Operation Planning and Execution System (JOPES)[34] and TRAC^{2}ES[21] can also be used for real-time casualty tracking. The mortuary affairs NCO, typically assigned to the staff of the BDE support BN, assists in the disposition of deceased soldiers.[35]

Sick Call Operations

Sick call is an assembly of sick and injured soldiers held each day at a designated time and place, usually at the Soldier-Centered Medical Home (SCMH) or unit aid station, for the purpose of providing routine medical examination and treatment. After examination by the senior medical officer (usually the unit PA or surgeon), soldiers who are medically unfit are either referred to the hospital or provided quarters (returned to unit or home for medically directed self-treatment) for up to 72 hours. All others are returned to either full duty or duty with specific limitations. Some clinics are moving away from sick call and going to an "appointment only" system.

The establishment of specific sick call procedures is at the PA's discretion; however, hours and procedures should be coordinated with the unit command sergeant major. For example, if the PA determines that specific sick call hours must be set to account for limited medical personnel, create appropriate sleep/work cycles, or simply consolidate resources, input should be sought from the command team. The PA should recognize that sick call is designed to enhance the unit's mission readiness, not hinder it.

It is the responsibility of the BN/SQN PA to provide care to unit personnel whether in the aid station or the garrison environment. While in the field, the PA or their medics should conduct sick call rounds (ie, taking an aid bag full of sick call supplies and checking on soldiers) for individuals who have competing requirements and cannot leave their posts. Examples include tactical operations center personnel, who may be working 12- or 14-hour shifts, and command teams, who may be unable to dedicate time to sick call.

Triage During Sick Call

Triage during sick call is managed according to the algorithm-directed troop medical care (ADTMC) system described in Medical Command (MEDCOM) Pamphlet 40-7-21.[36] This system is designed to allow providers to quickly evaluate the urgency of a soldier's acute conditions and, if possible, effectively treat the soldier for return to duty. ADTMC provides a medical complaint-based algorithm for the medical screener, usually a senior medic, to follow to determine the level of care each soldier requires.[36] Once the soldier is triaged using ADTMC, based on the complexity of the medical problems, the screener can either (*a*) treat the acute condition, (*b*) educate the patient on medications and treatment options they may use at home, (*c*) refer the patient to a physician or PA for immediate evaluation, or (*d*) set up an appointment with the physician or PA, who may then refer the patient for specialty care if needed.

"Sick Call Slip"

DD Form 689, known as a "sick call slip," is a communication tool between unit leadership and the medical team for accountability and visibility of duty status.[37] Before reporting to sick call, soldiers should have a sick call slip signed by their unit leadership (usually a platoon sergeant or above). The sick call slip can be found at the unit orderly room or wherever the local SOP dictates. After the soldier is examined by the medical officer, the soldier's disposition is indicated on the sick call slip, which is returned to the unit commander or other leader. The sick call slip should provide duty status recommendations, such as return to duty or quarters (with both duration and expiration date), and time released from sick call (physical limitations should be entered on DA Form 3349, not DD Form 689). The DD Form 689 may also be used by the commander to request medical evaluations, such as fitness for duty evaluations, by the unit medical provider.[23,37]

Training Medics During Sick Call

The PA is responsible for developing and implementing programs that encourage and teach medics to conduct patient assessments, perform physical exams, and develop proper treatment plans. Sick call is an ideal opportunity to conduct training and teach medics to evaluate patients, especially to prepare for situations when the medic is the only provider available (eg, during a MASCAL at a location distant from the aid station, in which the line medic is the only medical personnel in the immediate area). Medics respond best to hands-on training with actual patients. A focus on identifying "red flags" (conditions that require immediate attention by, or evacuation to, a medical provider) is a good starting point for training new medics. A medic assigned only to take vitals (blood pressure, temperature, pulse, and pain level) and write the subjective portion of a report (what the patient tells the medic) at sick call will not learn to function when separated from medical providers. In addition, cultivating the responsibilities of a medic in the presence of unit soldiers will instill a sense of confidence throughout the unit in their medical personnel.

Clinical Operations

BN/SQN PAs will be in a clinical setting during much of their time at the BDE Combat Team level. The PA is the primary leader in establishing the efficient performance of clinical duties. The medics and SCMH staff will seek guidance from the PA on how to manage schedules, perform procedures, handle medication refills, and conduct unit physicals (ie, the processes for completing each part of the various types of examinations for schools, retirements, chapter separations, periodic health assessments, etc).

In the past, nearly all aspects of primary patient care were completely under the PA's control because most units operated nearly all medical operations out of an aid station. However, over the last few years, the Army has transitioned to the SCMH model and has required PAs to see patients in troop medical clinics operated by MEDCOM.[38] Therefore, PAs must know which aspects of health care delivery are determined by MEDCOM and which they can influence at the BN/SQN level to ensure the needs of the unit are met. Establishing a good working relationship with MEDCOM soldiers, civilians, and contractors helps in coordinating unity of effort.

To start practicing medicine at a given duty station, the PA must receive appropriate credentials from the local MTF. This process can be lengthy and unique for each MTF, so it should be initiated as soon as the next duty station is known. The BDE PA, BDE surgeon, or MTF staff can provide information about the credentialing process and how to expedite the process. The PA should be very familiar with the expectations and limitations of their role as a provider. Further guidance and expectations for PA performance are available in AR 40-501[3] and AR 40-68, *Clinical Quality Management*.[8]

Although clinical operations are largely affected by the policies set forth by MEDCOM, PAs must remember they answer to the BN/SQN commander and their primary mission is to meet the operational needs of the unit. The PA must also be proactive in communicating clinic schedules and policies to the units within the BN or SQN. For example, units must know sick call times and procedures, the process and schedule for completing periodic health assessments, physical examinations, and audiology and vision screenings. The medical operations officer or platoon sergeant can assist with this. A one-page "smart card" outlining the times, locations, and procedures for these tasks is also an efficient way to ensure all units have the information. The smart card serves as a quick reference and is easily posted in unit areas as a reminder for soldiers. Helpful information includes topics such as separation physical procedures, annual periodic health assessment requirements, or the necessity to complete Department of Veterans Affairs separation history and physical examination forms on the Medical Readiness Portal prior to disability appointments.[39]

Logistical Operations and Property Accountability

Property and Accountability

As the primary provider for the unit, responsible for the health care of its soldiers, the PA should quickly assess the Class VIII (medical) supply level of readiness upon arrival at a new duty station. The PA must know which medical assets the section has and which it lacks. If the unit has a Medical Service Corps officer, he or she should be the primary hand receipt holder for the section and sub-hand receipt various items to the primary user. However, many units have no assigned Medical Service Corps officer, and in these units the medical platoon sergeant may also manage the hand receipt and supply. Here are some things to consider upon arrival at a duty station:

- When was the last 100% inventory completed?
- Have sub-hand receipt holders been assigned to primary users of all equipment?
- What are the deficiencies of durable, non-durable, and expendable items? Has action been taken to fill the shortages? Shortages should be reflected on a shortage annex (DA Form 2062) and funding verified to requisition replacement supplies.
- When was the last time medical equipment sets (MESs) were inventoried? MESs should be inventoried after every field training exercise or every 6 months, whichever comes first.[40,41] No more than 3% of excess durable and nonexpendable Class VIII items should be maintained.[41] See "Sets, Kits, and Outfits and Medical Equipment Sets" below for more information on how to determine what should be in an MES.
- Has an inventory been completed since the last field training exercise? Inventories should be part of recovery operations and should be documented.[41]
- If not done already, a binder should be made that accounts for all hand receipt items and the national stock number (NSN), authorized quantity, quantity on hand, and an accompanying picture for each item. This will greatly facilitate change of command, cyclic, or expendable Class VIII inventories.

PAs should also ensure a method is in place to track expiration dates of medical supplies with limited shelf lives, typically referred to as "Ps & Ds" (potency and dated items). Medical equipment is unique in that items expire relatively quickly and must be reordered on a regular basis. Two key mechanisms to manage medical supplies are the Medical Materiel Mobilization Planning Tool (M3PT) and the Defense Medical Logistics Standard Support (DMLSS) Customer Assistance Module (DCAM).

M3PT is the approved system for management of MES inventory.[41] Although it requires an investment in time up front to enter all the section's Class VIII items into M3PT, the system can be used to keep track of when items expire; send a notification 30 days before expiration (to allow reordering before items expire); quantify percent fill in accordance with AR 220-1, *Army Unit Status Reporting and Force Registration–Consolidated Policies*; and generate a list of shortages that need to be reordered.[42] If used correctly, M3PT can support the medical platoon's equipment readiness and rapid deployability. Another benefit is M3PT's ability to quantify (in both amount and cost) a unit's Class VIII shortages. For example, a commander may choose to assume risk by underfunding Class VIII replenishment to fund other requirements. The PA should be prepared to provide the commander visibility of the costs (in dollars, capability, and readiness) of this decision. Using reports from M3PT, this data can be rapidly queried to provide such information to the command.

DCAM is a medical logistics ordering tool that enables operational units to order Class VIII and replenish levels when required. It automates the medical materiel supply requisition process at lower levels of care and allows non-logisticians to electronically view and order from their supplier's catalog.[43] DCAM can interface with other Department of Defense medical logistics systems, including the Joint Medical Asset Repository (JMAR), the Theater Army Medical Management Information System (TAMMIS), and the Theater Enterprise-Wide Logistics System (TEWLS). Each section should have two soldiers with access to and training on DCAM.[43]

Sets, Kits, and Outfits and Medical Equipment Sets

One of the most important concepts the PA needs to know is how the Army assigns and accounts for medical equipment in their unit. First, the PA should work with the medical platoon leadership (the platoon leader and platoon sergeant) to identify the numbers and types of equipment authorized on the medical section's modified table of organization and equipment (MTOE). Next, it is important to establish the correct version of components or contents for that equipment.

All equipment is issued from the commander's property book to a sub-hand receipt holder. Most equipment sets are known as sets, kits, and outfits (SKOs); MESs are medical-specific SKOs. The medical section is authorized and issued multiple MESs based on its required medical capability. The MES's line item number (LIN) identifies a specific medical capability that the unit must be able to accomplish (eg, sick call, tactical combat medical care, ground ambulance).

The number and type of authorized MESs for each unit can be found on the unit's MTOE. The Force Management System website, or FMSWeb (https://fmsweb.army.mil)[44] is the repository for every Army unit's MTOE (Attachment 1). After requesting access from the homepage, the PA can search the website by the unit identification code (UIC, a six-digit alphanumeric code assigned to each Army unit) or unit type (infantry, armor, etc). It is important to note that the MTOE only shows what the unit is authorized. The medical section's actual equipment on hand is on the section's sub-hand receipt from the unit commander. Variation from authorizations may exist.

While every item of equipment on the MTOE (rifle, truck, computer, etc) has an LIN, the specific item assigned to the unit to meet that LIN's required capability is represented by a unique NSN (eg, LIN C06935 is a requirement for an individual weapon, and a Carbine 5.56 mm M4A1 has a different NSN than a Rifle, 5.56 mm M16A4). The specific NSN assigned to each MES LIN represents a "version" of that MES. For example, the addition of new equipment or medication (eg, junctional tourniquets and ketamine) results in a new version of the contents list, and thus a new NSN. This new content list and NSN is associated with a unit assemblage code (UAC).

To determine which version of the MES is issued to the medical section, identify the associated NSN on the medical section's sub-hand receipt and cross reference that NSN to the US Army Medical Materiel Agency (USAMMA) Medical Materiel Information Portal (MMIP) assemblage lists (https://a01.usamma.amedd.army.mil/mmip/).[45] The MESs can be searched under the "Unit Assemblage Search" tab. The USAMMA assemblage list for each UAC also provides a hyperlinked listing of additional information for every item on the list, which includes the subcomponents of each item (eg, the durable and expendable items needed for a blood warmer or a ventilator). It is important to note that if the PA does not correctly identify which UAC (by NSN) the unit is issued, then it is impossible to know exactly what supplies (by item, quantity, and sub-component) are supposed to be maintained within the MESs.

Packing Lists

Packing lists are essential to ensuring appropriate readiness within the section. They can and should be applied to aid bags, ambulances, aid stations, individual chests within the MES, and load plans. The PA should be very involved in managing packing lists to ensure medics and the entire section are properly prepared to treat casualties and that aid stations are set up in an efficient and organized manner. The PA should explicitly state how each item should be packed. A soldier or NCO should then develop a standardized packing list and load plan (Attachment 2) with pictures to incorporate into the section SOP.

Although opinions differ about how and what medics should carry in their aid bag, a minimum packing list should be established (Attachment 3) to provide a certain level of accountability for readiness, while allowing some personal preferences. Whatever the approach, a clear standard should be established and incorporated into the section SOP, and medics' aid bags should be inspected regularly by leadership.

Narcotics Management

Narcotics are a useful and potentially necessary part of patient care in and out of the aid station. However, they can also become a liability to the unit when not managed appropriately. Narcotics are sensitive items and should be treated as such. Each unit or MTF will have its own SOP for safeguarding, storing, managing, drawing from storage, and disposing of narcotics. PAs must become familiar with how to access these medications and the process of turning them back in. In deployment situations, while operating under predefined protocols, junior personnel (eg, line medics) can administer these medications in the absence of direct supervision. It is the PA's responsibility to ensure that the acquisition, storage, inventory, and use of narcotics are in accordance with current regulations, TCCC guidelines, SOPs, and organizational requirements.[33] It is also the unit PA's responsibility to know which narcotics are used forward of the aid station. Furthermore, the BN/SQN PA, in coordination with the supervising physician, must approve the medications their combat medics are authorized to carry and ensure the medics are trained in their proper use. The unit PA, and any medic carrying opioids, should also carry and know how to use naloxone hydrochloride to counter the effects of an opioid overdose.

In a deployed setting, units may be required to adhere to theater-specific policies in addition to Army regulations. It is critical for the PA to verify current standards with higher levels of command. PAs should become familiar with narcotic SOPs as early as possible to ensure they can quickly support the unit's operational needs. Training should also be started early, before deployment (eg, during field training exercises and Combat Training Center rotations) on how the medical platoon and treatment teams will manage narcotics (Figure 12-4). The BDE surgeon cell, BDE medical supply officer, and Role 3 (eg, combat support hospital) pharmacy are excellent sources of information concerning these policies and procedures in a deployed environment. For further guidance refer to the unit SOP and ARs 40-3, *Medical, Dental, and Veterinary Care*[46]; 40-61, *Medical Logistics Policies* (chapter 3)[40]; 190-51, *Security of Unclassified Army Property* (chapter 4)[33]; and AR 735-5, *Property Accountability Policies*, chapter 2-8.[47] The following list describes a few key components of appropriate narcotic management.

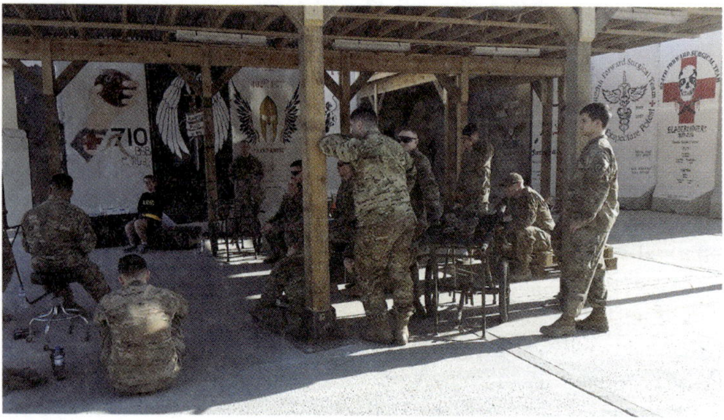

Figure 12-4. Medical platoon, 1st Battalion, 501st Infantry Regiment, 4th Brigade, 25th Infantry Division (Airborne), conducts narcotics refresher training while deployed to Jalalabad, Afghanistan, February 10, 2018.
Photograph courtesy of Major Devon Greer.

- To request controlled medications, a physician or PA must sign a DA Form 1687 (Delegation of Authority/Signature Card).
- A disinterested officer (E-7 or higher) must be appointed by the commander to perform monthly inventories.
- Narcotics must be tracked on a DA Form 3949 (Controlled Substances Record). Any change in the quantity on hand (medication given,destroyed, turned in, or lost) must be documented immediately. Lost medication should trigger an immediate investigation.
- The PA must perform weekly inventories at the hand receipt holder level and document supplies accordingly on DA Form 3949.
- The PA must ensure proper securing of narcotics per unit SOP. AR 190-51 requires a double lock and key.[33] One way to prevent problems is to let the PA have one key and the noncommissioned officer in charge (NCOIC) have the other, so no one can access narcotics by themselves.
- Narcotics issued to a medic must be on the medic's person at all times and under their constant supervision when not locked in an approved narcotics storage container.[33,41,46]
- The PA or NCOIC should provide written counseling to all personnel who will be handling narcotics to clearly communicate their expectations and the consequences of failing to meet those expectations.

Deployment

Prior to deploying, the unit PA should inquire about the Class VIII resupply process to find out how long supplies take to be delivered, what type of storage is available, what the turn-in process is for equipment and narcotics, and how regulated medical waste is disposed of. They must also know what theater-provided equipment is available (there will likely be some if the theater is well-established and other units deploy there on a rotating basis). If the deployment is to an austere environment (eg, the first units into Afghanistan or Iraq), then what the unit brings is what it will have until the supply system is established.

In addition to day-to-day management of supplies, BN/SQN PAs must be aware of the operational tempo and timelines within their unit and other supported elements. They must know when the unit will be executing missions and what type of medical support each might require. Unit PAs must resource the medics and soldiers with appropriate Class VIII supplies and knowledge of medical assets on hand. For example, units or medics may request a medical "speedball"—a standardized package of Class VIII supplies that is prepackaged, staged, and rapidly dispersible to units in the field when needed. These supplies can be packed per unit SOP (based on the anticipated mission needs) and strategically placed (eg, with a quick reaction force or air medevac team) to facilitate rapid resupply to units in the field.

Combat Medic Training

Combat medic specialists (68W) have several requirements they must meet to maintain their MOS qualification.[48] Most non-medical units are unfamiliar with the requirements and amount of time necessary to complete this training; therefore, the PA must ensure that command teams are aware of these requirements and allow appropriate time in the training schedule to accomplish them.[49]

Tracking all the required medical training can be a laborious process. Proof of all the training conducted must be maintained in a competency assessment file (CAF) and should be given to the medic upon leaving the unit. "Documents that reflect the individual's employment history, education, and assessment of competence will be maintained in the CAF for a minimum of 3 years and may be purged according to local policy."[8] The CAF is best maintained in a brown, six-sided folder (its assembly is outlined in Appendix C of AR 40-68[8]). Below are medic requirements for MOS recertification and validation:

- biennial Emergency Medical Technician (EMT) recertification by the National Registry of Emergency Medical Technicians in accordance with AR 40-68[8,49];
- Basic Life Support certification at the health care provider level;
- 24 hours of continuing education equivalency refresher training;
- 48 hours of additional continuing education;
- verification of skills validation (Table VIII training), an annually required hands-on skills test (refer to Figure 1.1 of TC 8-800, *Medical Education and Demonstration of Individual Competence*[49]); and
- role-based TCCC training every 3 years and within 12 months before deployment.[6,7]

Refer to TC 8-800 for more detailed information on MOS requirements for combat medics (Figure 12-5).[49]

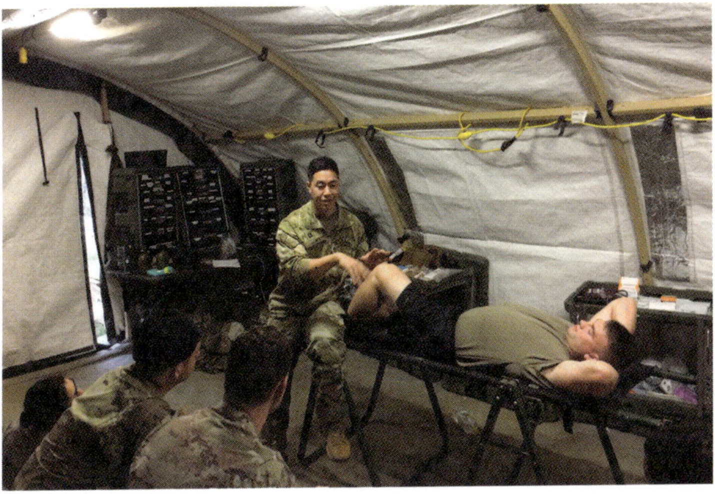

Figure 12-5. Captain Bryan Jow, Regimental Engineer Squadron, 2nd Cavalry Regiment, trains medics on orthopedic physical exams using a simulated patient (First Lieutenant Connor Fink), October 4, 2019.
Photograph courtesy of Staff Sergeant William Maldonado.

When training medics, it is important to remember that requirements for 68W certification may differ from requirements for preparation to provide medical care in combat according to TCCC guidelines.[6] TCCC guidelines have been proven to reduce both morbidity and mortality in combat and are the most effective way to reduce the 25% of battlefield deaths that are potentially preventable.[50] The Committee on TCCC, made up of leading experts in the field of combat and tactical medicine, constantly updates TCCC guidelines as new information and equipment become available.[6] In the past, some medical providers have determined that a skill or medication recommended by the committee was too complex or dangerous for medics to use[50]; however, soldiers on the battlefield deserve the best evidence-based care that the TCCC guidelines provide. If the TCCC guidelines recommend anything medics are not regularly trained in, the PA must develop a training program to fill that knowledge or skill gap. PAs are the subject matter experts in the application of TCCC for their unit, and it is up to them to ensure the following[50]:

- TCCC is the standard of care for prehospital medical care in their unit.
- Commanders and unit leaders are aware of the TCCC guidelines so they can be integrated into training exercises at all levels. Initial casualty response (from point of injury to the casualty collection point) is both a tactical and medical problem. Therefore, it is a maneuver unit, not a medical, responsibility, and must be trained until its practice is automatic.
- Unit medics are trained and resourced to provide care in accordance with the most current TCCC guidelines.

Modified Table of Organization and Equipment Assigned Personnel

With the transition to the Defense Health Agency, the Army eliminated the Professional Filler System (PROFIS). PROFIS providers held assignments in an MTF and deployed in support of Forces Command (FORSCOM) units, filling critical deployment shortages when needed.[51] To replace PROFIS and increase readiness, the MTOE Assigned Personnel (MAP) system was created. With MAP, providers are assigned to FORSCOM units and perform their clinical duty in MTFs. This reorganization makes MAP providers accountable to the unit they are assigned to, instead of the MTF they work in. With MAP, the unit can train and deploy with their organic providers, thus decreasing the likelihood of provider changeover and anonymity.

The unit PA should understand this system because MAP providers are an integral part of the unit's medical team. A MAP provider is likely to be the PA's supervising physician, but they are not always collocated at the same duty station or MTF. Requests for MAP providers stationed elsewhere to attend training must be submitted at least 90 days before the training begins.[51] Because the training (ie, medical specialty) and military experience of MAP personnel will vary, the PA should be prepared to assist with their orientation and integration into the unit. The PA should contact a new MAP provider as early as possible after they are identified and ensure they have needed information (packing lists, points of contact, timelines, etc) to make a smooth transition into the unit.

Combat Lifesaver Training

The unit PA is also ultimately responsible for the success of the unit's CLS program.[9] NCOs in the medical section will likely have experience conducting CLS training, but the unit PA is charged with ensuring the training is relevant, realistic, and applicable to the combat environment. The PA should have an active role in the training while still providing ample opportunity for medics to take charge. CLS competency is an ongoing process, not just a certificate, and the PA should create opportunities for soldiers to revisit CLS principles and procedures during training.

Initial Certification

The 40-hour CLS certification course includes both didactic and practical training, in addition to a 40-question test and a hands-on test. After successful completion of the course, soldiers are considered CLS qualified for 1 year. Unit independence in conducting this training will facilitate flexibility in adjusting to the unit's training calendar.[52]

Recertification

Recertification of combat lifesavers via an 8-hour class must occur annually. Hands-on skills and a written test are required for recertification. Validation and recording of recertification is maintained at the unit level. It is important to monitor the recertification and training needs of the unit combat lifesavers; it is much easier to recertify combat lifesavers in smaller numbers over time than it is to wait until the unit requires a large number to be trained just before deployment, a Combat Training Center rotation, or a command inspection. Training in smaller numbers also makes it easier for the unit medical team to fit this requirement into the unit's training schedule.[52]

"Battle Rhythm"

The following section lists some of the regular day-to-day aspects of being a BN/SQN PA.

Daily

- Sick call: see "Sick Call Operations" earlier in this chapter.
- Clinic: PAs must work a minimum of a 0.5 full-time equivalent day (dependent on MTF and unit leadership guidance).
- Administrative duties: as required, including completing paperwork for physical exams and medical clearances for training.

Weekly

- Command and staff: PAs should be prepared to answer command questions about the unit's medical readiness and training requirements.
- Non-deployable profile reviews: meetings with command teams to review and discuss soldiers in non-deployable status and outline the way forward for these soldiers. These meetings provide an opportunity to educate leaders on medical trends that are adversely affecting their units and answer questions about medical concerns. BN/SQN, BDE, and senior mission commanders must review profiles that exceed 120, 180, and 240 days, respectively.[17]
- Medical platoon huddle: this meeting ensures that unit PAs who work primarily in SCMHs stay in touch with the needs of the platoon and their BN/SQN.
- Medic training meetings: unit PAs must be sure to spend adequate time with their medics. Treatment administered by medics to unit personnel is ultimately the responsibility of the PA. Clinic and leader responsibilities must not prevent PAs from keeping medics trained on both clinical and emergency medical care skills.
- Other regular meetings.

Reserve Component and National Guard

Unit Medical Readiness and Soldier Tracking

In most states, reserve and National Guard unit medical readiness (immunizations, periodic health assessments, etc) is maintained at the state level during annual soldier readiness processing events, in which the entire unit designates one drill period for getting all soldiers ready to deploy. Unit PAs should still know the medical readiness status of their unit, identify deficiencies and trends, and be able to brief the commander on how the unit can get and stay healthy. This may require coordination and communication with state medical assets.

PAs in the reserve component (RC) face different challenges in tracking non-deployable soldiers in their unit and providing a way forward to command teams. Because many RC units do not have an organic PA, and most RC soldiers are not treated within the military system, staying up to date on their injuries and treatment progress can be difficult. In addition, the PA must rely on each soldier to provide their most recent medical records from non-military medical providers. As stated in AR 40-501:

- It is the responsibility of RC soldiers to maintain their medical and dental fitness. This includes correcting remedial defects, avoiding harmful habits, and controlling weight. RC soldiers are responsible for seeking medical advice and treatment quickly when they believe their physical well-being is in question. RC soldiers must report any change in their health status that impacts their readiness status to their unit commander.
- All RC soldiers are responsible for providing the unit commander all medical documentation, including civilian health records, and for completing the annual physical health assessment. Civilian health records documenting a change which may impact their readiness status will be placed in the soldier's military health record.[3]

RC soldiers get their health care from civilian medical providers, who cannot write profiles. It is possible that the only military medical providers writing soldier profiles are consolidated at the state level and have no interface with command teams. To overcome this communication gap, command teams must pay close attention to their Commander Portal account to keep track of soldiers' medical conditions. The provider writing the profile also has the responsibility to clearly state the recommended next step in the patient's care, which will allow the commander to conduct proper follow-up.

However, given the time constraints on RC units, this close tracking often does not occur. Additionally, RC soldiers may have ongoing, untreated medical conditions because they might not participate in the daily physical training or activities performed by active duty soldiers. Untreated conditions may only become an issue when it is time to perform the Army fitness test, attend a field training exercise, or deploy. There may be soldiers who are not ready to deploy, yet lack a profile. As a result, command teams may have a false sense of security regarding the readiness of their unit. Thus it is important that RC providers be familiar with AR 40-501 and the requirements for being medically fit.[3]

As soon as a medical condition is identified, a profile must be written. It can be helpful to outline a treatment plan on the profile as permitted by HIPAA. Command teams must track these soldiers closely because there is often no follow-up with a military medical provider once the soldier's profile expires. Soldiers and leaders must remember that RC soldiers have the same maximum 12 months to rectify an ailment as do active duty soldiers. Beyond the 12 months, or as soon as the medical retention decision point has been met, a permanent profile should be completed if the soldier can perform basic soldier functions and the duties of their MOS per DA PAM 611-21.[3,24] If not, the RC soldier should be referred to a MAR2 or IDES as appropriate.

Line of Duty

The line of duty (LD, or LOD, as it is often referred to) determination is a tool commanders can use to determine if an injury, illness, disease, or death occurred while a service member was in an authorized duty status. This determination is used to decide if the Department of Defense is responsible for covering the resulting costs and associated entitlements. AR 600-8-4, *Line of Duty Policy, Procedures, and Investigations*, chapter 2, states, "The Army LOD Program is a commander's program which essentially protects the interest of both the Soldier and the U.S. Government where service is interrupted by injury, disease or death."[53(p6)] The frequency of required LD determinations is higher in the RC because its soldiers are not on duty continuously.[54] LD determinations can have significant financial and professional impacts on soldiers and their families. Although initiating an LD determination is a command responsibility, both active duty and RC PAs should be familiar with the process, and advise command when its use is appropriate. It is especially important when an RC soldier is medically evacuated from theater because a determination that an injury or other condition was incurred in the line of duty is required for admission into a warrior transition unit or BN/SQN.[54]

Deciding whether an injury, illness, or death occurred on duty may or may not require an investigation. If warranted, investigations "are conducted essentially to arrive at a determination of whether misconduct or negligence was involved in the disease, injury, or death and, if so, to what degree. Depending on the circumstances of the case, an LOD investigation may or may not be required to make this determination."[53(p6)] AR 600-8-4, section 2-2 lists the conditions when an LD investigation must be performed. Investigations are imitated on DA Form 2173 and can be performed informally or formally by the chain of command.[53]

LD determinations for the National Guard must be input into the Electronic Medical Management Processing System (eMMPS). Without a completed LD investigation in eMMPS, the service member will not be authorized for any benefits associated with the incident. PAs should check their unit SOP to determine who is responsible for entering this information into eMMPS.

Incapacitation of Reserve Component Soldiers

When an RC soldier sustains an injury or aggravates a preexisting injury, illness, or disease while on active duty, or on inactive duty training orders, that either restricts performance of military duties or causes a loss of income from a civilian job, the soldier can submit an incapacitation pay claim to help supplement lost financial income.[55,56] AR 135-381, *Incapacitation of Reserve Component Soldiers*,[55] and DA PAM 135-381, *Incapacitation of Reserve Component Soldiers Processing Procedures*,[56] provide further details regarding incapacitation of RC soldiers.

Being a Good Steward of the Army Profession

The term "stewardship" expresses the Army's responsibility to strengthen the soldier's profession. "It includes caring for the people and resources entrusted to [us] by the American people, ensuring Army forces are ready, now and in the future, to accomplish the Army's missions."[57] Officers and leaders have a duty to teach, coach, and mentor their subordinates to groom the next generation of Army leaders. Good stewardship is about investing in people and the organization before oneself. PAs should always strive to leave their BN, SQN, medical platoon, or unit better than they found it. Ways to do this include:

- improving SOPs and continuity books to establish best practices for future PAs and MAP providers[58];
- teaching medics and encouraging those who have the desire and aptitude to become PAs;
- mentoring soldiers and NCOs to assist them in performing their assigned duties or preparing for positions of increased responsibility;
- focusing on long-term sustainability over short-term success by establishing systems to accomplish routine tasks that are sustainable in the future; and
- ensuring the medical platoon honors traditions such as military customs and courtesies, the "hail and farewell," and recognition of good performance (awards, certificates of achievement, coins, etc) (Figure 12-6).

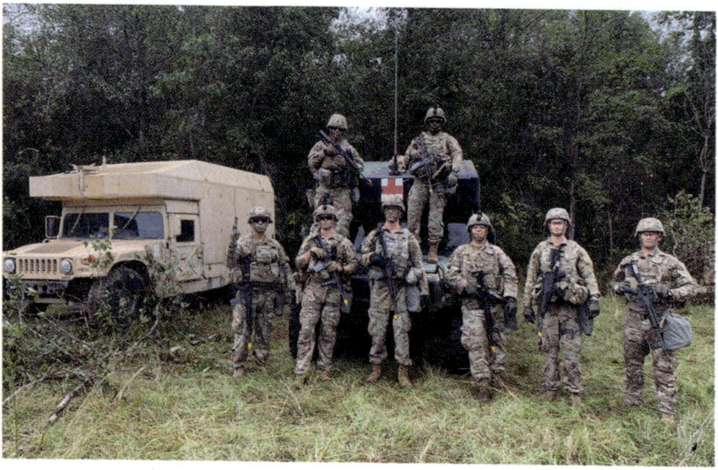

Figure 12-6. Medical platoon, 2nd Battalion, 377 Parachute Field Artillery Regiment, 4th Brigade, 25th Infantry Division (Airborne), poses for a group photo after completing a month-long rotation at the Joint Forces Training Center, Camp Shelby, Mississippi, October 15, 2019.
Photograph courtesy of Captain Isaias Lopez.

Lessons Learned

The most fundamental responsibility of the BN/SQN PA is understanding their role in the unit. The unit PA is the commander's medical advisor, responsible for providing informed decisions regarding the health, welfare, and readiness of the unit. As such, their primary duty is working to meet the commander's readiness goals. To effectively do this, they must work in conjunction with the unit's physical therapist, behavioral health officer, nurse case managers, and the specialty clinics, both on post and in the surrounding area. The role and responsibilities of the PA are detailed in ATP 4-02.3, *Army Health System Support to Maneuver Forces*.[29] A thorough understanding of this publication is integral to the PAs success in the BN/SQN.

When arriving at the unit, the PA must become familiar with the base hospital, its clinics, its referral guidelines, and the civilian trauma centers soldiers are likely to be transferred to. The unit's mission and upcoming training events should be discussed with the BN/SQN executive officer, BDE PA, and BDE surgeon. Each person should be seen as a mentor and resource to evaluate performance. Relationships should be built with the other providers in the clinic. It is likely the PA will need their help while assigned to the BDE. The PA should cultivate a good working relationship with the medical platoon sergeant, clinic staff, and medical operations officer (if allocated in the MTOE). The more the PA is integrated into the team, the better they are able to support the unit (Figure 12-7). The PA should take part in organization days, unit/formation runs, hail and farewells, unit balls, family readiness group meetings, and other events. Be a part of the unit!

The BN/SQN PA must also take time to improve their medical practice through continuing their medical and military education, training the unit's medics, and mentoring the medical operations officer, platoon sergeant, and junior medics. The better trained these individuals are, the more the PA is able to focus on providing excellent medical care to the unit's soldiers. Patients should be educated on medical diagnoses, the clinic's procedures, and SOPs to increase understanding and decrease clinic return rates. If soldiers are transferred to civilian emergency rooms or admitted to off-post hospitals, the PA should take the opportunity to visit them during

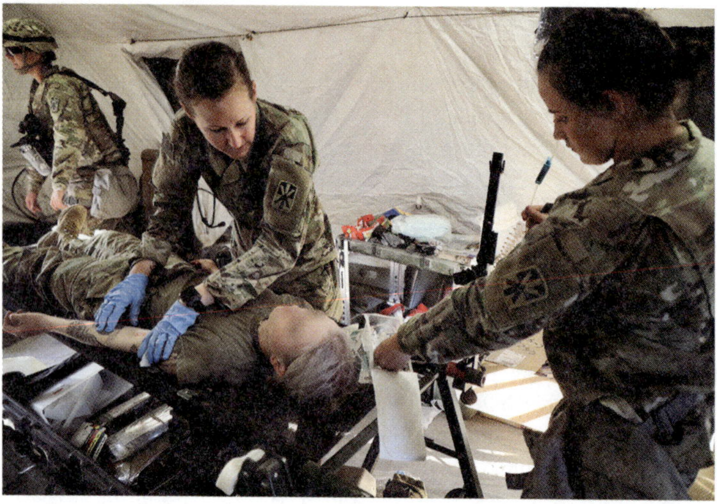

Figure 12-7. First Lieutenant Danielle Hicks, a battalion physician assistant with the 2-43 Air Defense Artillery Battalion from Fort Bliss, Texas, treats a patient as combat medic Private First Class Jenna Andrada assists during a deployment in Al Asad Air Base, Iraq, in February 2020.
Photograph courtesy of First Lieutenant Danielle Hicks.

their recovery. Without violating HIPAA, the PA should be available to speak with spouses, relatives, or other family members about a soldier's disposition. It must be understood that evaluating patients in clinic may come second to soldier readiness processing, PHAs, or immunization rodeos specified by the commander to increase deployability. Readiness is the first priority!

Conclusion

The PA is the linchpin in the Army Medical Department's mission to conserve the fighting strength. PAs proactively shape their unit's medical readiness by providing mentorship and direction to medical personnel, conducting expert patient care, advising unit commanders, and planning for an array of real-world operations. The unit PA is intimately involved in the aid station, the most forward location providing an MTF. They also serve as liaison between soldiers and their leaders in matters of health protection, combat health readiness, and preventive care. The discussions outlined in this chapter are an effort to ensure that future BN/SQN PAs are educated and trained in the management of their duties and responsibilities in this critical role.

References

1. Department of the Army. *The Army Body Composition Program*. HQDA; 2019. AR 600-9. Accessed August 31, 2020. https://armypubs.army.mil/epubs/DR_pubs/DR_a/pdf/web/ARN7779_AR600-9_FINAL.pdf
2. Individual Critical Task List. 65D Physician Assistant–Readiness Requirements. US Army Central Army Registry (CAR) database. Approved July 19, 2019. Accessed August 31, 2020. https://atiam.train.army.mil/catalog-ws/view/100.ATSC/13A27D39-E81E-4A3A-8040-931D71E60A7D-1563544535147/report.pdf
3. Department of the Army. *Standards of Medical Fitness*. HQDA; 2019. AR 40-501. Accessed August 31, 2020. https://armypubs.army.mil/epubs/DR_pubs/DR_a/pdf/web/ARN8673_AR40_501_FINAL_WEB.pdf
4. Department of the Army. *Medical Readiness*. HQDA; 2019. AR 40-502. Accessed August 31, 2020. https://armypubs.army.mil/epubs/DR_pubs/DR_a/pdf/web/ARN8680_AR40_502_FINAL_WEB.pdf
5. Department of the Army. *Medical Readiness Procedures*. HQDA; 2019. DA PAM 40-502. Accessed August 31, 2020. https://armypubs.army.mil/epubs/DR_pubs/DR_a/pdf/web/ARN8672_P40_502_FINAL.pdf
6. Joint Trauma System, Committee on Tactical Combat Casualty Care. *Tactical Combat Casualty Care Guidelines*. Defense Health Agency; 2019. Accessed August 31, 2020. https://deployedmedicine.com/market/31/content/40
7. Department of Defense. *Medical Readiness Training*. DOD; 2018. Department of Defense Instruction 1322.24. Accessed August 31, 2020. https://www.esd.whs.mil/Portals/54/Documents/DD/issuances/dodi/132224p.pdf?ver=2018-03-16-140510-410

8. Department of the Army. *Clinical Quality Management.* HQDA; 2004. AR 40-68. Accessed August 31, 2020. https://armypubs.army.mil/epubs/DR_pubs/DR_a/pdf/web/r40_68.pdf

9. Department of the Army. *Army Training and Leader Development.* HQDA; 2017, 182. AR 350-1. Accessed August 31, 2020. https://armypubs.army.mil/epubs/DR_pubs/DR_a/pdf/web/ARN18487_R350_1_Admin_FINAL.pdf

10. Defense Health Agency. Military Health System GENESIS fact sheet. Accessed August 31, 2020. https://health.mil/Reference-Center/Fact-Sheets/2019/07/30/MHS-GENESIS

11. US Army Medical Department. Medical Operational Data System (MODS) website. Accessed August 31, 2020. http://www.mods.army.mil/

12. Department of the Army. *Personnel Readiness Processing.* HQDA; 2018. AR 600-8-101. Accessed August 31, 2020. https://armypubs.army.mil/epubs/DR_pubs/DR_a/pdf/web/ARN2088_AR600-8-101_final_Web.pdf

13. US Army Medical Department. Medical Readiness Portal. Medical Operational Data System (MODS) website. Accessed August 31, 2020. https://medpros.mods.army.mil/portal/

14. US Army Medical Department. Healthcare portal user guide. Medical Readiness Portal website. Accessed August 31, 2020. https://medpros.mods.army.mil/Portal/SPA/Shared/Components/HelpCenter/portal/ViewDocument.axd?id=17

15. US Army Medical Department. e-Profile user guide. Medical Readiness Portal website. Accessed August 31, 2020. https://medpros.mods.army.mil/Portal/SPA/Shared/Components/HelpCenter/portal/ViewDocument.axd?id=43

16. US Army Medical Department. Commander portal user guide. Medical Readiness Portal website. Accessed August 31, 2020. https://medpros.mods.army.mil/Portal/SPA/Shared/Components/HelpCenter/portal/ViewDocument.axd?id=12

17. Secretary of the Army. *Redesign of Personnel Readiness and Medical Deployability.* DA; 2016. Army Directive 2016-07. Accessed August 31, 2020. https://armypubs.army.mil/epubs/DR_pubs/DR_a/pdf/web/ad2016_07.pdf

18. US Army Medical Department. Admin portal user guide. Medical Readiness Portal website. Accessed August 31, 2020. https://medpros.mods.army.mil/Portal/SPA/Shared/Components/HelpCenter/portal/ViewDocument.axd?id=31

19. US Army Medical Department. MEDPROS web data entry (MWDE) user guide. Medical Operational Data System (MODS) website. Accessed August 31, 2020. https://medpros.mods.army.mil/MEDPROSNew/Documents/MWDE

20. US Army Medical Department. Medical Health Assessments (MHA) user guide. Medical Operational Data System (MODS) website. Accessed August 31, 2020. https://rc.mods.army.mil/MHA/Documents/MHA%20User%20Guide.pdf

21. Department of the Army. Transportation Command (TRANSCOM) Regulating and Command & Control Evacuation System (TRAC^{2}ES) website. Accessed August 31, 2020. https://trac2es.transport.mil/

22. US Army Medical Protection System (MEDPROS) website. Accessed August 31, 2020. https://medpros.mods.army.mil/MEDPROSNew

23. Department of the Army. *Army Physical Readiness Training.* HQDA; 2012. FM 7-22. Accessed August 31, 2020. https://armypubs.army.mil/epubs/DR_pubs/DR_a/pdf/web/ARN7938_FM%207-22%20INC%20C1%20Final.pdf

24. Department of the Army. *Military Occupational Classification and Structure*. HQDA; 2018. Smartbook DA PAM 611-21. Accessed August 31, 2020. https://login.milsuite.mil/?goto=https%3a%2f%2fwww.milsuite.mil%3a443%2fbook%2fgroups%2fsmartbookdapam611-21%2f

25. Department of the Army. *Disability Evaluation for Retention, Retirement, or Separation*. HQDA; 2017. AR 635-40. Accessed August 31, 2020. https://armypubs.army.mil/epubs/DR_pubs/DR_a/pdf/web/ARN6811_AR635-40_ADMIN_WEB_Final.pdf

26. US Army G1 website. US Army Soldier Leader Risk Reduction Tool (USA SLRRT). Accessed August 31, 2020. https://www.armyg1.army.mil/hr/suicide/spmonth/risk_assessment_tool.asp

27. Department of the Army. *Active Duty Enlisted Administrative Separations*. HQDA; 2016. AR 635-200. Accessed August 31, 2020. https://armypubs.army.mil/epubs/DR_pubs/DR_a/pdf/web/AR635-200_Web_FINAL_18JAN2017.pdf

28. Department of the Army. *Pathfinder Operations*. HQDA; 2006. FM 3-21.38. Accessed August 31, 2020. https://armypubs.army.mil/epubs/DR_pubs/DR_a/pdf/web/fm3_21x38.pdf

29. Department of the Army. *Army Health Systems Support to Maneuver Forces*. HQDA; 2014. ATP 4-02.3. Accessed August 31, 2020. https://armypubs.army.mil/epubs/DR_pubs/DR_a/pdf/web/atp4_02x3.pdf

30. Department of the Army. *Casualty Evacuation*. HQDA; 2013:4-1. ATP 4-25.13. Accessed August 31, 2020. https://armypubs.army.mil/epubs/DR_pubs/DR_a/pdf/web/atp4_25x13.pdf

31. Department of the Army. *Medical Evacuation*. HQDA; 2019. ATP 4-02.2. Accessed August 31, 2020. https://armypubs.army.mil/epubs/DR_pubs/DR_a/pdf/web/ARN17834_ATP%204-02x2%20FINAL%20WEB.pdf

32. Department of the Army. *Army Health System Support Planning*. HQDA; 2020:2–10. ATP 4-02.55. Accessed August 31, 2020. https://armypubs.army.mil/epubs/DR_pubs/DR_a/pdf/web/ARN21532_ATP_4-02x55_FINAL_WEB.pdf

33. Department of the Army. *Security of Unclassified Army Resources (Sensitive and Nonsensitive)*. HQDA; 2019. AR 190-51. Accessed August 30, 2020. https://armypubs.army.mil/epubs/DR_pubs/DR_a/pdf/web/ARN5636_AR190_51_FINAL_WEB.pdf

34. Department of Defense. *User's Guide for JOPES (Joint Operation Planning and Execution System)*. DOD; 1995. Accessed August 31, 2020. https://www.jcs.mil/Portals/36/Documents/Doctrine/Other_Pubs/jopes.pdf

35. Department of the Army. *Contingency Fatality Operations*. HQDA; 2014. ATP 4-46. Accessed August 31, 2020. https://armypubs.army.mil/epubs/DR_pubs/DR_a/pdf/web/atp4_46.pdf

36. US Army Medical Command. *ADTMC: Algorithm-Directed Troop Medical Care (ADTMC)*. MEDCOM; 2019. MEDCOM Pamphlet 40-7-21. Accessed August 31, 2020. https://mitc.amedd.army.mil/sites/DC/MEDCOM%20Publications/Pam%2040-7-21.pdf

37. Department of the Army. *Medical Record Administration and Healthcare Documentation*. HQDA; 2008/Rapid action revision date 2010. AR 40-66. Accessed August 31, 2020. https://armypubs.army.mil/epubs/DR_pubs/DR_a/pdf/web/r40_66.pdf

38. US Army Medical Command. *Army PCMH SCMH Manual: Leaders Guide to Army Soldier Centered Medical Home Transformation*. MEDCOM; 2014. Accessed August 31, 2020. http://www.usafp.org/wp-content/uploads/2013/12/ARMY-SCMH-Leaders-Guide-FINAL-13Feb-14.pdf

39. US Army Medical Department. Separation history and physical examination user guide. Medical Readiness Portal website. Accessed August 31, 2020. https://rc.mods.army.mil/MHA/Documents/SHPE%20User%20Guide.pdf

40. Department of the Army. *Medical Logistic Policies*. HQDA; 2005. AR 40-61. Accessed August 31, 2020. https://armypubs.army.mil/epubs/DR_pubs/DR_a/pdf/web/r40_61.pdf

41. Department of the Army. *Army Medical Department Supply Information*. HQDA; 2018. SB 8-75-11. Accessed August 31, 2020. https://www.amlc.army.mil/USAMMA/Logistics/Publications/

42. Department of the Army. *Army Unit Status Reporting and Force Registration—Consolidated Policies*. HQDA; 2010. AR 220-1. Accessed August 31, 2020. https://armypubs.army.mil/epubs/DR_pubs/DR_a/pdf/web/r220_1.pdf

43. Department of Defense. Defense Medical Logistics Standard Support (DMLSS) customer assistance module (DCAM) website. Accessed August 31, 2020. http://www.mc4.army.mil/apps/DCAM

44. US Army Force Management Support Agency. Force Management System website (FMSWeb). Accessed August 31, 2020. https://fmsweb.army.mil/

45. US Army Medical Materiel Agency. Medical Materiel Information Portal (MMIP). Accessed September 9, 2020. https://a01.usamma.amedd.army.mil/mmip [CAC access required]

46. Department of the Army. *Medical, Dental, and Veterinary Care.* HQDA; 2013. AR 40-3. Accessed August 31, 2020. https://armypubs.army.mil/epubs/DR_pubs/DR_a/pdf/web/r40_3.pdf

47. Department of the Army. *Property Accountability Policies.* HQDA; 2016. AR 735-5. Accessed August 31, 2020. https://armypubs.army.mil/epubs/DR_pubs/DR_a/pdf/web/r735-5_Web_Final.pdf

48. US Army Medical Department. 68W Combat Medic Specialist website. Accessed August 31, 2020. https://www.milsuite.mil/book/groups/68w-combat-medic

49. Department of the Army. *Medical Education and Demonstration of Individual Competence.* HQDA; 2014. Training Circular 8-800. Accessed August 31, 2020. https://armypubs.army.mil/epubs/DR_pubs/DR_c/pdf/web/tc8_800.pdf

50. Sauer SW, Robinson JB, Smith MP, et al. Saving lives on the battlefield (part II)–one year later. *J Spec Oper Med.* 2015;15(2):25–41. Accessed August 31, 2020. https://pdfs.semanticscholar.org/5ed6/29f4ebf70ef1cae577667aff2d87c531eecf.pdf

51. Department of the Army. *Army Medical Department Professional Filler System.* HQDA; 2015. AR 601-142. Accessed August 31, 2020. https://armypubs.army.mil/epubs/DR_pubs/DR_a/pdf/web/r601_142.pdf

52. Department of the Army. *Army Training and Leader Development*. HQDA; 2017: 182. AR 350-1. Accessed August 31, 2020. https://armypubs.army.mil/epubs/DR_pubs/DR_a/pdf/web/ARN18487_R350_1_Admin_FINAL.pdf

53. Department of the Army. *Line of Duty Policy, Procedures, and Investigations*. HQDA; 2019. AR 600-8-4. Accessed August 31, 2020. https://armypubs.army.mil/epubs/DR_pubs/DR_a/pdf/web/ARN5227_AR600_8_4_FINAL.pdf

54. Department of the Army. *Warrior Care and Transition Program*. HQDA; 2015. AR 40-58. Accessed August 31, 2020. https://armypubs.army.mil/epubs/DR_pubs/DR_a/pdf/web/r40_58.pdf

55. Department of the Army. *Incapacitation of Reserve Component Soldiers*. HQDA; 2006. AR 135-381. Accessed August 31, 2020. https://armypubs.army.mil/epubs/DR_pubs/DR_a/pdf/web/r135_381.pdf

56. Department of the Army. *Incapacitation of Reserve Component Soldiers Processing Procedures*. HQDA; 2008. DA Pamphlet 135-381. Accessed August 31, 2020. https://armypubs.army.mil/epubs/DR_pubs/DR_a/pdf/web/P135_381.pdf

57. Department of the Army. *Army Leadership*. HQDA; 2019. ADP 6-22. Accessed August 31, 2020. https://armypubs.army.mil/epubs/DR_pubs/DR_a/pdf/web/ARN20039_ADP%206-22%20C1%20FINAL%20WEB.pdf

58. Nascimento L. *Building a Useful Continuity Book*. Center for Army Lessons Learned; 1999. Accessed August 31, 2020. https://call2.army.mil/toc.aspx?document=2531

ATTACHMENT 1: BASIC MEDICAL EQUIPMENT SET INFORMATION

120 - MEDICAL TREATMENT SQUA

PARNO	LIN	ERC	NOMENCLATURE	REQ EQ	AUTH EQ	PARENT UNIT REQ EQ	PARENT UNIT AUTH EQ	RMK 1	RMK 2	CDUIC	MOD PATH	SUBCO
120	A05034	A	AUTOMATIC EXTERNAL DEFIBRILLATOR (AED) :	2	2	2	2				SAM288	
120	A79381	A	ANTENNA GROUP: OE-254()/GRC	2	2	2	2				CAM378	
120	C05002	A	COMPUTER SYS DIGITAL: AN/PYQ-10(C)	1	1	1	1				CAM304	
120	C05036	A	COMPUTER SET DIGITAL (JBC-P): AN/UYK-128B(V)3	2	2	2	2				FAM006	
120	C06935	A	CARBINE 5.56 MILLIMETER: M4A1	6	6	6	6				IAM151	
120	C07506	A	CHEMICAL- BIOLOGICAL PROTECTIVE SHELTER (CBPS): M8	1	1	1	1				GAM048	
120	C18345	A	COMPUTER SET: DIGITAL AN/TYQ-106(V)1	2	2	2	2				SAM211	
120	E05008	A	ENCRYPTION-DECRYPTION EQUIP: KGV-72	2	2	2	2				FAM024	
120	G18358	A	GEN SET: DED SKID MTD 3KW 60HZ	1	1	1	1	TEB			OAM926	
120	J00697	A	JOINT CHMCL AGENT: DETECTOR	1	1	1	1				GAM024	
120	M12986	A	MASK CHEMICL BIOLOGICL JOINT SERVICE GENERAL PURPOSE: FIELD M50	8	8	8	8				GAM002	
120	M23673	A	MEDICAL EQUIPMENT SET CHEMICAL AGENT PATIENT PROTECTIVE WRAP:	1	1	1	1				SAM171	
120	M25865	A	MEDICAL EQUIPMENT SET PATIENT DECONTAMINATION & CHEM TREATMENT:	1	1	1	1				SAM172	
120	M30499	A	MEDICAL EQUIPMENT SET TACTICAL COMBAT MEDICAL CARE:	2	2	2	2				SAM080	
120	N05482	A	NIGHT VISION: GOGGLE	8	8	8	8				IAM059	
120	N96248	A	NAVIGATION SET: SATELLITE SIGNALS AN/PSN-13	2	2	2	2				CAM005	
120	P05043	A	PISTOL, MODULAR : XM-17	2	2	2	2				IAM051	
120	P40750	A	POWER SUPPLY: PP-6224/U	1	1	1	1				CAM102	
120	P99881	A	PROC DATA CAISI 2.0:	1	1	1	1				NAM006	
120	R20684	A	RADIAC SET: AN/VDR-2	1	1	1	1				GAM013	
120	R31061	A	RADIAC SET: AN/UDR-13	1	1	1	1				GAM021	
120	R44999	A	RADIO SET: AN/VRC-89F(C)	2	2	2	2				CAM006	
120	S60288	A	SIGHT: REFLEX COLLIMATOR	6	6	6	6				IAM064	
120	T56383	A	TRUCK UTILITY EXPANDED CAPACITY ENHANCED 4X4: M1165A1	1	1	1	1				TEM299	
120	T95992	A	LIGHT TACTICAL TRAILER: 3/4 TON	1	1	1	1				TAM056	
120	W69528	A	TOWBAR MOTOR VEHICLE: WHEELED VEHICLE	1	1	1	1				OAM461	

Here is the FMSWeb-generated Modified Table of Organization and Equipment (MTOE) as an example of identifying the Medical Equipment Set Tactical Combat Medical Care (MES TCMC) line item number (LIN) M30499 in the red box. The medical platoon sergeant, company supply sergeant, and battalion S-4 (logistician) are the subject matter experts on property, equipment, and sub-hand receipts and can assist in navigating FMSWeb to find the specific equipment authorized and issued to the medical section. Non-medical supply specialists may not be aware of US Army Medical Materiel Agency (USAMMA) unit assemblage codes (UACs) for the medical equipment sets (MESs).

LIN Characteristics

Equipment Characteristics

LIN	Class	Cargo Cat	Pieces	Length	Width	Height	Weight	Sq Feet	Cube
M30499		138	6	30 in	18 in	6 in	134	4	2

LIN Properties

Documentable on MTOE	YES
Documentable on TDA	YES
4610R Current Requests	2
AMC Life Cycle Mgmt. Command (LCMC)	Not Applicable, Supply Class not BCE MAP?
TWV Tactical Wheeled Vehicle	Not Applicable
NTV Non Tactical Vehicle	Not Applicable
CSLA Comm. Sec. Logistics Activity	Not Controlled
TAT (To Accompany Troops)	Not Qualified
BOIP	SA8080
SB 700-20 Sub LINs	No Substitutes Found
SB 700-20 Convert/TCO	No Conversions or TCO Found

HQDA Managed LIN Information

Agency (HQDA Record)	G8
HQDA Cost (as reported by eQuip/SLAMIS)	$78,648.00
Synchronization Staff Officer (SSO) Name	Christian Duback

Current ModPath Information

Mod Path	ModPath Title	BOIP Base	LIN	Term FY
SAM080	MES TACTICAL COMBAT MEDICAL CARE (TCMC)	SA8080	M30499	50

National Stock Number (NSN) Information

NSN	LCC	CIIC	Supply Class	ARC	Cost	Nomen
6545-01-228-1087	B	2	84	2	$30,395	MES TRAUMA FIELD (2)
6545-01-490-2338	B	2	84	2	$35,017	MES TRAUMA FL(2)2003 B69-2
6545-01-534-6135	S	2	84	2	$101,448	MES TRAUMA FIELD-2004B69-2
6545-01-585-3507	B	2	84	2	$145,278	MES TACT CBT MED CARE
6545-01-605-1778	B	2	84	2	$117,925	MES TACTICAL COMBATME
6545-01-647-5649	A	2	84	2	$169,884	MEDICAL EQUIPMENT SET

In Latest SB-700-20 (Chap. 2/4/6)	Yes

LIN Family

Portfolio	Combat Service Support Sustainment

On this MTOE, there are different national stock numbers (NSNs) issued to meet line item number (LIN) authorizations. In this example, six different NSNs are issued for the LIN M30499. The MESs have NSNs that correlate to a specific UAC, which can be located on the USAMMA website via the MMIP, as identified in the previous example.

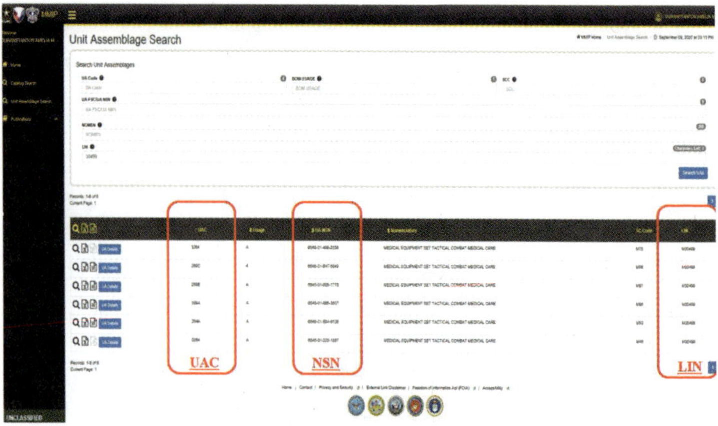

In this example of a USAMMA MMIP search for LIN 30499 (MES Tactical Combat Medical Care [TCMC]), six UACs and the associated NSNs are shown, each representing a different version of the list of equipment contained within the TCMC MES. Additionally, the hyperlinked UAC will provide the assemblage list, and each item on the list is hyperlinked to additional information including the subcomponents of each item on the list, both durable and expendable.

ATTACHMENT 2: EXAMPLE OF BATTALION AID STATION LOAD PLANS

VEHICLE LOAD CARD

(TB 55-46- 1 & 2) and (FORSCOM Reg 55-1)

UNIT UIC	VEH LIN NO	NOMEN / MODEL NO	SEC / PLT	SHIPMENT UNIT NO	DATE COMPILED
WAJRT0	HQ-10	M1078	MED/TMT		21-May-10

LENGTH OF VEH		WIDTH OF VEH		HEIGHT OF VEH		VEH EMPTY WT
OPERATIONAL	REDUCED	OPERATIONAL	REDUCED	OPERATIONAL	REDUCED	

CARGO AREA			CARGO AREA CUBIC FEET	
LENGTH	WIDTH	HEIGHT	OPERATIONAL	REDUCED

NOT COMPUTED FOR HS TO MS		TEST LOAD VERIFIED BY	DATE
CB/CG IS	INCHED FROM		

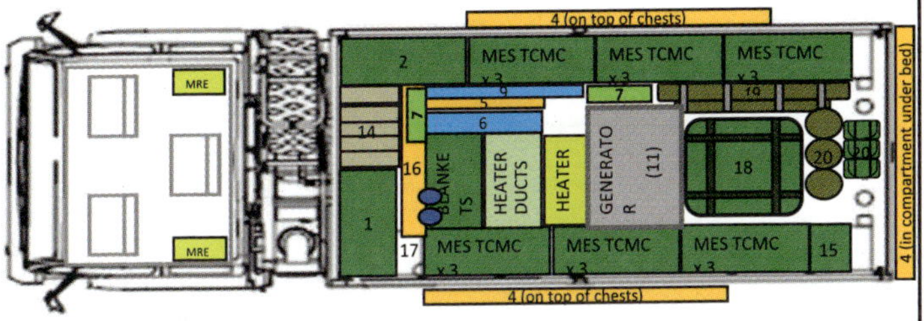

CARGO LOC NO	CARGO DESCRIPTION & TYPE PACK	NO OF ITEMS	PC CUBIC FEET	TOTAL CUBIC FEET	TOTAL WT
1	*MES CHEM PATIENT DECONTAMINATION	4.5			
2	*MES CHEM PATIENT TREATMENT	3			
3	*MES TACTICAL COMBAT CASUALTY CARE	25			
4 / 5 / 6	LITTERS REG / RAVEN LITTERS / LITTER STANDS	10 / 2 / 4			
7	SUCTION APPARATUS	1			
8	OXYGEN TANKS	2			
9	SPINE BOARDS	2			
10	HEATER	13			
11	GENERATOR - HQ10G	1			
12	OLD MC4 COMPUTERS (GREEN CASE)	3			
13	NEW MC4 PRINTER (BLACK CASE)	1			
14	HYPOTHERMIA MANAGEMENT KITS (HPMK)				
15	MED DRAWER CHEST	1			
16 / 17	PLASTIC ROLLS (CHEM DECON) / DECON BUCKETS	1			
18 / 19	CAMO NET / POLES	1 / 1 SET			
20	PERSONAL BAGS (1 RUCK / 1 DUFFEL EA)	6			

FORSCOM Form 285-R 1 Mar 93 EDITION OF 1AUG80 MAY BE USED

VEHICLE LOAD CARD

(TB 55-46- 1 & 2) and (FORSCOM Reg 55-1)

UNIT UIC	VEH LIN NO	NOMEN / MODEL NO	SEC / PLT	SHIPMENT UNIT NO	DATE COMPILED
WAJRT0	HQ-85	M998	MED/TMT		20-May-10

LENGTH OF VEH		WIDTH OF VEH		HEIGHT OF VEH		VEH EMPTY WT
OPERATIONAL	REDUCED	OPERATIONAL	REDUCED	OPERATIONAL	REDUCED	

CARGO AREA			CARGO AREA CUBIC FEET	
LENGTH	WIDTH	HEIGHT	OPERATIONAL	REDUCED

NOT COMPUTED FOR HS TO MS				TEST LOAD VERIFIED BY	DATE
CB/CG IS		INCHED FROM			

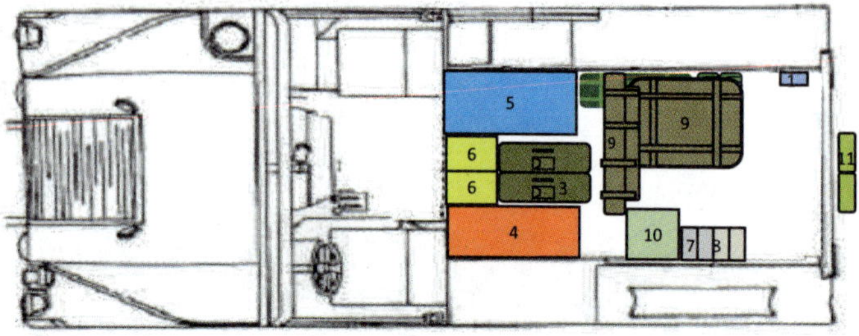

CARGO LOC NO	CARGO DESCRIPTION & TYPE PACK	NO OF ITEMS	PC CUBIC FEET	TOTAL CUBIC FEET	TOTAL WT
1	LZ MARKING KIT	1			
2	OE-254	1			
3	PERSONAL BAGS (1 RUCK / 1 DUFFEL EA)	4			
4	TRAINING FILES/SOPs/FMs	1			
5	CLASS II SUPPLIES	1			
6	MREs	2			
7	MC4 LAPTOP	2			
8	NIPR LAPTOP	2			
9	CAMO NET W/ POLES	1 EA			
10	MC4 PRINTER	1			
11	FUEL CAN	2			

FORSCOM Form 285-R 1 Mar 93 **EDITION OF 1AUG80 MAY BE USED**

VEHICLE LOAD CARD

(TB 55-46- 1 & 2) and (FORSCOM Reg 55-1)

UNIT UIC	VEH LIN NO	NOMEN / MODEL NO	SEC / PLT	SHIPMENT UNIT NO	DATE COMPILED
WAJRT0	HQ-11T	M1101	MED / TMT		

LENGTH OF VEH		WIDTH OF VEH		HEIGHT OF VEH		VEH EMPTY WT
OPERATIONAL	REDUCED	OPERATIONAL	REDUCED	OPERATIONAL	REDUCED	

CARGO AREA			CARGO AREA CUBIC FEET	
LENGTH	WIDTH	HEIGHT	OPERATIONAL	REDUCED

NOT COMPUTED FOR HS TO MS		TEST LOAD VERIFIED BY	DATE
CB/CG IS	INCHED FROM		

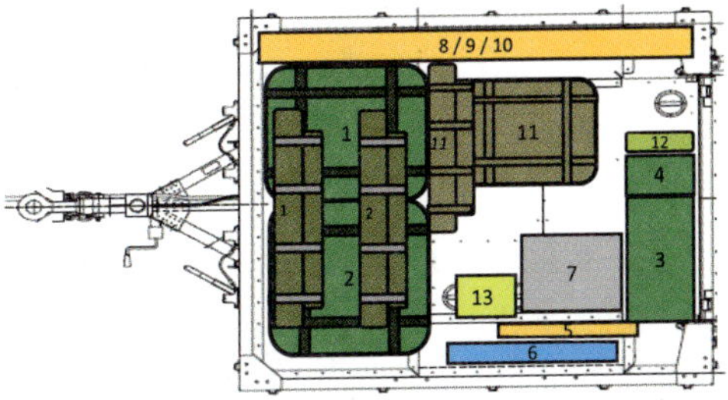

CARGO LOC NO	CARGO DESCRIPTION & TYPE PACK	NO OF ITEMS	PC CUBIC FEET	TOTAL CUBIC FEET	TOTAL WT
1	TENT, MGPTS, SMALL (BAS) W/ POLES	1 EA			
2	TENT, MGPTS, SMALL (SLEEP/CP) W/ POLES	1 EA			
3	*MES TCMC CHESTS (1A AND 1B)	2			
4	*MED DRAWER CHEST (1D)	1			
5	*RAVEN FOLDING LITTERS	2			
6	*LITTER STANDS	2 PR			
7	PRINTER/COPIER/SCANNER	1			
8	TABLE, FOLDING	2			
9	MAP BOARD	1			
10	DRY ERASE BOARD	1			
11	CAMO NET W/ POLES	1 EA			
12	*OXYGEN TANK	1			
13	CASE OF MRE's	2			
	* Denotes Tailgate Medicine Equipment				

FORSCOM Form 285-R 1 Mar 93 **EDITION OF 1AUG80 MAY BE USED**

ATTACHMENT 3. M9 AID BAG PACKING LIST

OUTSIDE (THREADED THROUGH OR BANDED TO MOLLE WEBBING WITH HEAVY DUTY RUBBER BANDS)

- □ 1PR. - SCISSORS W/ RETRACTABLE LANYARD
- □ 1 EA. - STRAP CUTTER W/ RETRACTABLE LANYARD
- □ 2 EA. - SHARPIE MARKER
- □ 1 EA. - CARABINER
- □ 1 EA.- BACKROLLED GORILLA TAPE ON PVC TUBING

LOWER COMPARTMENT

- □ 1 EA. IV SET CONSISTING OF THE FOLLOWING:
  - □ 1 GALLON ZIP LOCK BAG
  - □ 1 PENROSE DRAIN (WRAPPED AROUND THE ZIP LOCK BAG)
  - □ 1 EA. - 500ML BAG OF HEXTEND
  - □ 3 EA. - 18 GA 1.25" ANGIOCATHETERS
  - □ 2 EA. - SALINE LOCKS
  - □ 4 EA. - ALCOHOL PREPS
  - □ 2 EA. - TAGEDERM/TRANSPARENT DRESSINGS
  - □ 2 EA. - 18 GA. 1.5" NEEDLES
  - □ 2 EA. - 10ML PRE-FILLED SYRINGES (NORMAL SALINE FLUSH)
  - □ 4 EA. - 4X4 GAUZE
  - □ 1 PR. - EXAM GLOVES
- □ 1 EA. – FAST IO KIT CONSISTING OF THE FOLLOWING:
  - □ 1 EA. – QUART ZIP LOCK BAG
  - □ 1 EA. - FAST IO DEVICE AND ACCOMPANYING EQUIPMENT
  - □ 1 EA. - SALINE LOCK

- □ 2 EA. - ALCOHOL PREPS
- □ 1 EA. - 10 ML PRE-FILLED SYRINGES (NORMAL SALINE FLUSH)

□ 1 EA. – 500 ML BAG HEXTEND

□ 1 EA. – 100 ML BAG 0.9% NACL (for TXA/ABX)

□ 1 EA. – PRESSURE INFUSER

□ 1 EA. – SHARPS SHUTTLE

MAIN COMPARTMENT

□ 1 EA. - CRIC SET

□ 1 EA. - BVM

□ 1 EA.- NONIN PULSE OXIMETER

□ 1 EA.- BLIZZARD BLANKET

□ 1 EA.- ABDOMINAL DRESSING (W/ SMALL TRASH BAG AND DONUT)

□ 1 EA.- PETZL TIKKA TACTICAL PLUS HEADLAMP

□ 1 EA. - SIGNAL PACK CONSISTING OF THE FOLLOWING:

- □ 1 EA. – SILK SIGNAL PANEL (for example MPIL Mk 1 by BattleSystems,LLC)
- □ 3 EA.- BLUE MINI-CHEMLIGHTS
- □ 1 EA. - SIGNAL MIRROR
- □ 5 EA. - AAA BATTERIES

□ 1-2 EA. - BATTLE PACKS IN 1 GALLON ZIP LOCK BAGS CONSISTING OF THE FOLLOWING:

- □ 1 EA. – TRAUMA DRESSING
- □ 1 EA. – 6" ACE WRAP
- □ 2 EA. – COMPRESSED GAUZE
- □ 2 EA. – CRAVATS
- □ 2 EA. – - OCCLUSIVE DRESSINGS (at least 1 vented)

- ☐ 2 EA. – 14 GA. 3.25″ ANGIOCATHETERS (NCD)
- ☐ 1 EA. – NASAL TRUMPET (NPA)
- ☐ 2 EA. – TOURNIQUETS
- ☐ 1 EA. – 3″ SILK TAPE
- ☐ 1 EA. – SHARPIE MARKER
- ☐ 1 PR. – EXAM GLOVES
- ☐ 1 EA. – RED MINI-CHEMLIGHT
- ☐ 1 EA. – GREEN MINI-CHEMLIGHT
- ☐ 1 EA. – TCCC CARD (DD FORM 1380)

BOTTOM OF BAG (BENEATH NETTING)

- ☐ 1 EA. – READY-HEAT BLANKET
- ☐ 1 EA. – SAM SPLINT
- ☐ 1 EA. – PRESSURE BOARD
- ☐ 1 EA. – POLELESS LITTER

Reproduced from: Compton S. Tiered Class VIII course handout, Tactical Combat Casualty Course, Army Medical Department Center and School Health Readiness Center of Excellence, Joint Base San Antonio–Fort Sam Houston, Texas; 2011: 153–162.

Chapter 13

ROLE OF THE SECURITY FORCE ASSISTANCE BRIGADE PHYSICIAN ASSISTANT

Christopher L. Torres, PA-C, MPAS; Stephen A. Karagosian, PA-C, MPAS; and Jacob W. Rouse, PA-C, MPAS

Introduction

The US Army Security Force Assistance Brigades (SFABs) are the US Army's dedicated conventional organizations for conducting security force assistance (SFA) around the world. The SFABs support US security objectives and warfighting combatant commanders, while strengthening US ally security capacity and proficiency.[1]

Security Force Assistance

SFA has played an essential role in US history since revolutionary times. One of the notable examples of SFA occurred in the early 1960s, when the US Army sent approximately 11,000 advisors to assist the pro-western government of Vietnam. More recently, the US Army has been engaged alongside foreign security forces in south central and southwest Asia for the greater part of two decades.

Due to an evolving worldwide threat, the need for a supporting, professionalized advisor force became necessary. The National Security Strategy redirected the brigade combat teams (BCTs) to prepare for conflict in multi-domain operations. SFABs enable the US Army to bolster the lethality of a foreign security force while freeing up BCTs.

Security Force Assistance Brigade

There are currently five active duty SFABs and one National Guard SFAB (Figure 13-1). Each SFAB has six battalions. Four PAs are assigned to each SFAB, with one allocated to each of the two maneuver battalions, one to the cavalry squadron, and one to the brigade support battalion as the brigade senior PA. Each SFAB is filled to a slightly higher capacity than in a maneuver battalion in a conventional BCT.

Employment

SFABs are employed in teams of 12 soldiers. The brigade headquarters exercises mission command from the home station, with larger echelons deploying and controlling operations in-country, unless the entire brigade deploys into a theater.[2]

The 12-soldier SFAB advisor team is modeled with small team functionality in mind. The SFABs work with conventional partner security forces to improve their capabilities and capacity to provide security.

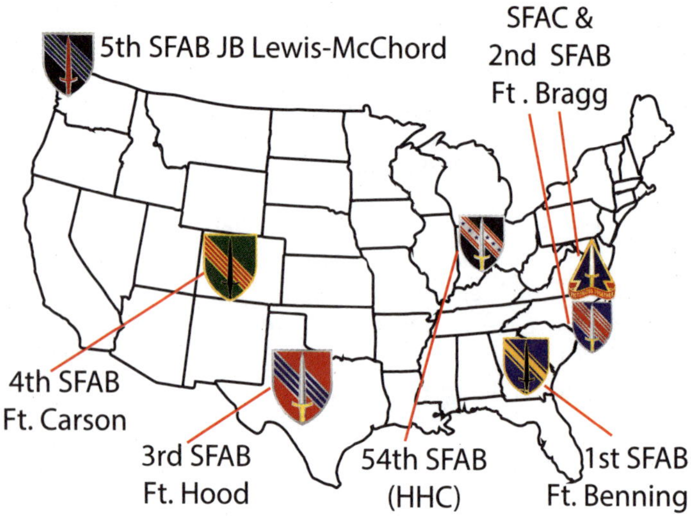

Figure 13-1. The security force assistance brigades are based in several locations around the United States, as depicted by their distinctive unit crests. The Army National Guard's 54th SFAB has battalions in Illinois, Indiana, Ohio, Georgia, and Texas. The Security Force Assistance Command is based at Fort Bragg, North Carolina.

The first SFAB deployed in 2018. It supported Operation Resolute Support in Afghanistan. In early 2019, the second SFAB deployed to continue the "train, advise, and assist" mission in Afghanistan and Iraq. The second SFAB was replaced by the third SFAB in late 2019.

Command and Control

Each SFAB has a command group structure similar to that of a traditional BCT headquarters, with the addition of a deputy commander. Contrary to most conventional BCTs, soldiers within an SFAB are already sergeants (E-5/SGT) or above, giving the ability to advise partner forces two echelons higher.

In addition to SFAB command and control, there is a Security Force Assistance Command (SFAC) at Fort Bragg, North Carolina. This one-star command maintains training and resourcing authority and functionally coordinates the employment of the SFABs (see Figure 13-1).

Duties and Responsibilities

SFAB PAs are unlike most conventional BCT PAs and are expected to conduct numerous duties, some exceeding the traditional PA responsibilities. SFAB PAs must be versatile in a dynamic environment. In a garrison setting, maneuver PAs spend approximately 1 to 2 days in clinic when the brigade is fully staffed with providers. These relatively small clinical requirements are due in part to the roughly 0.25 full-time equivalent requirement, based on patient population size and increased health and physical standards of the SFAB.

While unit readiness is still a top priority, SFAB PAs spend a great deal of time training advisor medics. This training includes refining their basic medical skills, while also focusing on more advanced medical skill sets such as prolonged field care and whole blood transfusion.[3,4] In addition to clinic responsibilities and medical training, the PAs also have a primary staff function as the senior medical advisor to the commander. SFAB PAs will work alongside the rest of the staff sections, attend meetings, and collaborate on product and plan development as prescribed by the battalion commander.

Skills and Attributes

Historically, SFAB PAs attended courses such as Tactical Combat Casualty Care, Prolonged Field Care, Mountain Medicine, Army Trauma Training, 70H (health services plans, operations, intelligence security and training), and numerous others that were applicable to their known deployment areas of operation. While there are no pipeline courses immediately required for SFAB PAs outside of Combat Advisor Training Course (CATC) and Tactical Combat Medical Care (TCMC), battalion PAs should communicate with their commander and brigade surgeon to ensure appropriate training is afforded when feasible.

PAs must also be comfortable supporting partner nation and subordinate medics through face-to-face and telemedicine encounters. While SFAB PAs have relatively little clinical time, they should expect significantly increased staff work. Unlike medical platoons in a BCT, SFAB battalions are not assigned an organic medical operations officer (MEDO) and the PA will fulfill these responsibilities.

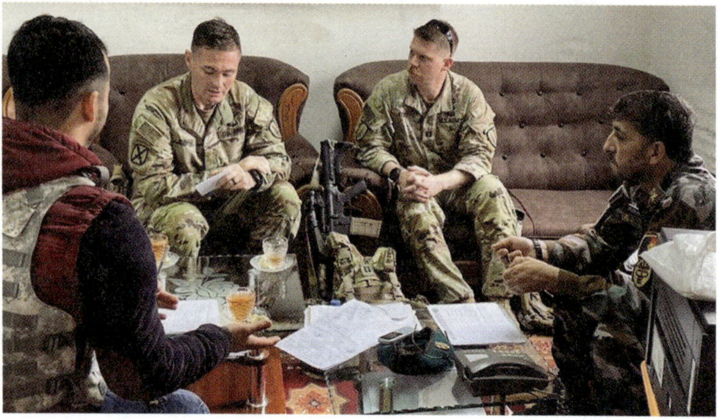

Figure 13-2. Captain Christopher Torres (right) and Major Russ Burnham (left) discussing medical evacuation during combat operations in the multinational Train Advise Assist Command-East with an Afghan Army corps surgeon. Meetings like this would occur twice weekly at a minimum, based on current operations within the region.
Photograph courtesy of Captain Christopher Torres.

During deployments, field training, and live-fire exercises, SFAB PAs must maintain the medical integrity of their formation and also support foreign security force medical counterparts on all things medical. This means PAs need to be subject matter experts in medical logistics, operations, patient evacuation, preventive medicine, and field sanitation. All of these can be leveraged to enhance the medical readiness of the foreign security force. SFAB PAs must thoroughly comprehend the military decision-making process (MDMP). They are expected to create and review medical concepts of operation, medical common

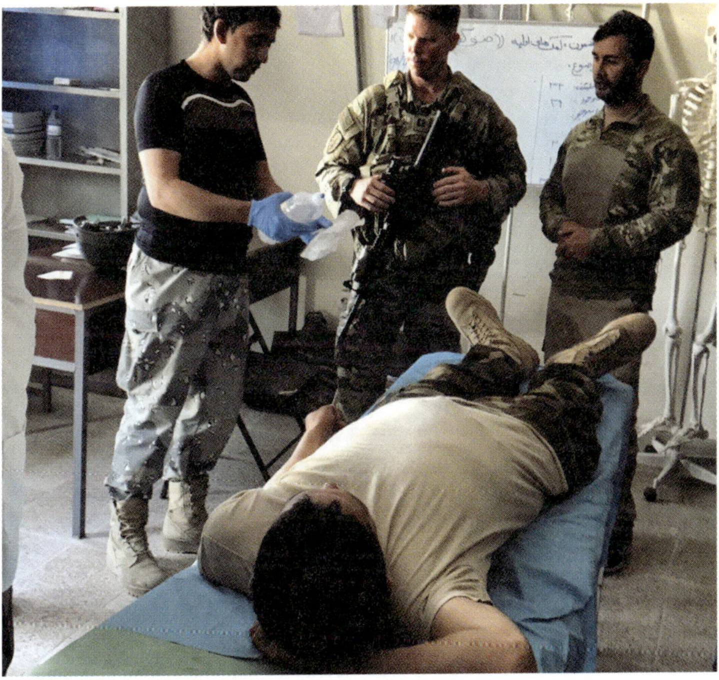

Figure 13-3. Captain Christopher Torres (center) being back briefed by an Afghan Army medic (left) following an intravenous infusion train-the-trainer class. The Afghan senior medic will take the skills learned and train fellow medics within his battalion. Instead of teaching medics the basic skills of combat medicine, advisors now focus on enabling and empowering this current generation of Afghan medics to become more self-reliant and independent. Photograph courtesy of Captain Christopher Torres.

operation pictures, and estimates. They must effectively integrate medical intelligence to enable operations. Being able to develop and implement medical support that ties into operations is key to being a successful SFAB PA (Figures 13-2 to 13-4).

Training and Requirements

Requirements for SFAB battalion PAs include mandatory attendance of the Combat Advisor Training Course (CAT-C) and the ability to maintain a security clearance. SFAB PAs must be free of duty-limiting physical

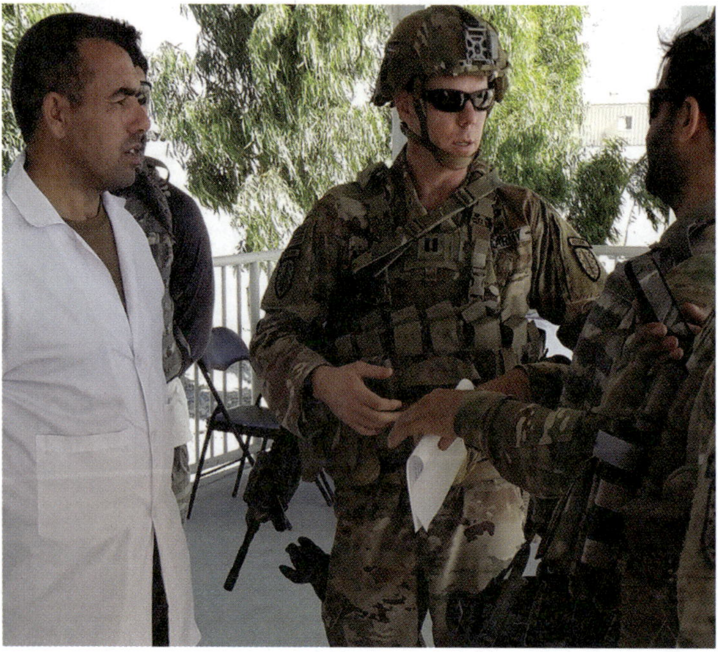

Figure 13-4. Captain Christopher Torres (center) on site at a culminating training event held by a corps-level Afghan Army combat medic program. This training event is held three times per year, ultimately leading to the graduation of the participating Afghan combat medics. Captain Torres and his team worked to align the Afghan tactics, techniques, and procedures with tactical combat casualty care standards.
Photograph courtesy of Captain Christopher Torres.

profiles and able to score a minimum of 240 on the APFT, with at least 70 points in each event, and have a PULHES of at least 111221.[1] There is currently no requirement for the Army Combat Fitness Test.

The SFAB PA is a job for those with experience as a battalion PA who also have a comprehensive understanding of a battalion medical officer. The SFAB PA is one who has mastered the basics and can apply their knowledge and experience to ambiguous and complex problem sets.

SFAB PA candidates must complete a DA 4187, Personnel Action form, and volunteer via the Assignment Interactive Module 2.0 portal. It is best if PAs attended the Captains Career Course prior to selection to an SFAB to facilitate a shared understanding of the MDMP. Additionally, PAs can expect to interview with the SFAB commander and the brigade surgeon or brigade senior PA. The final hiring authority is the SFAB Commander.

Lessons Learned and Tips for Success

The following are lessons learned and tips for success for the SFAB PA:

- The SFAB PA must anticipate training all advisors across their formation in a more deliberate version of the Combat Lifesaver program,[4] and be prepared to create a program if joining one of the newer SFABs.
- The SFAB PA must prioritize battlefield whole blood transfusion certification. They must learn to teach this critical skill. Medics in the first three SFABs are already being certified, and SFAB commanders expect their PAs to have this skill set.
- The SFAB PA must add medical occupational specialty 68W (combat medic) sustainment training to the long-range training calendar. This should be a top priority. Line medics are allocated under their line company, rather than under the headquarters company. This can make sustainment training difficult because the medics are pulled in many directions. If the PA captures this training on the calendar early, it will not be an issue later.
- The SFAB PA must canvass the installation (and other connections) for expired and excess Class VIII medical supplies to support rigorous training in the SFAB. This is especially important if assigned to one of the newer SFABs that have not yet been fitted with their sets, kits, and outfits.

Conclusion

While SFAB utilization is still a very new concept, the deployment of SFAB teams across Afghanistan and Iraq has shown great promise. The NCOs and officers in the SFAB are highly trained, mature self-starters who can operate independently. SFAB PAs work alongside other battalion staff and train medical advisors on the newest combat medical skills. If seeking a new career challenge like this, contact the Human Resources Command through the Assignment Interactive Module 2.0 portal for SFAB consideration.

References

1. Go Army website. Security Force Assistance Brigade (SFAB). Updated November 19, 2019. Accessed July 2, 2020. www.goarmy.com/careers-and-jobs/current-and-prior-service/advance-your-career/security-assistance-brigade.html
2. US Department of the Army. *Security Force Assistance Brigade*. DA; 2018. ATP 3-96.1.
3. US Department of Defense. *Medical Readiness Training (MRT)*. DOD; 2018. DOD Instruction 1322.24.
4. Deployed Medicine website. Accessed July 2, 2020. https://www.deployedmedicine.com/

Additional Sources

- South T. The next Army SFAB deployments might look a whole lot different from recent ones. *Army Times*. May 8, 2019. Accessed July 8, 2020. https://www.armytimes.com/news/your-army/2019/05/08/the-next-army-sfab-deployments-might-look-a-whole-lot-different-from-recent-ones/
- Remfer K. Army SFAB troops will be dispatched to Colombia next month. *Army Times*. May 28, 2020. Accessed August 8, 2020. https://www.armytimes.com/news/your-army/2020/05/28/army-sfab-troops-will-be-dispatched-to-colombia-next-month/

Chapter 14

ROLE OF THE US SOUTHERN COMMAND AND JOINT INTERAGENCY TASK FORCE–SOUTH PHYSICIAN ASSISTANT

Brian Gomez, APA-C, MPAS

Introduction

The US Southern Command (USSOUTHCOM) is one of six geographic combatant commands (CCMDs). USSOUTHCOM's area of influence includes every nation in the Western Hemisphere south of Mexico, including the Caribbean. South America by landmass constitutes one-sixth of the planet, with over 15.6 million square miles, 31 countries, and 16 dependencies. The region holds more than 45 million indigenous people, over 260 million Spanish speakers, and 200 million Portuguese speakers. While predominantly peaceful, the region faces ongoing sociopolitical and environmental challenges. Because of corruption in many countries, government officials are complicit in illicit activities and public trust in government institutions is eroded. For these reasons, the US government maintains security cooperation activities in the region to promote shared values and prevent instability and foreign adversary influence.

Background

USSOUTHCOM is the nation's military instrument of power in the region and is charged with the mission of countering threat networks and enabling rapid response to natural and manmade disasters common to the region, in order to build and strengthen South American partnerships. Weak governance and corruption are among the most critical challenges that impede strategic objectives. Corruption allows threats to flourish and provides opportunities for malign regional and external state actors to expand their influence. Corruption also increases vulnerability to environmental shocks, including natural disasters. Transnational criminal organizations and violent extremist organizations threaten citizen safety, regional stability, and the national security of the United States and its allies. The use of bribery, fraud, and violence by illicit networks disrupts legitimate economic opportunity and undermines the rule of law.[1] These illicit networks exploit the interconnected nature of transnational trade and transportation systems to smuggle people, drugs, bulk cash, weapons, and other contraband across borders.

The region is the largest source of illicit drugs and illegal migrants coming into the United States. Many transnational criminal organizations trafficking in drugs are better funded and organized than the security organizations that confront them. Their activities contribute to the challenges of violence, corruption, and poverty, which are also among the primary drivers of illegal migration. In order to curb these negative trends, USSOUTHCOM leverages traditional military capabilities, interagency organizations, and political-military relations in building a framework for success (Figure 14-1).

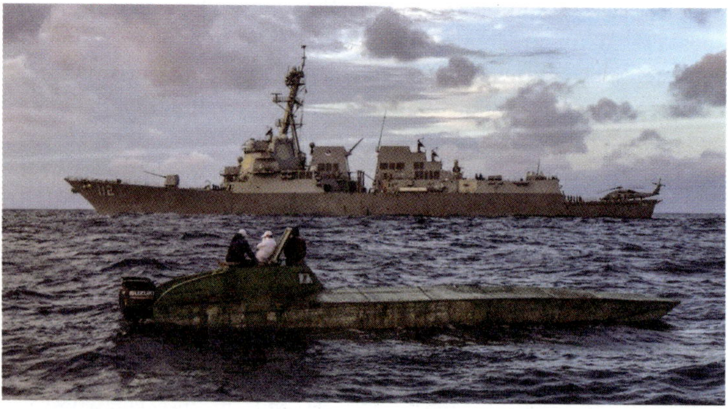

Figure 14-1. An interceptor team from the USS *Michael Murphy* (DDG 112) provides security from the ship's rigid-hull inflatable boat after a low-profile vessel was sighted by an MH-60R Sea Hawk. US Navy photo by Command Master Chief Jose Ramiro/Released.

Strategy

USSOUTHCOM is responsible for military-to-military relationships and the employment of US forces in its area of responsibility. The strengths and opportunities of the hemisphere are set against a complex array of threats and challenges. Governance and institutional capacity remain uneven across the region. USSOUTHCOM is part of a multinational and whole-of-government team working to advance security, governance, and economic opportunity in the region. While USSOUTHCOM exercises traditional military relationships, the command is intrinsically reliant on the expertise and cooperation from partner institutions to fulfill a whole-of-society approach to security operations.[2] A strong focus is placed on international partnerships, which include foreign partner militaries, academic institutions, and nonfederal entities, with efforts to achieve measurable and sustainable outcomes along three lines of effort: strengthen partnerships, counter threats, and build the team.[1]

Unit Structure

USSOUTHCOM headquarters is located in Doral, Florida. The command has three direct reporting units. The Joint Inter-Agency Task Force–South (JIATF-S), based out of Naval Air Station, Key West, is charged with the interdiction mission of illicit trafficking in the area of operations. Joint Task Force–Guantanamo oversees detainee operations and related intelligence operations at Guantanamo Bay, Cuba. Joint Task Force–Bravo is the forward staged execution arm of USSOUTHCOM. Based in Soto Cano, Honduras, its mission is to organize multilateral exercises, support humanitarian assistance/disaster relief operations in coordination with partner nations, and counter transnational organized crime to promote regional cooperation and security. USSOUTHCOM supports 24 security cooperation offices with 31 country teams out of 24 embassies in the region. Like all CCMDs, the Air Force, Army, Navy, Marines, and Special Operations are represented at USSOUTHCOM and play distinct roles in CCMD operations (Figure 14-2).

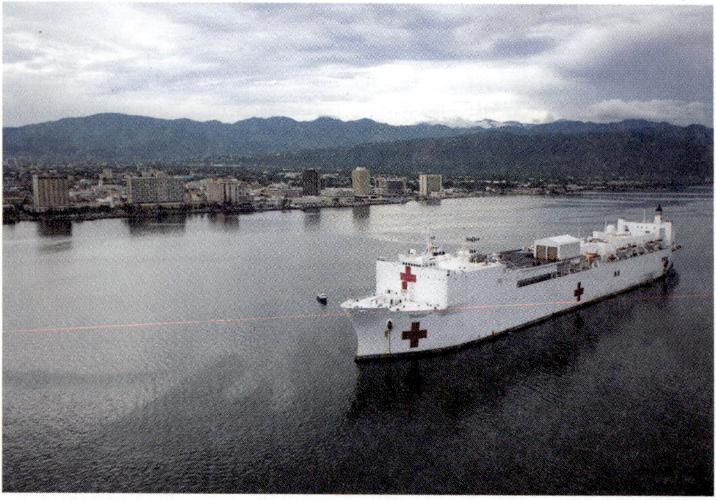

Figure 14-2. The hospital ship USNS *Comfort* (T-AH 20) is anchored off the coast of Kingston, Jamaica, as it prepares for a 6-day medical mission. US Navy photo by Mass Communication Specialist 2nd Class Morgan K. Nall/Released.

Roles and Responsibilities

The Army physician assistant (PA) is the chief of clinical operations for USSOUTHCOM, responsible for developing and recommending health care doctrine and policy for the command. In this role, the Army PA also provides clinical quality assurance (QA) and quality management (QM) of all medical operations in the area of responsibility (AOR) on behalf of the USSOUTHCOM command surgeon. QA/QM functions for Department of Defense (DOD) regulatory requirements include AOR medical entry standards, patient movement operations, secretarial designation requests, reciprocal health care agreements, partner nation capacity-building strategies, and clinical input to contingency plans. Additionally, the Army PA at USSOUTHCOM serves as the counter transnational organized crime/counter threat network medical planner and the detainee health care medical policy and compliance officer at Guantanamo.[3] The Army PA also serves as the JIATF-S surgeon, responsible for oversight of the health care of a multinational, multi-service, and multi agency task force. Lastly,

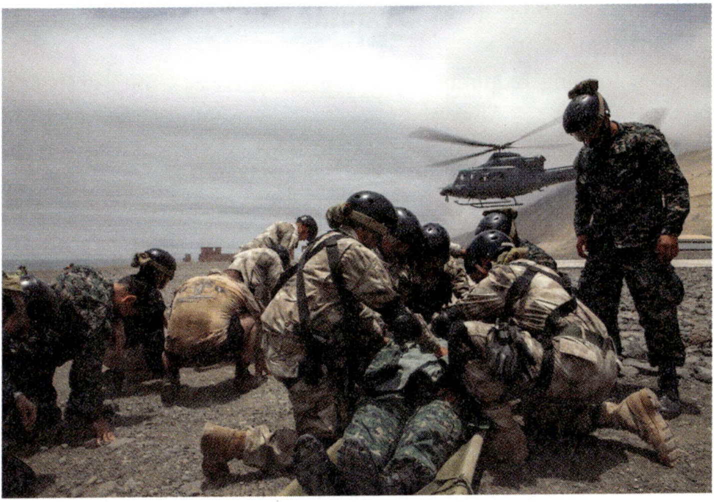

Figure 14-3. Tactical Combat Casualty Care subject matter expert exchange (training exercise) in Lima, Peru. US Army photo by Specialist Austin Carrillo/ Released.

the Army PA at USSOUTHCOM is expected to serve in an executive medicine function for senior ranking officers, including the four-star combatant commander (Figure 14-3).

Desired Skills and Attributes

Desired skills and attributes of the Army PA at SOUTHCOM include:

- field-grade officer,
- operational experience,
- experience in a senior staff role,
- special operations and interagency experience,
- outstanding written and oral communication skills,
- high-level executive and critical thinking skills,
- top secret clearance,
- fluency in Spanish and Portuguese, and
- familiarity with DOD Instruction 1322.24, *Medical Readiness Training,*[4] and DOD Instruction 6490.03, *Deployment Health.*[2]

Training

Desired training requirements of the Army PA at USSOUTHCOM include:

- Command and General Staff College graduate,
- dive medical officer qualified,
- flight surgeon qualified, and
- Joint Medical Operations Course graduate.

Other training courses available to the Army PA include several resident planning courses, crisis action training, media engagement training, and continuing medical education opportunities. One unique experience available to the PA is a trauma rotation at the Army Ryder Trauma Training Detachment at Jackson Memorial Hospital in downtown Miami.

Lessons Learned

A major lesson learned for the USSOUTHCOM and JIATF-S PA is to create systems. The volume of action items that will cross the PA's desk is not manageable otherwise. Creating products such as operating mail boxes, SharePoint sites, and procedural regulations will make or break the PA. Furthermore, not everything that is requested of the surgeon's cell is necessarily for the surgeon's action. Often, lines of responsibility are grey. Finding the "who" of the problem set is half of the recipe for success. Finally, the PA must not be afraid to have dissenting opinions. At the four-star level it is expected. That said, the PA must always have their facts in order and always have talking points prepared to brief at a moment's notice.

Tips for Success

In addition to lessons learned, here are tips for success in excelling as the USSOUTHCOM and JIATF-S PA:

- The PA must learn joint doctrine, beginning with reading Joint Publications 5-0, *Joint Planning*[5] and 4-02, *Joint Health Services*.[6]

- The interagency and civil affairs staff have a synergistic relationship with the surgeon's office, so the PA should get to know these personnel well.
- The PA has medical expertise that is often sought by high-ranking leaders. The PA must use these opportunities to get face time with their leaders, which builds trust and pays dividends when the PA is seeking support for a project.
- The PA should learn to communicate effectively; public speaking, official correspondence, and policy writing will be an enormous part of the PA's success.

Conclusion

The USSOUTHCOM PA position is an extremely rewarding job. The complexity of the mission and level of responsibility assumed makes this a unique position for Army PAs. It requires inherent maturity, initiative, and an understanding of operational art to develop approaches to complex military problems in sometimes unorthodox ways.

References

1. Faller CS. *United States Southern Command Strategy: "Enduring Promise for the Americas."* Headquarters, US Southern Command; May 8, 2019. Memorandum. Accessed September 8, 2020. https://www.southcom.mil/Portals/7/Documents/SOUTHCOM_Strategy_2019.pdf?ver=2019-05-15-131647-353
2. US Department of Defense. *Deployment Health*. DOD; June 19, 2019. DOD Instruction 6490.03. Accessed September 8, 2020. https://www.esd.whs.mil/Portals/54/Documents/DD/issuances/dodi/649003p.pdf
3. US Department of Defense. *Medical Program Support for Detainee Operations*. DOD; September 5, 2019. DOD Instruction 2310.08. Accessed September 8, 2020. www.esd.whs.mil/Portals/54/Documents/DD/issuances/dodi/231008p.pdf

4. US Department of Defense. *Medical Readiness Training*. DOD; March 6, 2016. DOD Instruction 1322.24. Accessed September 8, 2020. https://www.esd.whs.mil/Portals/54/Documents/DD/issuances/dodi/132224p.pdf?ver=2018-03-16-140510-410

5. US Department of Defense. *Joint Planning*. DOD; June 16, 2017. JP 5-0. Accessed September 8, 2020. https://www.jcs.mil/Portals/36/Documents/Doctrine/pubs/jp5_0_20171606.pdf

6. US Department of Defense. *Joint Health Services*. DOD; September 28, 2018. JP 4-02. Accessed September 8, 2020. https://www.jcs.mil/Portals/36/Documents/Doctrine/pubs/jp4_02ch1.pdf

Chapter 15

ROLE AS A COMMANDER

Amy L. Jackson, PA-C, MPAS; Curtis Aberle, RN, MSN; Avery J. Carney, PA-C, MPAS; John F. Detro, APA-C, MPAS, MSS, MEd; Robert S. Heath, APA-C, MPAS; David L. Hamilton, PA-C, MPAS, MPH; James G. Pairmore, APA-C, MPAS; Christopher Pase, APA-C, MPAS; Bill A. Soliz, APA-C, MPAS; and Richard A. Villarreal, APA-C, PhD, MPAS

Introduction

The diverse operational, clinical, and administrative backgrounds of Army physician assistants (PAs) give them a competitive edge for command. Command opportunities for PAs exist at all levels in nearly every type of medical unit. However, not every PA or officer is well suited for command. Neither is command an automatic path to promotion, although command will distinguish a PA from their peers. PAs must seriously consider the choice of taking command. The hours are long, the decisions are tough, and the risks may be high, but the personal and professional gratification is immeasurable. Army medicine needs great leaders, and PAs who are ready and willing should answer the call.

Why Command?

Serving as a commander has been the highlight of my military career. When you become a commander, you are given a great deal of authority and responsibility. You are charged with taking care of America's sons and daughters. Every decision you make or fail to make has an impact.

—Colonel John F. Detro
240th Forward Surgical Team, 2010–2012
187th Medical Battalion, 2016–2018

Command is about solving problems every day. No single person has a greater influence or effect on a soldier's life than the commander. Every decision the commander makes can result in great soldiers that will become future leaders. That is a legacy which will span years and generations. PAs have the experience and skills both medically and operationally to make a real difference for Army Medicine as commanders.

—Colonel James G. Pairmore (Figure 15-1)
Public Health Activity Hawaii, 2017–2019
14th Combat Support Hospital and Task Force Medical-Iraq, 2019–2021

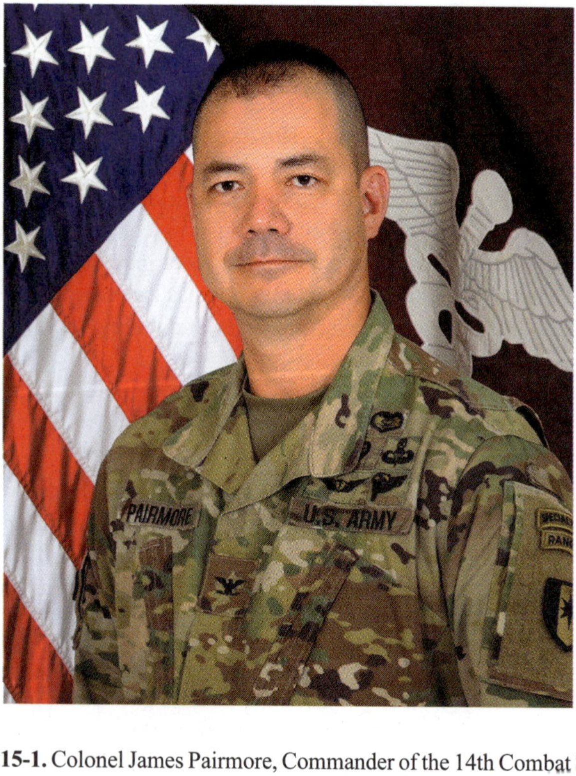

Figure 15-1. Colonel James Pairmore, Commander of the 14th Combat Support Hospital, Fort Benning, GA, 2019–2021.

As a medic charged with helping teammates navigate through a convoluted military health care system, I became a PA to have more autonomy in helping soldiers with their care. However, as a 2LT PA, I found that others in health care leadership positions could propagate obstacles to access to care. Despite the bureaucracy, I was able to set up systems to improve soldier care. As a Major, I accepted the opportunity to be a "Charlie MED" commander in an Airborne Brigade Combat Team – only because I was at the right time and right place – no recruiting, just showing value as a PA and potential as a commander. The April Fool's Day change of command was simple, and then I had a seat in the tactical operation center (TOC). PA commanders can improve soldier care, evacuation, and return to duty. They do this by applying resources to streamline the systems and processes of pre- and post-deployment health processing, en route care, primary care, and readiness care from the perspective of a provider and line medic. In those 30 months of command, I experienced some of the most rewarding times of my Army career – developing and mentoring medics, NCOs, and officers to do better every day. Many of a commander's successes come from setting conditions to let others excel – usually by getting out of their way and allowing teammates to innovate and collaborate!

—Colonel David Hamilton (Figure 15-2)
Company C, 173rd Brigade Support Battalion,
Afghanistan, 2008–2010
Public Health Command District Fort Bragg, 2013–2016
9th Hospital Center, 2019–2021

All Army PAs possess the essential tools necessary to command successfully. Many of us were leaders, NCOs and officers alike, before becoming health care providers and leaders in medicine. The IPAP curriculum not only hones our medical knowledge, but that is just the start. Through invaluable operational experience, we refine the soft skills and personal attributes necessary to best care for the sick, ill, or wounded, and while serving on many staffs. The very basis of our profession as Army PAs requires mastery of three necessary clinical core qualities: genuineness, respect, and empathy, the same crucial building blocks for any commander, at any level.

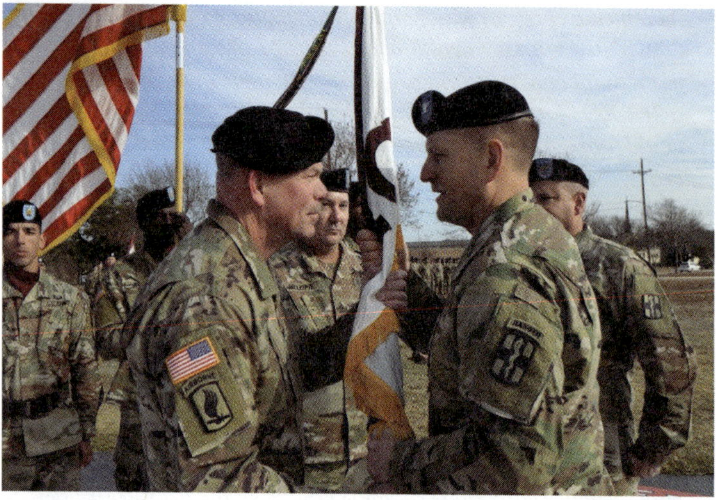

Figure 15-2. Colonel David Hamilton receives the 9th Hospital Center colors from Colonel Robert Howe II, Commander, 1st Medical Brigade, during the change of command of the 9th Hospital Center (formerly the 21st Combat Support Hospital), 1st Medical Brigade, Fort Hood, TX, from Colonel Jeffrey Yarvis, December 12, 2019.
Photograph courtesy of Corporal Yanira Green.

Long ago, in what seems like almost a different lifetime, my battalion commander, LTC Joe Martin (now, VSCA GEN Martin), planted the seed of command. In one of our mentorship sessions, as we decided on my next three broadening assignments, he told me something that I found profoundly inspiring. He said, "Doc, the essence of the Army and our profession is command." He went on to say that it was an absolute must that I pursue and seize any/all opportunities to command soldiers. Fast-forward to today, nearly 9 months into Battalion Command, and I know precisely what LTC Martin was telling me 16 years ago.

It is an awesomely powerful and deeply rewarding experience to command. To recognize and demonstrate to soldiers that they are our most precious commodity. To push and inspire soldiers to be the very best version of themselves. Likewise, I endeavor at all times to give soldiers in my command the very best of myself. My leadership philosophy is simple: to lead, you must first serve. This is how I view servant leadership – serving among those you lead. My company commanders understand this and that I expect them to do the same, because the best organization is only as good as its leader(s). Commanding is so much more about selflessness than I ever imagined, and it reinforces my belief that as Army PAs, we understand that more than anybody in the AMEDD. We need more PAs to understand this and trust in the robust, diverse, and rare amalgam of skills that they bring to the table. We need more Army PAs to seize the guidon and just lead!

—Lieutenant Colonel Christopher C. Pase
Troop Command, Martin Army Community Hospital, 2019–2021

Commanding soldiers is the very pinnacle of Army leadership and culture. After creating a vision and communicating a vivid picture of the desired end state, you have the privilege of serving, shaping, and mentoring them in the execution of your intent. Done correctly, the commander sets the organization's climate and cultivates the formation's talents towards mission accomplishment and success. Command and leadership precepts transcend either operational (TO&E) or fixed facility (TDA) domains.

Army PAs are well suited to command at all levels because we have medical knowledge and operational experience coupled with an innate perspective and understanding of Army medicine from its most pure and fundamental tactical origins. The tenants of leading, rallying, and developing young soldier medics in the field or around the Battalion Aid Station hold true at all levels and variants of command.

Command is not for the faint of heart nor those unwilling or unable to devote themselves to their teams. You will be expected to lead in and through times of both trial and triumph. In my experience, the greatest reward is to be empowered and purposed to create a space and format to facilitate the patriotic service of our nation's sons and daughters and having the honor to watch each of them grow, mature, and achieve in the process. For me it's the epitome of absolute purpose and fulfillment! It doesn't come easy, but what truly worthy in life does? As an Army PA if you are up to the task and provided the opportunity – don't hesitate! FROM THE LINE, FOR THE LINE!

—Lieutenant Colonel Avery Carney
601st Medical Company (Area Support), Iraq, 2007–2009
98th Medical Detachment (Combat Operation Stress Control), 2014–2016
US Army Health Clinic Grafenwoehr, 2019–2021

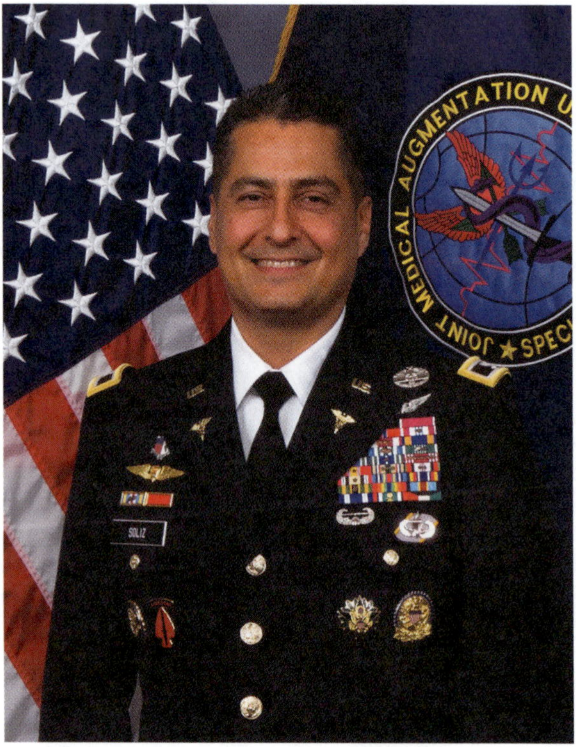

Figure 15-3. On June 13, 2019, Colonel Bill A. Soliz assumed command of the Joint Special Operation Center (JSOC) Joint Medical Augmentation Unit (Special Mission Unit Command Select List) at the JSOC Compound, Fort Bragg, NC.
Photograph courtesy of Joe Belcher, JSOC command photographer.

I thought I had the best job in the Army being a leader of soldiers and a PA as I was able to take care of people and lead change for the better. That was until I became a commander. Commanders are responsible for everything that happens and does not happen within your formation. You have the authority to set policy, the presence to inspire and instill a positive influence, and the ability to change people's lives for the better. All while accomplishing the mission of your command, which for most of us is saving lives in time of war. There is no better reward and self-gratification than to help others become better and save lives. People are your priority and relationships are everything.

—Colonel Bill A. Soliz (Figure 15-3)
California Medical Detachment and Presidio of Monterey
Army Health Clinic, 2015–2017
Joint Medical Augmentation Unit,
Joint Special Operations Command, 2019–2021

Requirements to Compete for Command

PAs may compete for command at any level; however, company and detachment command depends on being at the right place at the right time, and competing when opportunities arise locally or through the Assignment Interactive Module (AIM.2) for 05A Army Medical Department (AMEDD) immaterial positions. These 05A opportunities may include brigade support battalion medical companies and forward surgical teams or medical center and community hospital companies. Command candidates attend and graduate from the appropriate professional military education, such as Captains Career Course, Command and General Staff College, Intermediate Level Education, and Senior Service College, in addition to appropriate pre-command courses (local and major command-driven).

Competition for command is stiff. It takes incredible professional stamina to remain on active duty after 20 years of active federal service, which includes maintaining deployability, health, and fitness. Recent Army chief of staff guidance, reflected in military personnel (MILPER) messages,[1] requires commanders at the battalion, brigade, and above to be fully medically ready and able to participate in and lead unit physical training.[1] Candidates competing for command must attest to the ability to pass an Army Combat Fitness Test (ACFT) without an alternative event. Commanders must also be deployable worldwide without a waiver (medically and administratively).

Command Selection List Board Process

PAs most frequently enter the command path through competing within the command selection list (CSL) O-5 (lieutenant colonel) and O-6 (colonel) boards for battalion- and brigade-level commands (Table 15-1). CSL command is a formal Army selection process in which eligible personnel must request consideration (opt-in) and prepare their board file (similar to the process for a promotion board).[1] It is important to note that officers can only compete at the O-5 level during the first 3 years of eligibility. Commanders who have completed an O-5 level command are the most competitive for O-6 level commands. The types of CSL command fall into three subcategories: operations (eg, field hospital, multifunctional medical battalion, hospital center); strategic support (community hospitals, clinics, troop commands, public health activities, research facilities); and training and recruiting.

CSL boards are conducted 2 fiscal years before the command positions open. The command selection board opening is announced through a MILPER message and posted on the HRC website, alerting all officers in the zone of consideration (ie, those eligible to compete for the specific board). Within AIM.2, officers opt-in and indicate preference for commands. It is highly encouraged for those not interested to opt-out. Data collected from officers who opt-out informs Army senior

Table 15-1. Command selection list categories.

Code	Subcategories	Competitive grouping
M6AP	AMEDD operations	AN, MC, MS, SP, VC
M6AR	AMEDD strategic support	AN, MC, MS, SP, VC
M6AT	AMEDD recruiting/training	AN, MC, MS, SP, VC

AMEDD: Army Medical Department; AN: Nurse Corps; MC: Medical Corps; MS: Medical Service Corps; SP: Medical Specialist Corps; VC: Veterinary Corps leaders about the reasons for not competing and informs future boards. Candidates who opt-in should give preference to commands where they feel they will thrive and succeed. An officer does not need to command the most complicated organization to be successful and potentially obtain a next higher level of command, but they must be successful, and it should be enjoyable.

Candidates must attest in writing that they will take the command offered and that they are physically and mentally fit for command. Declining the slated command, once offered, is generally with prejudice (ie, preventing the officer from competing for future commands). When opting in for CSL, officers should be ready to move based on the needs of the Army, in the time frame defined by the MILPER CSL announcement.[1] It is vital to remember that if a PA does not get slated in the command of preference, success depends on pursuing excellence and doing one's best, no matter the circumstance.

To prepare for CSL consideration, officers should review their officer records brief (ORB) for correctness and currency. All pending officer evaluation reports (OERs) should be completed and submitted to HRC by the OER cutoff date in the MILPER message announcing eligibility for the CSL. Officers should obtain a current ACFT and be prepared to report the score and date in the fitness attestation. A current periodic health assessment is also recommended. In short, a competitive board file is current and validated, including an updated ORB, supporting documents from the interactive Personnel Electronic Records Management System (iPERMS), and slate of recent OERs that paint a picture of a motivated, well-balanced leader with the professional stamina to endure the demands of command.

HRC holds the CSL boards at the Department of the Army (DA) secretariat (a panel that puts together all DA boards). Board members vote to develop an order of merit list (OML), with both principal and alternate selections. There are twice the number of alternates as principals. The DA secretariat uses the preferences and OML to place officers within respective subcategories; for example, an officer who is first on the OML will get their subcategory of choice. The results are released in two stages, referred to as a split release. The names are released after being approved by the chief of staff of the Army (CSA), and several months later the slate of specific commands is released, as follows:

1. **By-Name Release**. Following the board and review by HRC's Leader Development Branch (LDB), Health Services Division (HSD), the list is forwarded to the CSA for approval. This approval allows for the release of the principal and alternate list. This early release provides some predictability to officers, who now know they will be taking command in 2 years. If activated, those positioned high on the alternate list of the OML could potentially take command up to 2 years before the principals.
2. **Slate Release.** Following CSA approval of the by-name release, the LDB assembles the AMEDD's six HRC branch chiefs to slate officers within their selected subcategories to specific commands, with guidance from the CSA and the surgeon general (TSG). The team begins with the first officer on the OML and works down the list until the last officer is slated. In addition to the OML, considerations include candidate preferences; the Exceptional Family Member Program and Married Army Couples Program; candidates' knowledge, skills, and attributes; and other factors. Following this process, the slate is briefed at multiple levels before being released. The LDB chief briefs, in the following order: the HSD chief, the director of the Officer Personnel Management Directorate, the HRC commander, Army G1/4/6 staff, TSG, the vice-CSA, and finally the CSA. Once the CSA approves the slate, it becomes official and is released through the HRC webpage. This year's colonel (O-6) CSL board met in August, and the slate will be release around March or April 2021.

Non-CSL Commands

PAs may choose to compete for non-CSL commands or commands not selected by a centralized process. In the past, the majority of these commands were filled locally. However, with the development of the AIM.2 marketplace, all officers who are eligible can compete. These opportunities include company commands (for captains [O-3]), forward surgical teams (majors [O-4]), and combat and operational stress control teams (majors [O-4]). PAs considering competing for command at the company level should first discuss this opportunity with their HRC assignment officer.

Additionally, TSG requested that the most complex commands be removed from the CSL process to allow senior AMEDD officers to better align talent for these organizations. These senior nominative commands (SNCs) include medical centers, medical brigades, and the largest research facilities. These commands were previously referred to as CSL Level II, requiring an officer to have commanded once at the colonel level to be eligible, but were removed from CSL in 2016. Today, a board composed of AMEDD general officers and one Army competitive category general officer choose these commanders in a single day. Board members establish the OML and then immediately discuss the principals and slate them using the same criteria as with the CSL. The slate is established and a General Officer Steering Committee (GOSC) meeting is established to brief TSG and gain their approval. Once the slate is approved, it is released by HRC. Currently, several Army PAs are completing CSL colonel-level

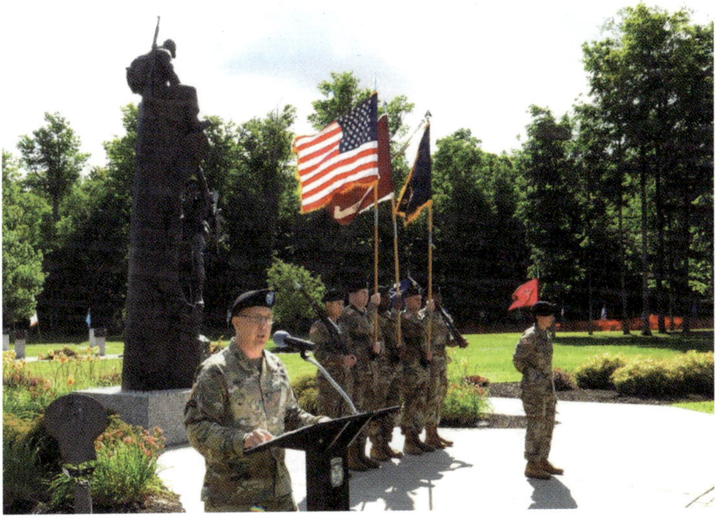

Figure 15-4. Colonel Robert Heath provides remarks upon receiving the colors as the Fort Drum Medical Activity commander from Brigadier General Michael Place (commanding general, Regional Health Command–Atlantic) during the change of command ceremony on August 9th, 2019, at Fort Drum, NY. Photograph courtesy of Colonel Robert Heath.

commands, making them eligible to compete for SNCs in fiscal year 2022 (Figure 15-4).

Ready for Command

PAs are not typically groomed to serve in command, so preparation can be a challenge. However, PAs possess a wealth of knowledge and experience that makes them ideal candidates for command. These experiences vary, but time as a primary and special staff officer, noncommissioned officer (NCO), and perhaps even first sergeant provides PAs with a sound foundation. Embracing the idea of commanding is a psychological process in which one crosses from a comfortable role (seeing patients every day, serving as a medical advisor, teaching) to a new, unfamiliar situation. To prepare for command, a PA must establish the mindset for command and stop thinking like a staff officer. It will also help for the PA to complete any unfinished personal and professional business, close out administrative issues from their last position, and get their family settled in the new environment.[2]

Command Preparation Assessment and Training

Recent changes in Army chief of staff policy require battalion and brigade commanders to attend the Pre-Command Course (PCC) through the School for Command Preparation at Fort Leavenworth, Kansas, before taking command, or shortly after, in cases of late notification or activation from an alternate list.[1] The following represents the phased approach to completing pre-command requirements: Phase I, Army Branch Immaterial; Phase II, Specific Command Training (recruiting, modified table of organization and equipment [MTOE] operational, initial military training, garrison); Phase III, Branch/Functional (AMEDD PCC); Phase IV, Senior Officers Legal Orientation course (for those eligible).[3]

Seasoned, recently retired brigade commanders are the small group leaders at PCC who provide and lead valuable presentations and discussions. Rare opportunities exist to meet and hear from principal Army senior leaders and the Army staff. Small group work allows commanders to share experiences and develop command products such as introductions, philosophy, training guidance, and terms of reference.

Advice from Brigadier General (Retired) Halstead

This section is adapted (with additions) from a typewritten document labeled "To: Future Commander, From: COL Becky Halstead, as of 04/19/01" (typed communication provided to then-MAJ Amy Jackson from COL Kirk Whitson, July 2014). The document describes command duties and includes useful advice.

Before Arrival

1. Make contact with your new unit and rater. To get acquainted with current issues and become familiar with key personnel prior to arrival, ask to be included in the distribution of pertinent email traffic.
2. Review biographies of key leaders; know who they are.
3. Review key briefs, including the last quarterly training brief, annual training guidance, current quarter training guidance, current review and analysis briefings, and command and staff briefings.
4. Prepare a change of command speech (incoming commanders should be very brief).
5. Draft a leadership philosophy, considering what matters to you and identifying expectations.[4] Consider having a shared command philosophy with your NCO counterpart (both may sign the document). This demonstrates that the command team of commander and senior NCO are in agreement. A commander should have a vision that identifies the organization's culture and provides a picture of its desired end state.[5]
6. Prepare an introductory brief, something that tells people who you are and where you come from. This can often result in finding common ground with people.

Duties: First 30 Days

1. Review and publish appropriate policy letters. Make command policies concise and direct. Research the various regulations that govern each policy subject and ensure that referenced regulations are current. It is also appropriate to look into higher headquarters' policies to ensure that your policies align with unit policy.
2. Request and review higher headquarters' CCIRs (commander's critical information requirements). Events such as death, injury, accident, incapacitation, or misconduct of key leaders; loss of

sensitive items; classified information breaches; sexual assault or harassment; or driving under the influence, arrests, and incidents with military police involvement often demand timely notification and reporting to various levels.

3. Commanders must understand public affairs and media relations. They need to tell the Army story in a timely and truthful manner while observing operational security measures. Public affairs officers can provide additional guidance to ensure appropriate and successful media relations.
4. Establish a "battle rhythm" that applies up and down in the organization. Be conscious that changes you make in the first 30 days may have second- and third-order effects. A battle rhythm will help organize the daily meetings, giving structure to the work week while also identifying "white space" (time that is available). It is critical to establish and stick to a predictable rhythm of meetings and times to manage specific recurring tasks. Incorporate battle rhythm events into your calendar and, if desired, allow your executive officer (XO), command sergeant major (CSM) or first sergeant, and personnel officer (S1) to manage access to your calendar. Having your staff and subordinates adhere to a routine schedule whenever possible will preserve your much-needed time to do things commanders must do: decide, proactively plan, guide, mentor, counsel, set policy, contemplate, write, predict, discipline, enforce, and communicate. Many other, routine tasks may be performed by the staff or XO.
5. A rating scheme is a published document that identifies the rater and senior rater for all officers, as well as the rater, senior rater, and reviewer of all NCOs. Civilians also have rating schemes. Have your administrative assistant establish the rating scheme for all, publish it for visibility, and review it regularly with your key staff to ensure it is accurate and appropriate.
6. Meet with the CSM (or first sergeant depending on type of command), the commander's "right hand," and the subordinate leaders (eg, company commanders and first sergeants in a battalion command, or platoon leaders and platoon sergeants in a company command). Provide them the command philosophy and discuss priorities. Remember to provide officer evaluation report support forms (DA Form 67-10-1A[6]), which define the officer's goals and objectives for the rating period and are later used to validate

contributions. Rated service members should receive the support forms from the two supervisors over them (rater and senior rater).

7. Ensure that all leaders in the organization conduct initial counseling of their subordinates on expectations and standards,[4] and discuss how each leader will support their subordinates in achieving their goals. Counseling, which may also be event-oriented, provides feedback for performance. Spot-check leaders to ensure they are completing all counseling.
8. Conduct both required command climate[7,8] and safety surveys[9] (your equal opportunity representative and safety officer, respectively, will assist you with this), followed by additional surveys in 12 months. Army command policy[7] states that a company-level unit will have a command climate survey conducted within 30 days of a new officer assuming command, followed by another 6 months after that and a third 12 months later. Above the company level, initial command climate surveys will be completed within 60 days. Command climate assessments assist commanders in establishing an effective organization and maintaining a positive, harassment-free environment. In conjunction, equal opportunity officers can conduct sensing sessions at various personnel levels: E-4 (specialist) and below; E-5 (sergeant) to E-6 (staff sergeant); E-7 (sergeant first class) and above; company-grade (second lieutenant, first lieutenant, captain, and warrant officers); and field-grade officers (majors). Sensing sessions can be conducted by the inspector general or equal opportunity officer. If the inspector general conducts a sensing session, any issue or allegation that arises during the meeting must be addressed by the inspector general.[10]
9. For key additional duties, put key individuals on written appointment orders and establish programs (see below).
10. Initiate and conduct key meetings (incorporating them into the battle rhythm) such as a training meeting, command and staff meetings, and legal briefs (in which the organization's legal advisor briefs all current and ongoing non-judicial and judicial punishment actions).

Advice: First 30 Days

1. Request and review all officer record briefs (a one-page summary of the career, assignments, overseas tours, demographics, etc, of an officer). This is a way of getting to know the officers under your

charge and also helps you assign the right officer to the right position, based on their experiences and expertise.

2. Develop and foster relationships. Key people to engage with are one level up and lateral XOs and staff officers, support personnel and support agencies such as the judge advocate general, medical providers and leaders, the chaplain, installation support leaders, Office of the Inspector General staff, and Criminal Investigations Division staff. Ensure you receive the blotter (a report of all crimes, property damage, and other incidents) from the provost marshal's office.
3. Make a point to visit subordinate units, going to their location, and allowing them to set the agenda.
4. Assess the environment and avoid major changes. Look for quick wins. Be open and flexible. Be positive and avoid overreacting when negative things happen. Discover the resources that are available. Use post agencies to assist soldiers.

Duration of Command

1. Always consult the legal advisor in matters involving money, financial liability, investigations of property loss, and Uniform Code of Military Justice (UCMJ) actions. When in doubt, CYA (contact your attorney).
2. Remember the roles of your leadership. The XO or deputy commander runs the staff. The CSM oversees the first sergeants. Good commanders support their staff and empower them to do their jobs, hence affording the commander the time to command. Delegation is a tool that commanders use to empower individuals. A clear and concise intent with left and right parameters (proper resourcing) can be enough for a good staff officer or subordinate commander to develop a concept and execution plan. For more information about mission command, refer to Army Doctrine Publication 6-0, *Mission Command*.[5]
3. People are watching to see how the new commander handles things. It is easy to command when no problems occur, but your subordinates will pay attention to what you do and say when things are difficult or stressful. Their acceptance and trust must be earned.
4. You should personally meet as many people as possible in your command and tell them they are trusted to do what they need to do on a daily basis. Attending training and observing your subordinates

performing their daily duties can give you an appreciation for what the soldiers and civilians are experiencing. A good leader will go to see soldiers where they live and work, which they will appreciate.

5. How one commands is an art; not everyone will do it the same way. The commander must, however, ensure that everyone in the command adheres to the organization's values and principles of legality, morality, and integrity. The intent is to build depth in the organization and develop leaders to make good decisions.
6. Be present and approachable. Have an open-door policy.
7. A good technique for ensuring good order and discipline is to establish policies that incentivize and reward good behavior.
8. Command team relationships are paramount. Nothing should be allowed to drive a wedge between the commander and their senior enlisted advisor; they should disagree behind closed doors and always be in agreement in public. Building a solid relationship with the first sergeant or CSM is essential.
9. Leadership is a privilege. Enjoy every day that this opportunity brings.

Thoughts Shared from Previous Battalion Commanders

What to expect for a new commander can be summed up in seven words: "you don't know what you don't know." How-to books and regulations are out there but until you go through it yourself as a commander, you do not know. In the first 90 days of being a commander, I had a suicide and a sexual assault in my command. Fellow commanders helped me realize what I didn't know and got me through those difficult times. So I recommend:

- *Make friends with fellow Commanders/Senior Enlisted Advisors (SEAs) of the same and higher levels; more than likely whatever you are going through at least one of them has been through and can offer advice.*
- *Make yourself available to your subordinate and peer Commanders/SEAs; the bonds that you form will help you out of tough situations.*
- *Remember when giving an order to a junior Soldier how you*

felt when an order was given to you at that rank; it will give you a perspective on commanding like nothing else.
- *Treat the E-1 and the O-6 the same, if all are treated the same (eg, awards, investigations, UCMJ), then there will never be a reason for your integrity to be called into question.*
- *Lastly, providing they are legal, ethical, and moral, carry YOUR superior commander's orders out to the best of your ability; this will create an environment for a successful command.*

—Colonel Richard A. Villarreal
Troop Command North,
Walter Reed National Military Medical Center, June 2013–July 2015

As a previous company and battalion commander, I want to pass along several thoughts about my experience, things to do and things to avoid. I hope that my notes may impart some concepts to hold to and ideas to consider that will help PAs be successful.

Do:

- *Start by communicating your vision and who you are, and keep delivering your message!*
- *Set goals early, know what you want to accomplish, and purposefully plan.*
- *Create your battle rhythm, guard time for administration, PT, and lunch!*
- *Be authentic. Be "all in" for your organization.*
- *Build trust in your organization through teambuilding and put it on the calendar.*
- *Be mindful of other people's time; keep meetings to an hour if possible for expectation management.*
- *Recognize NCOs as the backbone of the Army and allow them to do what they do best.*
- *Enable others to act through empowerment.*
- *Create space for the organization to create value for their organization and community.*
- *Go to the fringe of your unit footprint and see what life is like out there! Then look back and gain perspective on how things*

appear from that vantage point.

- *Gather with your people! Know your "squad," their passions, their talents, their personal and professional pursuits.*
- *Legal and Inspector General (IG) folks are inner circle-type, bring them into the fold.*
- *As a commander, your higher command wants your input on the packets (awards, legal, actions) that come from your desk. Give your recommendation, don't just pass it along.*

Do not:

- *Allow separation between you and your senior enlisted advisor. Be present together, and agree in the open, disagree behind closed doors.*
- *Command in fear of taking a risk; have courage, this is what you signed up for, lead.*
- *Spend most of your time in your office; get out and see the organization and the people. Take the opportunity for unscheduled one-on-one time as it presents itself.*
- *Delay legal packet processing. You should meet with the lawyer once a week if there are active legal cases and know the status of every one.*

Other thoughts:

- *If you are seeking to make a culture change in your organization, look to those doing positive things and doing it right. Recognize a squad or platoon that all passed their APFT. Recognize the unit for hitting a goal of days without driving under the influence (DUI). (One of my posts used to have the day counter for how many days the division had survived without a DUI . . . and we all knew that when we reached a certain point, it meant we would get a pass!)*
- *If you hear people say, "my commander" versus "the commander," you're doing something right.*
- *If you have young soldiers or trainees, you must have a presence in the barracks: leadership presence. Soldiers need to know that you are going to visit. The adage of "soldiers do what the commander checks" is a real thing. Monitor maintenance in the barracks and workplaces and engage when there*

is a critical need (electricity, water, heat, air conditioning) or when things are taking a tad too long.

These are not the "end all, be all" to a successful command; however, they will surely help you get started, along with all the other guidance from successful commanders in this chapter. Lead well!

—Colonel Amy L. Jackson
Echo Company, 704th Division Support Battalion, 2001–2002
Academy Battalion (Provisional), later designated as
188th Medical Battalion, 2015–2017
Keller Army Community Hospital, 2020–2022

These are the seven principles I apply when in command.

1. *Trust is the bedrock of any successful organization. The commander must allow for individual development by providing clear guidance while allowing subordinates to employ disciplined initiative within the commander's intent. As a commander, you must be willing to write off and taking responsibility for these mistakes. Only by allowing subordinates to make mistakes in training will they be ready for war.*
2. *Mission Command: Your subordinates must understand what is important to you for it to become important to them. Effective leadership requires that you establish a clear command philosophy while providing subordinates with an achievable vision and mission statement. Every member of the team must understand both and must be able to execute in your absence. Your vision and mission must be nested with your higher headquarters.*
3. *Balance: It is your calling to inspire the team to accomplish any mission while also balancing the individual and family needs of your Soldiers and Civilians. The mission must be accomplished, but as a leader you must balance completion of the mission with care of your team.*
4. *Command Climate: You will know when your unit has the right command climate when personnel are fighting to stay within it. The commander must set the right example for oth-*

ers to follow. Sergeant Major of the Army Richard Kidd once stated, "Soldiers learn to be good leaders, from good leaders." Timely recognition and discipline are important. When a Soldier/Civilian makes a mistake requiring discipline, my direction to subordinate commanders is to remain impartial and unemotional. Deal with the situation in a professional manner regardless of the eventual outcome. Even good Soldiers make mistakes.

5. *Key Enablers: It is important to quickly establish a positive repertoire with key enablers to include your legal team, Equal Opportunity Advisor, SHARP Advisor, and the Inspector General to name a few. If your organization includes GS or Contract employees then you should establish an early working relationship with the union representative and contract Contracting Officer's Representative. Your first engagement should not be during a crisis.*
6. *Support Your Boss: As a leader, it is important to be frank and honest with your Commander, but once the discussion is over, it is important to own the decision whether or not it aligns with your recommendations. Never disagree with your boss in front of your subordinates and never tell the team "we are doing this because the boss said so." Once the decision is made you own it.*
7. *Leader Development: The commander is responsible for ensuring the unit has both a formalized and informal leader development program. In many cases, informal mentorship will have the biggest impact. Leader development is an investment in the future of your organization and the Army.*

—Colonel John F. Detro
240th Forward Surgical Team, 2010–2012
187th Medical Battalion, 2016–2018

As a Commander, everyone will look to you for how you will set the tone. Everything you say and do will influence that tone. If you are positive, they will be positive. The command will get their energy from you. How you respond to bad news and crisis will have tremendous impact on the command and the people you lead. Trust is the foundation of relationships; you cannot lead effectively without it. Your people really just want to know the answer to three things about you: Are you competent, do you care, and can I trust you? Lead Well!

—Colonel Bill A. Soliz
California Medical Detachment and
Presidio of Monterey Army Health Clinic, 2015–2017
Joint Medical Augmentation Unit,
Joint Special Operations Command, 2019–2021

Conclusion

In closing, command is both a great opportunity and a privilege. It is key to remember that a command is a marathon, not a sprint. PAs bring a wealth of knowledge and experience that makes them ideal for command. Commanders should go into command prepared. They should let soldiers know what is important to them and what they expect. A commander's most important responsibility is to take care of their soldiers and their families. No one can command from behind a desk. Commanders should watch their soldiers train and work; they should delegate and empower subordinates to do their jobs; and they should ensure that their soldiers have everything they need to succeed and complete the unit's mission. Command is a vitally important position, both challenging and fulfilling, in which PAs can excel.

References

1. US Army Human Resources Command. Fiscal year 2022 (FY22) colonel (COL) Army Medical Department (AMEDD) centralized selection list (CSL) command/key billet board. Published April 3, 2020. Accessed August 24, 2020. https://www.hrc.army.mil/milper/20-096

2. Sheehan TJ, 165th Infantry Brigade Commander. Speech on preparing to transition into command. Presented at: Training and Doctrine Command Pre-Command Course; Fort Jackson, SC; July 24, 2015.

3. Department of the Army. *Pre-Command Course (PCC) and the Brigade Combat Team Commanders Development Program (BCTCDP)*. DA; April 2008. ALARACT 117/2008.

4. Department of the Army. *Army Leadership*. HQDA; July 2019. Army Doctrine Publication 6-22. Accessed August 26, 2020. https://armypubs.army.mil/ProductMaps/PubForm/Details.aspx?PUB_ID=1007609

5. Department of the Army. *Mission Command: Command and Control of Army Forces*. HQDA; July 2019. Army Doctrine Publication 6-0. Accessed August 24, 2020. https://armypubs.army.mil/ProductMaps/PubForm/Details.aspx?PUB_ID=1007502

6. Department of the Army. *Officer Evaluation Report Support Form*. DA Form 67-10-1A. Accessed August 24, 2020. https://armypubs.army.mil/pub/eforms/DR_a/pdf/ARN17086_A67_10_1A_FINAL.pdf

7. Department of the Army. *Army Command Policy*. HQDA; July 24, 2020. AR 600-20. Accessed August 26, 2020. https://armypubs.army.mil/epubs/DR_pubs/DR_a/ARN30132-AR_600-20-002-WEB-3.pdf

8. Defense Equal Opportunity Management Institute website. Accessed August 24, 2020. https://www.deomi.org

9. Department of the Army. Army Readiness Assessment Program website. Accessed August 24, 2020. https://arap.safety.army.mil/

10. Department of the Army. *Inspector General Activities and Procedures*. HQDA; March 23, 2020. Army Regulation 20-1. Accessed August 24, 2020. https://armypubs.army.mil/ProductMaps/PubForm/Details.aspx?PUB_ID=1004582

Chapter 16

ROLE OF THE AEROMEDICAL PHYSICIAN ASSISTANT

Joseph (Buck) Eddins, APA-C, MPAS; Andrea N. Gonzalez, APA-C, MPAS; Seth A. Grubbs, APA-C, DMO, MPAS; Jeffrey D. Morgan, APA-C, MPAS; Eric W. Pelkey, BS, NRP, FP-C; and John Joe Peña, APA-C, MPAS, MSIR

"There is a very interesting togetherness between medicine and aviation with which I have been fascinated over the years."

—Major General (Retired) Spurgeon Neel[1]

Introduction

The aeromedical physician assistant (APA) is an essential member of the aviation medicine health care team. While an APA performs their duties under the guidance and supervision of the unit's flight surgeon (FS), together they jointly manage the unit's aviation medicine program (AMP). The AMP is supported by a multispecialty and multidisciplinary team to provide the highest quality of medical support to Army aviation operations. The APA is considered a subject matter expert with an intimate knowledge and understanding of aviation medicine. APAs are relied on by the command and the FS to assist with managing the AMP. They ensure compliance with aeromedical requirements and the various Army regulations (ARs) governing aviators and aircrew members. By doing so, APAs ensure the medical readiness of aircrew members, help prevent aviation accidents, and safeguard the execution of aviation operations.[2,3]

Aviation Medicine Team Structure

The aviation medicine team (AMT) differs in the number of providers and medical specialties according to structure. A combat aviation brigade will typically contain eight medical personnel in the AMT, whereas general support aviation battalions and other aviation battalions will have five medical personnel in the AMT (Tables 16-1 and 16-2).[4] Providers in each medical discipline (except the combat medic sergeant and specialist) must complete aeromedical specialty training specific to their medical field before providing health care to assigned aircrew members. Aeromedical specialty training can only be completed at the School of Army Aviation Medicine (SAAM) at Fort Rucker, Alabama.[3,5]

Requirements

To serve in this position, a PA must:

- pass the Army Class 2 Flying Duty Medical Exam, with a "Qualified" or "Waiver granted" stamp by the US Army Aeromedical Activity, indicating they are fully qualified;
- be in the grade of captain (O-3) through colonel (O-6);
- be assigned or on orders to a modified table of organization and equipment or table of distribution and allowances as an APA; and
- complete the required utilization tour of at least 18 months following completion of the Army Flight Surgeon Course–Primary (AFSCP) training at the SAAM.

Table 16-1. Aviation medicine team in the combat aviation brigade structure.

AOC/MOS	Grade	Title	Branch	Quantity
61N	O-4	FS	MC	1
65DM3	O-3	APA	SP	1
73BN7	O-3	Aeromedical Psychologist	MS	2
68W30	E-6	Combat Medic Sergeant	NC	1
68X20	E-5	Behavioral Health NCO	NC	1
68W10	E-4	Combat Medic Specialist	EN	1
68W10	E-3	Combat Medic Specialist	EN	1

AOC: area of concentration; APA: aeromedical physician assistant; EN: enlisted; FS: flight surgeon; MC: Medical Corps; MOS: military occupational specialty; NC: noncommissioned; NCO: noncommissioned officer; SP: Army Medical Specialist Corps

Training

At the SAAM, APAs attend the 6-week AFSCP (Figures 16-1 and 16-2) and are awarded the M3 (aviation medicine PA) skill identifier upon graduation from the course. Completion of the AFSCP is required for the APA to be credentialed and privileged by the local military medical treatment facility to provide aviation-related medical services.[6] APAs who have not actively practiced or participated in an AMP for 3 years or more may attend the Operational Aeromedical Problems Course,[6-8] conducted annually at SAAM. Students can register for attendance by contacting the SAAM Operations Division.[7]

The APA's understanding and ability to teach and train medical tasks and skills to unit personnel is key to maintaining operational readiness. The APA must be intimately knowledgeable about the US Army Medical Evacuation (MEDEVAC) Standard Medical Operating Guidelines (SMOG) protocols and other standing orders used by critical care flight paramedics (CCFPs) holding the military occupational specialty and additional skill identifier 68WF2.[9,10] The AFSCP includes content on the SMOG but does not cover its administrative aspects in depth. It is important for APAs to understand that the SMOG protocols and other standing orders must be signed by the unit FS and commander. If a battalion or brigade FS is not available, the medical treatment facility commander assumes the responsibility for the SMOG protocols and other standing orders. APAs must also be skilled and proficient in the

Table 16-2. Aviation medicine team in the general support aviation battalion structure.

AOC/MOS	Grade	Title	Branch	Quantity
61N	O3	FS	MC	1
65DM3	O3	APA	SP	1
68W30	E6	Combat Medic Sergeant	NC	1
68W10	E4	Combat Medic Specialist	EN	1
68W10	E3	Combat Medic Specialist	EN	1

AOC: area of concentration; APA: aeromedical physician assistant; EN: enlisted; FS: flight surgeon; MC: Medical Corps; MOS: military occupational specialty; NC: noncommissioned; SP: Army Medical Specialist Corps

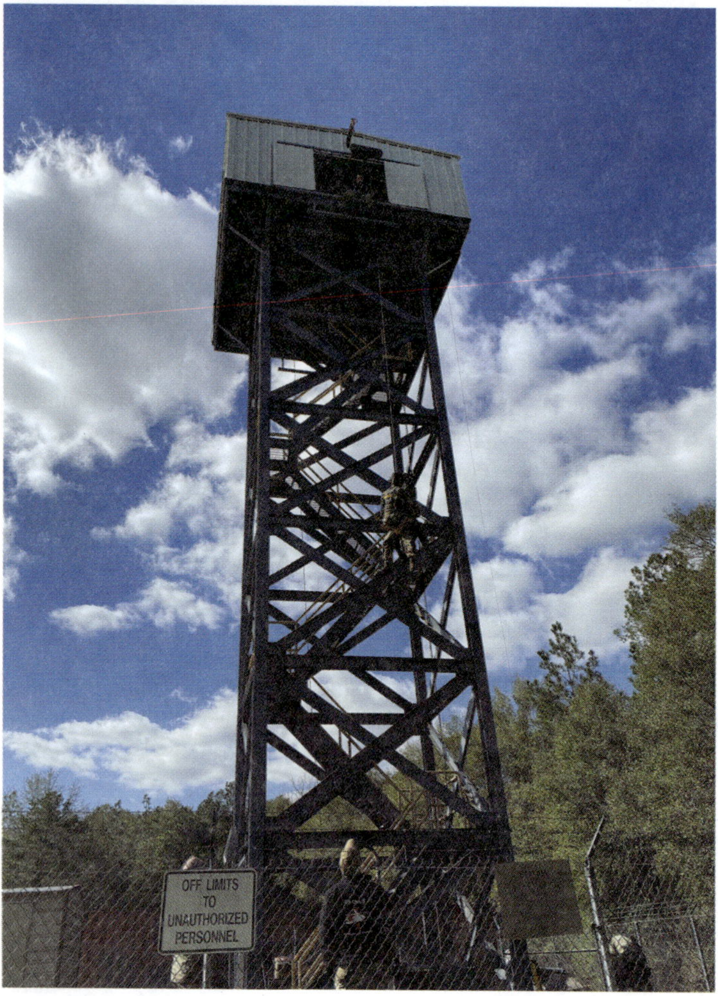

Figure 16-1. First Lieutenant John D. Howell practices hoist operations for an ambulatory patient at the Dust Off Training Complex at the School of Army Aviation Medicine, Fort Rucker, Alabama; January 14, 2020.
Photo courtesy of Major Timothy B. Pekari.

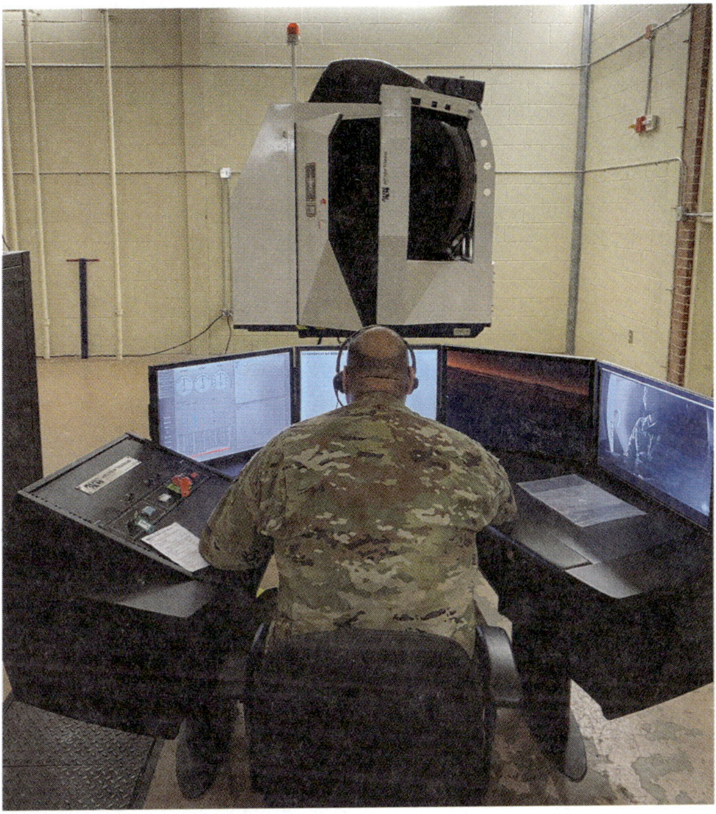

Figure 16-2. Captain Samuel Cheek sits inside a helicopter spatial disorientation simulator, preparing to experience the Coriolis effect, at the School of Aviation Medicine, Fort Rucker, Alabama; January 14, 2020.
Photo courtesy of Major Timothy B. Pekari.

required sustainment and deployment training as directed in Department of Defense Instruction (DODI) 1322.24, *Medical Readiness Training*,[11] and DODI 6040.47, *Joint Trauma System.*[12]

Aviation Medicine Program

Aviation commanders are ultimately responsible for establishing an AMP.[13] However, the FS is the medical director and medical authority responsible for the AMP's execution. The APA is considered a medical technical advisor to the commander and assists the FS in developing the commander's aeromedical training program, the commander's approved air ambulance clinical operations standing orders, and treatment guidelines based on the CCFP SMOG.[9,14]

The APA routinely assists the FS in completion of both clinical and nonclinical duties. Aviation medicine duties include all functions of health service support and force health protection. The APA should participate in all aspects of the Aviation Safety Program and assist the FS in developing and updating medical tasks and requirements of the pre-accident plan. Absent an FS, potentially due to operational requirements (aviation units split between rear and forward operations), the commander may require the APA to assume primary responsibility for all aviation medicine duties. However, the APA will need to coordinate for a supervisory FS at the next higher echelon or from an adjacent unit.[6]

Additional Duties

Although they may be authorized to conduct flight duties at command discretion, APAs have no regulatory obligation to do so. At this time, there is no established guidance for APAs to earn senior or master flight surgeon wings. This issue is known, and updating the current regulations will require concurrence from the aerospace medicine consultant. Otherwise, if an FS is operationally absent or not assigned, the APA is expected to participate in the commander's Aircrew Training Program (ATP). Therefore, the APA should meet all ATP requirements, successfully complete the annual proficiency and readiness testing, and attain the minimum flight hours to maintain currency for hazardous duty incentive pay for flying.[15,16] Completion of ATP requirements are documented on DA Form 7120, Commander's Task List, and DA Form 7122, Crew Member Training Record, for each aircraft the APA is considered qualified for and will fly regularly.[17] The APA may also assist with monitoring the aviation life support equipment (ALSE) program, including supervising the fitting and use of ALSE and crewmember personal safety equipment. However, it is important to note that the APA is not a substitute for an FS in these activities, per AR 40-68, *Clinical Quality Management.*[6]

Nor can the APA substitute for the FS in aircraft mishap investigations or flight evaluation boards (FEBs), or sign reports for these investigations or FEBs.[6] An FS must be on the accident investigation board if the accident involves injuries or problems with personal protective equipment, egress from the aircraft, MEDEVAC, or rescue or survival, per AR 385-10, *The Army Safety Program*, and AR 40-21, *The Medical Aspects of Army Aircraft Accident Investigation*.[18,19] The APA may assist in these investigations, but the FS must manage casualties, assist at the mishap site, and obtain any necessary lab specimens for biochemical testing.

Although stated otherwise in AR 40-68, there can be extenuating circumstances when an APA performs an aviation accident investigation[6]: in remote locations where an FS is physically unavailable and contingent on the aviation accident class (Table 16-3).[20] In these cases, the supervising FS must remotely guide the APA through conducting the initial mishap site assessment, evaluation, treatment, and specimen or data collection from crewmembers in the mishap.[18,19,21]

Aviation Medicine Team Timeline

As a crucial member of the AMT, the APA should coordinate with the FS to establish goals during the first 30, 60, and 90 days after arriving at a unit. AMT goals should be easily actionable and focused so they can be accomplished within the defined timeframe. Achieving the established goals ensures the success of the AMT's mission of supporting the aviation community. Several resources are available to assist APAs in accomplishing these goals, including the Joint Technical Data Integration (JTDI) website,[22] for viewing the US Army Forces Command commander's aeromedical-specific Aviation Resource Management Survey (ARMS) guide; the US Army Operational Aviation Medicine group in MilSuite, for examples of aviation medicine and other administrative standard operating procedures[7]; and the US Army Combat Readiness Center for additional specific guidance on safety regulations, procedures, and readiness information.[23,24] Table 16-4 lists suggested 30-, 60-, and 90-day AMT goals.

Lessons Learned and Tips for Success

APAs are key to ensuring the medical readiness of aviation units. With the inception of newly codified medical readiness guidance, it is important that aviators are not just fit for flight duties, but fully medically

Table 16-3. Army aviation accident classifications.

Class	Property damage and/or injury/occupational illness
A	$2M or more and/or Army aircraft, missile, or spacecraft missing, destroyed, or abandoned. Fatality or permanent total disability. NOTE: a destroyed, missing, or abandoned UAS will not constitute a Class A accident unless repair or replacement is >/= $2M.
B	>/= $500K, but < $2M. Permanent partial disability and/or three personnel are hospitalized as inpatients.
C	> $50K but < $500K. Nonfatal injury or occupational illness resulting in days away from work beyond the day/shift when the injury occurred.
D	> $2K but < $50K. Nonfatal injury or illness resulting in restricted work, transferal to another job, medical treatment more than first aid, needle stick injuries and cuts from sharps that are contaminated with another person's blood or other potentially infectious material, medical removal under medical surveillance requirements of an OSHA standard, occupational hearing loss, or a work-related tuberculosis case.
E	< $2K and/or an operational or maintenance mission is interrupted or not completed (intent for flight may or may not exist) due to fair wear and tear or malfunction of a component or part.
F	Unavoidable aircraft turbine engine damage as a result of internal/external FOD.

Data source: Headquarters, Department of the Army. *Army Accident Investigations and Reporting.* HQDA; March 18, 2015. DA Pamphlet 385-40 Accessed July 8, 2020. https://armypubs.army.mil/epubs/DR_pubs/DR_a/pdf/web/p385_40.pdf
FOD: foreign object damage
OSHA: Occupational Safety and Health Administration
UAS: unmanned aircraft system

ready to deploy, fight, and win in the multi-domain operational environment and large-scale operations. Conserving the flying force should not be a distraction from obtaining and sustaining the aviation unit's medical readiness standard.

The APA is not only a practitioner of aviation medicine for their unit, but is also considered a special staff officer. The APA assists with forming a bridge between the AMP and unit commanders. To optimize success, the APA should thoroughly understand the relationships and responsibilities of the FS, the AMT, and unit leadership, as well as the applicable regulations governing the AMP in order to successfully execute full-spectrum aviation operations.

Table 16-4. Aviation medicine team goals timeline.

Time period	Goals
Complete within 30 days	• Complete unit in-processing; become integrated into the unit headquarters, especially the operations (S3) staff, other unit leaders, and medical section personnel. Reinforce AR 40-8, *Temporary Flying Restrictions Due to Exogenous Factors Affecting Aircrew Efficiency*, requirements and understanding of individual responsibilities of all unit assigned aircrew members.[1] • Ensure physical and electronic system access training requirements are current and completed for medical personnel assigned.[2–4] • Gain and maintain access to electronic systems used for monitoring and documenting the medical care of aircrew members.[5,6] • Review medical supply and equipment inventory. Begin requisition process for replacing medical supplies.[7] • Update or establish an automated or manual tracking system for the medical equipment maintenance program; ensure all biomedical equipment is functional and calibrated in accordance with federal regulations, Army directives, manufacturer literature, or other applicable standards.[8,9] • Review previous aeromedical-specific FORSCOM ARMS results; maintain and reinforce best practices or develop and implement a plan to correct deficiencies over the next 60 to 90 days.[10]
Complete within 60 days	• Review, update, and correct deficiencies of the unit's individual flight records folders for applicable medical waivers and approval letters; electronic health records; medical readiness; and DD Form 2992s, Medical Recommendation for Flying or Special Operational Duty.[5,6,11,12] • Update or generate unit administrative, aviation medicine, and personnel recovery standard operating procedures.[10,13–15] • Participate in the unit's Pre-accident Plan Safety Council; schedule AAP surveys; record identified and corrected deficiencies in the unit hazard log.[16] • Continue to correct deficiencies of the aeromedical portion of the FORSCOM commander's ARMS guide. • Obtain a copy of flight duty appointment orders; participate in the commander's ATP.[17–20] • Begin making regular visits to aviation hangars, airfields, and other spaces to assess unit esprit de corps and safety consciousness of aircrew.

AAP: aviation accident prevention
ALSE: aviation life support equipment
ARMS: Aviation Resource Management Survey
ATP: Aircrew Training Program
FORSCOM: Forces Command
ICTL: individual critical task list

Table 16-4 *continued.*

Complete within 90 days	• Complete correction of deficiencies of the aeromedical portion of the FORSCOM commander's ARMS guide; review the entire ARMS checklist and ensure all additional requirements are accounted for and completed. • Maintain proficiency and currency with the deployment readiness training and the current 60 readiness requirements listed in the ICTL approved on July 19, 2019.[21–23] • Review and schedule, through the unit S3, medical-specific training requirements for assigned medical personnel.[22–23] • Collaborate and coordinate with the FS, the unit's aviation safety and standards officer, and the S3 to schedule quarterly safety stand-down lectures and briefs on potential in-flight stressors for aircrews to promote aviation safety and decrease potential for aircraft mishaps.[16,24] • Conduct frequent and regular aerial flights in all types of aircraft supported units as required.[17,19] • Assist the unit aircrew ALSE shop with Class VIII support and survival education.[25]

1. Headquarters, Department of the Army. *Medical Services: Temporary Flying Restrictions Due to Exogenous FactorsAffecting Aircrew Efficiency.* HQDA; May 16, 2007. Army Regulation 40-8.
2. Department of Defense. *DoD Information Security Program*. February 24, 2012. DOD Manual 5200.01. Accessed April 16, 2020. https://www.esd.whs.mil/Portals/54/Documents/DD/issuances/dodm/602518r.pdf
3. Department of Defense. *Security of Individually Identifiable Health Information in DoD Health Care Programs.* Under Secretary of Defense for Personnel and Readiness (USD[P&R]); August 12, 2015. DOD Instruction 8580.02. Accessed July 8, 2020. https://www.esd.whs.mil/Portals/54/Documents/DD/issuances/dodi/858002_2015_dodi.pdf
4. Department of Defense. *DoD Health Information Privacy Regulation*. January 24, 2003. 6025.18-R. Accessed July 8, 2020. https://deploymentpsych.org/sites/default/files/mc_resources/DoD%206025.18-R%20Health%20Information%20Privacy%20Regulation.pdf
5. Aeromedical Electronic Resource Office. AERO portal. Accessed July 8, 2020. https://vfso.rucker.amedd.army.mil/pls/aedrweb/aedrweb.downloads
6. Headquarters, Department of the Army. *Medical Record Administration and Healthcare Documentation*. HQDA; June 17, 2008. Rapid action revision issue date: January 4, 2010. Army Regulation 40-66. Accessed June 1, 2020. https://armypubs.army.mil/epubs/DR_pubs/DR_a/pdf/web/r40_66.pdf
7. Headquarters, Department of the Army. *Medical Services: Medical Logistics Policies*. HQDA; January 28, 2005. Army Regulation 40-61. Accessed July 8, 2020. https://armypubs.army.mil/epubs/DR_pubs/DR_a/pdf/web/r40_61.pdf
8. Code of Federal Regulations, Title 21, Subchapter J. Accessed July 8, 2020. https://www.accessdata.fda.gov/scripts/cdrh/cfdocs/cfCFR/CFRSearch.cfm?CFRPart=1020
9. Headquarters, Department of the Army. *Operating Guide for MTOE Medical Equipment Maintenance*. HQDA; November 1, 2006, Technical Bulletin MED 750-2. Accessed July 8, 2020. https://armypubs.army.mil/epubs/DR_pubs/DR_a/pdf/web/tbmed750_2.pdf
10. Society of US Army Flight Surgeons. Best practices website. Accessed July 8, 2020. https://sites.google.com/site/societyofusarmyflightsurgeons/resources/best-practices
11. Headquarters, Department of the Army. *Medical Services: Standards of Medical Fitness.* HQDA; June 27, 2019. Army Regulation 40-501. Accessed July 8, 2020. https://armypubs.army.mil/epubs/DR_pubs/DR_a/pdf/web/ARN8673_AR40_501_FINAL_WEB.pdf
12. Headquarters, Department of the Army. *Medical Services: Medical Readiness.* HQDA; June 27, 2019. Army Regulation 40-502. Accessed July 8, 2020. https://armypubs.army.mil/epubs/DR_pubs/DR_a/pdf/web/ARN8680_AR40_502_FINAL_WEB.pdf

Table 16-4 *continued.*

13. Headquarters, Department of the Army. *Aircraft Recovery Operations*. HQDA; April 16, 2018. Army Techniques Publication 3-04.13. Accessed July 8, 2020. https://armypubs.army.mil/epubs/DR_pubs/DR_a/pdf/web/ARN8264_ATP%203-04x13%20FINAL%20WEB.pdf
14. Headquarters, Department of the Army. *Military Operations: Army Personnel Recovery*. HQDA; March 5, 2010. Army Regulation 525-28. Accessed July 8, 2020. https://armypubs.army.mil/epubs/DR_pubs/DR_a/pdf/web/r525_28.pdf
15. Joint Chiefs of Staff. *Personnel Recovery*. JCS; October 2, 2015. Accessed April 16, 2020. Joint Publication 3-50. https://jdeis.js.mil/jdeis/new_pubs/jp3_50.pdf
16. Headquarters, Department of the Army. *Safety: Army Aviation Accident Prevention Program*. HQDA; August 28, 2007; Rapid action revision issue date: February 24, 2010. DA Pamphlet 385-90.
17. US Army Aviation Center of Excellence, Directorate of Evaluation and Standardization. *Clarification of TC 3-04.11, Flight Surgeon and Aeromedical Physician's Assistant ATP Integration*. USAACE; August 28, 2018. Standardization communications (STACOM) message 18-05.
18. Headquarters, Department of the Army. *Commander's Aviation Training and Standardization Program*. HQDA; January 2, 2019. Training Circular 3-04.11. Accessed July 8, 2020. https://armypubs.army.mil/epubs/dr_pubs/dr_a/pdf/web/arn14459_tc%203-04x11%20c1%20incl%20final%20web.pdf
19. Headquarters, Department of the Army. *Personnel—General: Flying Status for Nonrated Army Aviation Personnel*. HQDA; March 12, 2018. Army Regulation 600-106. Accessed July 8, 2020. https://armypubs.army.mil/epubs/DR_pubs/DR_a/pdf/web/ARN2863_AR600_106_Final.pdf
20. US Army Aviation Center of Excellence. *UH-60 Series Aircrew Training Module*. USAACE; September 1, 2019.
21. Army Aviation Medicine Physician Assistants. MilSuite portal. *65DM3 Aviation Medicine Physician Assistant–ICTL*. Army Medical Center of Excellence; July 19, 2019. Accessed July 8, 2020. https://www.milsuite.mil/book/docs/DOC-654303
22. Department of Defense *Medical Readiness Training (MRT)*. Under Secretary of Defense for Personnel and Readiness (USD[P&R]). March 16, 2018. DOD Instruction 1322.24. Accessed July 8, 2020. https://www.esd.whs.mil/Portals/54/Documents/DD/issuances/dodi/132224p.pdf?ver=2018-03-16-140510-410
23. Officer of the Under Secretary of Defense for Personnel Readiness. *Joint Trauma System (JTS)*. Department of Defense; 2016 (Change 1 effective August 5, 2018). DOD Instruction 6040.47. Accessed June 15, 2020. https://www.esd.whs.mil/Portals/54/Documents/DD/issuances/dodi/604047p.pdf?ver=2018-08-06-124902-047
24. Headquarters, Department of the Army. *Aeromedical Training for Flight Personnel*. HQDA; August 1, 2018. Training Circular 3-04.93. Accessed July 8, 2020. https://armypubs.army.mil/epubs/DR_pubs/DR_a/pdf/web/ARN14652_TC%203-04x93%20C1%20INC%20FINAL%20WEB.pdf
25. Headquarters, Department of the Army. *Aviation: Flight Regulations*. HQDA; March 22, 2018. Army Regulation 95-1. Accessed July 8, 2020. https://armypubs.army.mil/epubs/DR_pubs/DR_a/pdf/web/ARN5966_AR_95-1_WEB_FINAL.pdf

Conclusion

The duties of the APA are vital to the operational aspects of their assigned unit's AMP. An APA has a unique role in which clinical and nonclinical duties are interwoven. The main mission of the APA is to support the AMP in order to achieve mission success. This is accomplished by ensuring medical readiness and emphasizing the importance of aviation safety to prevent personnel injuries and fatalities.

References

1. Whitcomb D. *Call Sign "Dustoff": A History of U.S. Army Aeromedical Evacuation From Conception to Hurricane Katrina.* Borden Institute; 2011:vii.
2. Radi J, Brisson M, Line M. The aeromedical physician assistant. *JAAPA*. 2016;29(12):42–44. doi:10.1097/01.jaa.0000502864.20975.f5.
3. Peña JJ, Lawson PG, Pavelites JJ. Aviation medicine orientation. Presented at: Initial Entry Rotary Wing Course; January 14, 2020; School of Army Aviation Medicine, Fort Rucker, AL.
4. Headquarters, Department of the Army. *Army Health System Support to Maneuver Forces*. HQDA; June 9, 2014. Army Techniques Publication 4-02.3. Accessed July 8, 2020. https://armypubs.army.mil/epubs/DR_pubs/DR_a/pdf/web/atp4_02x3.pdf
5. Headquarters, Department of the Army. *Personnel Selection and Classification: Military Occupational Classification and Structure*. HQDA; July 19, 2018. DA Pamphlet 611-21 (Smartbook). Accessed July 8, 2020. https://armypubs.army.mil/epubs/DR_pubs/DR_a/pdf/web/ARN8940_P611_21_FINAL.pdf
6. Headquarters, Department of the Army. *Medical Services: Clinical Quality Management.* HQDA; February 26, 2004; Rapid action revision issue date: May 22, 2009. Army Regulation 40-68.
7. US Army Operational Aviation Medicine. MilSuite portal. Accessed July 8, 2020. https://www.milsuite.mil/book/groups/us-army-operational-aviation-medicine/pages/aeromedical-home
8. Army Aviation Medicine Physician Assistants. MilSuite portal. *65DM3 Aviation Medicine Physician Assistant–ICTL*. Army Medical Center of Excellence; July 19, 2019. Accessed July 8, 2020. https://www.milsuite.mil/book/docs/DOC-654303
9. Medical Evacuation Concepts and Capabilities Division (MECCD). Army Aeromedical Evacuation Ops (MEDEVAC). MilSuite Portal. MEDEVAC Enterprise Portal. Accessed July 8, 2020. https://www.milsuite.mil/book/docs/DOC-565891

10. Headquarters, Department of the Army. *Army Health System*. HQDA; August 26, 2013. Field Manual FM 4-02 (ATTP 4-02). Accessed July 8, 2020. https://armypubs.army.mil/epubs/DR_pubs/DR_a/pdf/web/fm4_02.pdf

11. Department of Defense. *Medical Readiness Training (MRT)*. Under Secretary of Defense for Personnel and Readiness (USD[P&R]). March 16, 2018. DOD Instruction 1322.24. Accessed July 8, 2020. https://www.esd.whs.mil/Portals/54/Documents/DD/issuances/dodi/132224p.pdf?ver=2018-03-16-140510-410

12. Officer of the Under Secretary of Defense for Personnel Readiness. *Joint Trauma System (JTS)*. Department of Defense; 2016 (Change 1 effective August 5, 2018). DOD Instruction 6040.47. Accessed June 15, 2020. https://www.esd.whs.mil/Portals/54/Documents/DD/issuances/dodi/604047p.pdf?ver=2018-08-06-124902-047

13. Headquarters, Department of the Army. *Safety: Army Aviation Accident Prevention Program*. HQDA; August 28, 2007; Rapid action revision issue date: February 24, 2010. DA Pamphlet 385-90.

14. Headquarters, Department of the Army. *Aeromedical Training for Flight Personnel*. HQDA; August 1, 2018. Training Circular 3-04.93. Accessed July 8, 2020. https://armypubs.army.mil/epubs/DR_pubs/DR_a/pdf/web/ARN14652_TC%203-04x93%20C1%20INC%20FINAL%20WEB.pdf

15. Headquarters, Department of the Army. *Aviation: Flight Regulations*. HQDA; March 22, 2018. Army Regulation 95-1. Accessed July 8, 2020. https://armypubs.army.mil/epubs/DR_pubs/DR_a/pdf/web/ARN5966 AR_95-1_WEB_FINAL.pdf

16. US Army Aviation Center of Excellence, Directorate of Evaluation and Standardization. *Clarification of TC 3-04.11, Flight Surgeon and Aeromedical Physician's Assistant ATP Integration*. USAACE; August 28, 2018. Standardization communications (STACOM) message 18-05.

17. Headquarters, Department of the Army. *Commander's Aviation Training and Standardization Program*. HQDA; January 2, 2019. Training Circular 3-04.11. Accessed July 8, 2020. https://

armypubs.army.mil/epubs/dr_pubs/dr_a/pdf/web/arn14459_tc%203-04x11%20c1%20incl%20final%20web.pdf

18. Headquarters, Department of the Army. *Safety: Army Safety Program*. HQDA; May 23, 2008. Army Regulation 385-10. Accessed July 8, 2020. https://armypubs.army.mil/epubs/DR_pubs/DR_a/pdf/web/ARN16777_ARN16343_AR385_10_FINAL.pdf

19. Headquarters, Department of the Army. *Medical Services: Medical Aspects of Army Accident Investigation*. HQDA; June 7. 2019. Army Regulation 40-21. Accessed July 8, 2020. https://armypubs.army.mil/epubs/DR_pubs/DR_a/pdf/web/ARN17699_R40_21_FINAL.pdf

20. Headquarters, Department of the Army. *Army Accident Investigations and Reporting*. HQDA; March 18, 2015. DA Pamphlet 385-40 Accessed July 8, 2020. https://armypubs.army.mil/epubs/DR_pubs/DR_a/pdf/web/p385_40.pdf

21. Armed Forces Medical Examiner System, Division of Forensic Toxicology. *Guidelines for the Collection and Shipment of Specimens for Toxicological Analysis*. AFMES; April 2012. Accessed July 8, 2020. https://www.cs.amedd.army.mil/FileDownloadpublic.aspx?docid=974a5682-4268-4bae-bf3c-90bc8367ffa0

22. Joint Technical Data Integration website. Accessed July 8, 2020. https://www.jtdi.mil/group/forscom/home

23. US Army Combat Readiness Center. Accident Investigation Advice website. Accessed July 8, 2020. https://safety.army.mil/REPORTING-INVESTIGATION/Accident-Investigation-Advice-AIA

24. US Army Combat Readiness Center. *Accident Investigators Handbook*. USACRC; August 2015. Accessed July 8, 2020. https://safety.army.mil/Portals/0/Documents/REPORTINGANDINVESTIGATION/REPORTINGANDINVESTIGATIONHOME/Standard/Accident_Investigators_Handbook.pdf

Chapter 17

THE ARMY NATIONAL GUARD PHYSICIAN ASSISTANT

Michael Korczykowski, APA-C, MPAS; J. Brandon Atkins, PA-C, MPAS; and Robyn L. Mason, APA-C, MS

Introduction

The Army National Guard (ARNG) is one component of the total Army, which consists of the active Army, the ARNG, and the Army Reserve. The ARNG is composed primarily of civilians serving their country, state, and community on a part-time basis. The ARNG is responsible for Role 1 and Role 2 care at the battalion level. The physician assistant (PA) is a critical member of the ARNG medical team, accountable for a multitude of missions. This tactical role represents the cornerstone of the care provided by the PA in the ARNG. As a part-time provider, the ARNG PA aids the local community during times of natural disasters, performs counterdrug and border control missions, participates in overseas state partnerships programs, and deploys to support Department of Defense (DOD) missions.

Unit Structure

The ARNG is an operational force that serves as a primary combat reserve of the Army and provides ready units that support global and domestic requirements. Because of this, the ARNG will replace an active Army unit structure in combat, necessitating a unit structure that mirrors the Army. When an ARNG unit deploys, it must be able to operate in the same capacity as its active duty counterparts.

Basic Duty Types

Traditional Guard

The vast majority of ARNG PAs are part-time members who serve one weekend each month and an additional 2 weeks per year (usually during the summer). These traditional ARNG members may also mobilize to support state or federal missions.

Active Guard Reserve

Although ARNG PAs usually support Army health services on a part-time basis, the Active Guard Reserve (AGR) program provides some full-time opportunities as well. The AGR program increases overall readiness in a National Guard force that primarily trains and operates part time. AGR PAs who serve full time enjoy the same benefits and entitlements as active component PAs. This includes an active duty retirement after 20 years of active federal service.

US Code identifies two categories of AGR positions available for ARNG PAs, Title 10 and Title 32.[1,2] Title 10 AGR PAs work at the federal level in support of the DOD, Department of the Army, National Guard Bureau, and the 54 states, territories, and federal district. Title 10 positions typically necessitate permanent change of station moves to assignment locations within or outside the continental United States (CONUS or OCONUS). The Title 32 AGR PA's duty assignment is linked to a specific state. It is usually a fixed position, but permanent change of station moves within the confines of the state border might be required.[2]

Career Opportunities

ARNG assignments vary from state to state due to differences in force structure and individual state operating requirements. There are multiple posts and opportunities for the PA (area of concentration 65D) serving in the ARNG. Generally, part-time PAs are assigned to ARNG TOE (table of organization and equipment) units that mirror the TOE structure of the active Army (eg, the composition of a brigade combat team). The following PA positions are examples of the assortment of opportunities that are available to both traditional and AGR PAs.

Brigade or Battalion Physician Assistant

There are numerous ARNG 65D TDA (table of distribution and allowances) positions at joint force headquarters in each state and territory. PAs are responsible for overall medical readiness. The PA participates in all soldier readiness processing and performs statewide periodic health assessments as part of the medical readiness mission. A thorough understanding of DOD health care policy and relevant Army regulations is crucial for the joint force headquarters PA because these positions are primarily engaged in administrative medical duties.

Civil Support Team Physician Assistant

Civil support teams (CSTs) are unique to the ARNG. These rapidly deployable teams support civil authorities in response to chemical, biological, radiological, or nuclear threats or hazards. There are 57 operational National Guard teams spread across the states and territories.

The role of the CST PA extends beyond the clinic to subject matter expertise on biological and chemical weapon exposure treatment. The CST PA provides technical and clinical expertise as the principal medical advisor to the CST commander. The CST PA's primary mission is to respond to and assess suspected chemical, biological, radiological, or nuclear events. The CST PA also advises civilian responders regarding appropriate actions and facilitates requests to expedite the arrival of additional state and federal assets to help save lives, prevent human suffering, and mitigate property damage. Additionally, the CST PA manages the occupational health program for the 22 assigned HAZMAT (hazardous materials) technicians and is responsible for providing emergency medical treatment for CST members during incident responses. CST PAs often speak and instruct at disaster management and preparedness conferences statewide.

Aeromedical Physician Assistant

The ARNG is home to 21 air ambulance companies and 27 Charlie medical companies (housed in a general support aviation battalion), and is responsible for approximately 60% of the Army medevac capability, providing numerous part-time APA opportunities. There are multiple ARNG AGR Aeromedical PA positions across the National

Guard. These positions include Title 32 assignments at the following locations:

- 49th Missile Defense Battalion, at Fort Greely, Alaska;
- Eastern ARNG Aviation Training Site (EAATS) at Fort Indiantown Gap, Pennsylvania;
- High-Altitude ARNG Aviation Training Site (HAATS) at Gypsum, Colorado; and
- Western ARNG Aviation Training Site (WAATS) at Marana, Arizona.

An aeromedical physician assistant (APA) works along with the supervising unit flight surgeon to function as an aviation medicine team. They jointly manage their assigned unit's aviation medicine program to help prevent aviation accidents and ensure that all aircrew members are trained and fit for flying duty.

Deputy State Surgeon

Deputy state surgeons (DSSs) plan, coordinate, direct, and implement the medical readiness programs of the state. They serve as the state surgeon's full time representative to the adjutant general, the chief of staff, and other directorate-level staff elements. They function as a liaison between the state, the National Guard Bureau, and federal organizations concerning matters relevant to medical readiness and medical support missions. Direct responsibilities include command health programs, and medical and dental readiness requirements for mobilization and deployment. Additional DSS duties include operations, medical education, sustainment, clinical proficiency training, credentialing of state health care providers, and the fiscal management of the state's medical readiness funding.

Army Medical Department (AMEDD) branch qualification is required for this position. Medical Service Corps (MS), Medical Specialist Corps (SP), and Nurse Corps (NC) officers frequently compete for the DSS position.

Special Operations Physician Assistant

The ARNG special forces (SF) PA has additional training requirements due to the nature of the mission. They typically go through an extensive, demanding training cycle that meets active duty standards. They train with their units 3 or 4 days per month, plus an additional 2 to 4 weeks per year. The ARNG special forces group (SFG) headquarters are in Alabama (19th SFG) and Utah (20th SFG). However, company elements are located in Texas, California, Washington, Colorado, Florida, South Carolina, Indiana, Ohio, West Virginia, Maryland, Rhode Island, Mississippi, and Massachusetts.

The missions undertaken by National Guard SF encompass a broad spectrum of capabilities, including unconventional warfare, counter-terrorism, foreign internal defense, and special reconnaissance. The Florida element developed a Rapid Impact Assessment Team (RIAT). Their mission is to rapidly mobilize and deploy to a disaster area and, in coordination with local officials, determine and report immediate victim needs (food, water, shelter, medical, and security) following a major or catastrophic disaster. SF soldiers from 3rd Battalion, 20th SFG, make up the RIAT and perform the RIAT missions.

Duty Locations

Each state has its own Guard, as required by the Constitution. No other branch of the military exists by constitutional requirement. In addition to a presence in the 50 states, today's ARNG is based in the District of Columbia and the US territories of Guam, Puerto Rico, and the US Virgin Islands, collectively referred to as the "54." Traditional and Title 32 PA assignments are established throughout the 54 states and territories. The Title 10 PA jobs primarily exist in the national capital region; the regional health commands; US Army Forces Command; and the Medical Center of Excellence, Joint Base San Antonio–Fort Sam Houston, Texas. There are multiple positions in the national capital region, at the Pentagon, the Office of the Surgeon General, and the National Guard Bureau.

PAs considering a transition from active duty to the ARNG and civilian PAs interested in serving with the ARNG should contact the state's Army Medical Department recruiter.

Lessons Learned and Tips for Success

Career development for the ARNG PA is crucial. Professional military education is integral to career progression for the ARNG PA, and completing the appropriate military schools is important to progressing through the ranks on time.[3] Although Intermediate Level Education is not required, it makes officers more competitive for the Department of the Army lieutenant colonel promotion board.[3,4]

The ARNG PA must be proactive as their own career manager. They must work with their unit S1 (personnel staff officer) to maintain and regularly update their officer record brief. They should also seek educational and career broadening opportunities.

Conclusion

The majority of ARNG PA positions at the brigade level and below emphasize the critical function of PAs in Role 1 and Role 2 missions. ARNG battalion PAs should understand their responsibility in mentoring and training unit combat medics, and recognize their duty as advisors to unit commanders in matters of combat health readiness and preventive care.

Regardless of position, the central task of the ARNG PA is primary medical officer of the state medical command, infantry battalion, or one of the many other combat arms or combat support units. Specialty assignments, with different professional requirements, provide additional opportunities for PAs.

References

1. US Department of the Army. *The Active Guard Reserve Program.* DA; 2017. Army Regulation 135-18.
2. National Guard Bureau. *The Active Guard Reserve (AGR) Program Title 32 Full Time Guard Duty (FTNGD) Management.* NGB; 2015. NGBR 600-5.
3. Jackson A. Career management. In: *US Army Physician Assistant Handbook.* Borden Institute; 2018:Chap 12.
4. US Department of the Army. *Army Medical Department Officer Development and Career Management.* DA; 2007. DA PAM 600-4.

Chapter 18

PHYSICIAN ASSISTANTS IN TACTICAL MEDICINE TRAINING PROGRAMS

Robert D. Blume, APA-C, MPAS; David W. Broussard, PA-C, MPAS; Walter Engle, PA-C, MPAS; Felipe Galvan, PA-C, MPAS; Christopher Gonzalez, PA-C, MPAS; Michael Holloway, APA-C, MPAS; Todd P. Kielman, PA-C, MPAS; Robert M. Levesque, PA-C, MPAS; James S. Lorenz, PA-C, MPAS; and Johnny Wayne Paul, APA-C, DMSc, MPAS

Introduction

To support the US Army warfighter, physician assistants (PAs) provide primary instruction and oversight to tactical medicine training programs in multiple organizations. Medics, nurses, PAs, and physicians receive training on initial entry to the military or as part of deployment or sustainment training. The branch assignments officer selects PAs for the training programs based on their qualifications and combat experience.

Unit Structure

The Department of Operational Medicine (DoOM) of the Medical Center of Excellence (MEDCoE) at Joint Base San Antonio–Fort Sam Houston (JBSA-FSH), Texas, is the parent organization for the tactical medicine training programs PAs serve in. This organization is newly aligned, and currently has a proposed unit structure. The DoOM encompasses the Department of Combat Medic Training (DCMT), the Brigade Combat Casualty Course (BCT3), the Tactical Combat Medicine Training (TCMC) program, the Defense Medical Readiness Training Institute (DMRTI) Combat Casualty Care Course (C4), and the Combat Paramedic Program (CPP). Each of these training programs has one to five PAs assigned in dual instructor and leadership roles.

Department of Combat Medic Training

The DCMT annually trains up to 6,500 soldiers to become combat medic specialists (military occupational specialty [MOS] 68W). This makes DCMT the second largest military occupational specialty training program in the US Army (after infantry), and the largest medical training program in the world. The training curriculum is 16 weeks, divided into 6 weeks of Emergency Medical Technician-Basic (EMT-B) training and 9 weeks of tactical medicine training, followed by a culminating field training exercise (FTX).

The EMT-B training is taught by 80 Defense Health Agency (DHA) civilian EMT-B and paramedic instructors, in conjunction with the Academic Standards Department of DCMT, utilizing the National Registry of Emergency Medicine Technicians (NREMT), the national certifying and accrediting agency for prehospital care providers through the Army Emergency Medical Services program. The didactic and hands-on instruction is tested by the administration of six written tests, two hands-on culminating tests, and the NREMT national examination. All medics must pass the NREMT examination prior to proceeding to the FTX. Soldiers who cannot pass the NREMT exam on the third attempt are reclassified in needs-of-the-Army MOSs (those with personnel shortages). The tactical medicine segment is subdivided into limited primary care training (used during sick call) and tactical combat casualty care (TCCC) training. The culminating FTX is a rigorous, 72-hour event held in an austere field environment at the Soldier Medic Training Site (SMTS) at JBSA-Camp Bullis.[1]

Organization Structure and Role of the Physician Assistant

The 68W program is led by a team of military and civilian PAs. The program is administered under the Medical Education and Training Campus (METC) through the DHA.[2] Under METC, the program's senior leader is the department chair, who is an O-5 (lieutenant colonel) PA. The department chair is responsible for the program's nearly 300 civilian and military instructors, academic administration, and management. The chair is dual-hatted as the Combat Medical Specialist Training Branch chief through MEDCoE, which provides service-specific strategic guidance for the 68W MOS. The program director is a civilian PA who provides the program's day-to-day administration and acts as the chief of staff. The director also frequently assists with the capabilities assessment of related equipment and practice innovations. He or she works with training team leaders, critical care and emergency room nurses, instructors, noncommissioned officers (NCOs), and paramedic-certified civilians to ensure students receive optimal training experiences.

Duties and Responsibilities of the Field Craft Physician Assistant

The three field craft PA O-3 (captain) positions, also known as the "Whiskey team officer in charge (OIC)," are responsible for the overall instruction and conduct of field craft training during all scheduled training events for their specific team. Team OICs must be credentialed providers to maintain proficiency and support Brook Army Medical Center and satellite clinics. The OIC's duties include, but not exclusively, periodically reviewing and rewriting lesson plans, reviewing training schedules, serving as subject matter expert on all medical matters and training, counseling up to 35 NCOs and Army civilians, reviewing physical profiles of all initial entry training (IET) soldiers to determine their ability to safely conduct training, and teaching classes of up to 420 IET soldiers.

The OIC actively works with the field craft chief to deconflict resource obstacles and support other field craft and EMT training teams for high-demand instructor events. The OIC must stay current on TCCC guidelines and impending changes to best practices in trauma treatment. He or she develops recommended changes to the curriculum and ensures all instructors are aware of TCCC updates and ways to implement them into the field craft curriculum. The Whiskey team OIC must be prepared to support MEDCoE, DHA, and Army deployments to Central Command, Africa Command, or European Command theaters, as well as local Tank-Automotive and Armaments Command tests for feasibility of replacement or new military technologies.

The successful team OIC will support key MEDCoE instruction by networking with TCMC, the Interservice Physician Assistant Program (IPAP), the Basic Officer Leader's Course (BOLC), and the Captains Career Course (CCC) to augment high-demand instructor training and testing and potentially becoming credentialed as an associate professor to teach IPAP on an as-needed basis. It is also possible to apply for long-term health education and training (LTHET) to obtain a DMSc in PA studies or clinical education during the assignment because this position also meets the requirements for a utilization tour. Whiskey team OICs may also transition to a company command position if available.

Duties and Responsibilities of the Field Training Exercise Officer in Charge

The 68W FTX branch chief is an O-3 or O-4 65D PA who is responsible for the overall instruction and management of the SMTS. Additionally, they continuously update the FTX to align it with current doctrine and simulate large-scale ground combat.

Desired Skills and Attributes

The desired skills and attributes for a field craft or FTX PA are leadership, trauma experience, medical and tactical competence and experience, and the ability to be a thorough and resourceful planner and team builder.

Brigade Combat Team Trauma Training

The MEDCoE BCT3 is a 5-day course that teaches advanced point-of-injury care to combat medic specialists (68W) and flight medics within their 90-day predeployment window, in accordance with Department of the Army EXORD (execute order) 096-09, *Mandatory Pre-Deployment Trauma Training (PDTT) for Specified Medical Personnel and the Regionally Aligned Forces (RAF).*[3] Annually, the BCT3 conducts an average of 7 courses at Camp Bullis, and approximately 20 courses at 10 different Forces Command (FORSCOM) installations using a mobile training team (MTT), training units of over 2,000 combat medics in approximately 20 separate iterations.

BCT3 training focuses on saving lives and addressing the four most common causes of preventable death on the battlefield: massive hemorrhage from junctional and extremity wounds, airway compromise, tension pneumothorax, and hypothermia.[1] BCT3 also teaches current tactics, techniques, and procedures (TTPs) derived directly from lessons learned in the operational environment, and provides an introduction to prolonged field care. In addition to conducting training, all members of the team must remain current on emerging point-of-injury trauma techniques and recommendations from the Committee on Tactical Combat Casualty Care and the Joint Trauma System.[1]

Organization Structure and Role of the Physician Assistant

The BCT3 branch chief is an O-4 PA OIC. A second O-3 PA position serves as the MTT leader (though either PA can perform this role as needed), providing the capability for simultaneous training events. The training team cadre consists of active duty NCOs in the rank of staff sergeant and sergeant first class and two DHA civilians. The PAs and senior NCOs must have at least two combat tours each. The PA is supervised by the chief of the Tactical Medicine Readiness Division, who assists with guidance on training and efficiency ratings of the team NCOs.

Prerequisites

Those seeking a position as a BCT3 PA team leader require:

- the rank of captain with completion of the Army Medical Department (AMEDD) CCC;
- a history of assignment to a battalion, squadron, or team PA position for 4 years or more; and
- two or more combat deployments with trauma experience.

Roles and Responsibilities

- Serves as OIC and program director for the BCT3 course.
- Responsible for course direction, improvement, coordination, and guidance of the mandatory predeployment trauma training for 68W combat medics and flight medics.
- Ensures didactic curriculum and practical exercises are current and relevant for Role 1 and 2 medical care on the battlefield.
- Responsible for leading, mentoring, developing, training, instructing, and supervising the MTT's 20 NCOs and 2 civilians.
- Responsible for equipment and supplies worth over $3 million.

Desired Skills and Attributes

A successful BCT3 OIC will:

- have excellent communication and interpersonal skills;

- be able to conduct operations with minimal oversight or guidance, especially during MTT missions;
- be comfortable interacting with brigade and division staff and command teams;
- builds relationships with other MEDCoE programs such as TCMC, IPAP, and BOLC, and be prepared to assist as needed; and
- be a highly competent medical provider and maintain credentials at Brooke Army Medical Center and outlying clinics.

Pertinent Program Resources

- The milsuite.mil BCT3 organizational webpage provides administrative and course content information.[4]
- The deployedmedicine.com website provides current TCCC guidelines, evidence-based medicine explanations, and classes.[1]
- The prolongedfieldcare.org website provides additional resources to assist deploying personnel.[5]
- The Joint Trauma System provides common practice guidelines and tools for deployed medical personnel.[6]

Tactical Combat Medical Care Course

The TCMC course provides the PA, physician, nurse practitioner, and senior medical NCO with a practical working knowledge of how to manage injured patients in a combat environment from point of injury to Role 1 or Role 2. The course information is based on TCCC, known trauma resuscitation methods, lessons learned from combat, and newly developed technology. Training consists of didactic lecture and hands-on practical training conducted at JBSA-FSH, where combat casualty management is taught in a simulated tactical environment. The course lasts 5 days and has 22 to 24 iterations per year.[7]

Organization Structure and Role of the Physician Assistant

Initially created by active duty PAs, TCMC currently employs two active duty PAs and three civilian PA instructors who plan, coordinate, and instruct the course. The senior active duty PA is also the section OIC.[7]

Prerequisites

Those seeking a PA position at the TCMC course require:

- the rank of captain with completion of the AMEDD CCC for those seeking the position of instructor;
- the rank of major for those seeking the position of OIC;
- a history of assignment to a battalion, squadron, or team PA position for 4 years or more; and
- 2 or more years of experience in combat trauma.

Defense Medical Readiness Training Institute Combat Casualty Care Course

DMRTI's C4 program, a faculty affiliate of the National Association of Emergency Medical Technicians, trains 750 triservice and international medical officers annually in the TCCC curriculum, supporting prolonged field and prehospital care training and education. C4 is an 8-day course consisting of a classroom-based professional program and a prolonged FTX. The course also requires prerequisite distance learning through the Joint Knowledge Online Emergency Preparedness Response Course–Clinician Course.

The professional program is targeted according to the student's medical field: physicians, dentists, and some PAs receive Advanced Trauma Life Support–Operational Emphasis; nurses receive Trauma Nursing Core Course–Operational Emphasis; all others receive Pre-Hospital Trauma Life Support.

The FTX is conducted in a forward operating base environment, in which C4 students must demonstrate medical proficiency in all three phases of TCCC (care under fire, tactical field care, and tactical evacuation care) while conducting mission-oriented exercises based on current combat theater scenarios or potential scenarios in other threat locations. Hands-on chemical, biological, radiologic, and nuclear training is included. The exercise integrates mission-oriented medical care in the following contexts: military operations in urban terrain, village stability operations, and tactical evacuation care on a Sikorsky UH-60 Black Hawk helicopter simulator, a simulated Role 2 facility, a tactical medicine obstacle course, and a mass casualty situation.

Organization Structure and Role of the Physician Assistant

DMRTI is under the DHA, which reports directly to the Assistant Secretary of Defense for Health Affairs. Its director is an Army, Navy, or Air Force physician. An Army PA serves as the C4 branch chief or deputy branch chief, and the staff consists of medics and corpsmen from the Army, Navy, and Air Force. The triservice role allows for joint staffing, training, and equipping to meet the requirements of TCCC training.

Prerequisites

Those seeking a position as the C4 PA require:

- the rank of major;
- completion of Intermediate Level Education training;
- a history of assignment and deployment in a brigade or regiment PA position for 2 years; and
- experience in combat trauma.

Combat Paramedic Branch

The Combat Paramedic Branch falls within the Combat Medic Division of the MEDCoE's DoOM. The branch is responsible for the annual total force generation of the Army's flight medic (68WF2) populations within all service components. This requirement includes initial training for 190 to 210 soldiers, as well as recertifying over 160 flight medics annually. Initial training for flight medics includes the 30-week CPP (Combat Paramedic Program), the 8-week Critical Care Course, and the 6-week AMEDD Aviation Crew Member Course (which falls within a separate MEDCoE department, the Department of Aviation Medicine at Fort Rucker, Alabama). The Combat Paramedic Branch also conducts the 2-week recertification course nine times annually.

Organization Structure and Role of the Physician Assistant

There are several opportunities for active duty PAs in the Combat Paramedic Branch, and more specifically the CPP. The chief of the Combat Paramedic Branch is an O-5 (lieutenant colonel) 65D and functions as both the OIC/branch chief and the CPP program director. In addition to the program director, the CPP has three O-4 (major) PAs who act as OICs for each block of instruction. Each OIC is responsible for the instruction in either block I, II, or III within the 30-week curriculum.

The CPP is a redesigned pilot course utilizing lessons learned and best practices from the previous Expeditionary Combat Medic program, as well as the legacy paramedic course, which was focused on civilian emergency medical services. The new course integrates paramedic curricula into an Army training program designed to meet the requirements of multi-domain operations and large-scale combat operations. The desired outcome is to produce operationally focused paramedics trained in prehospital medicine, as well as TCCC (to preserve life), prolonged care (to sustain life), force health protection (to protect the force), and focused primary care (to sustain the force). The course is expected to grow to include ground evacuation medics and austere duty medics (eg, security force assistance brigades and FORSCOM civil affairs battalions). Current graduates will proceed to the second and third courses of flight paramedic training.

Roles and Responsibilities

Responsibilities of the branch chief include:

- management, direction, oversight, and control of the flight paramedic program to meet the requirements of current and future operating environments, as well as the National Defense Authorization Act of 2013 (NDAA),[8] which stipulated all flight medics be paramedic certified and critical care trained;
- CPP direction, oversight, improvement, and coordination to meet requirements in TCCC, prolonged care, primary care, and force health protection;
- ensuring evidence-based didactic curricula and practical exercises are current, relevant, and rigorous to prepare medics for the challenges of multi-domain operations and large-scale combat operations;
- leading, mentoring, developing, training, instructing, and supervising a team of three PAs, two critical care nurses, six civilians, and eighteen senior NCOs; and
- accountability and execution of over $5 million in equipment and supplies annually.

Responsibilities of team chiefs include:

- management, direction, oversight, and control of 7 to 10 weeks of assigned instruction, including the continuous use of the TRADOC "analysis, design, develop, implement, evaluate" (ADDIE) model to identify course requirements and ensure evidence-based didactic curricula and practical exercises are current, relevant, and rigorous to prepare medics for the challenges of multi-domain operations and large-scale combat operations; and
- leading, mentoring, developing, training, instructing, and supervising a team five or six personnel, comprised of experienced senior NCOs and civilians.

Prerequisites

Those seeking a position as the Combat Paramedic Branch chief require:

- the rank of major (promotable) or lieutenant colonel with completion of the Army's Intermediate Level Education;
- a history of assignment to a battalion, squadron, or team PA position for 4 years or more; and
- a minimum of 1 year's experience serving as an aeromedical PA (65DM3).

Those seeking a position as a CPP team chief require:

- the rank of major (promotable) or lieutenant colonel (completion of the Army's Intermediate Level Education preferred); and
- a history of assignment to a battalion, squadron, or team PA position for 4 years or more.

For both positions, experience in combat trauma, certification as a paramedic, experience as an AMEDD special operations officer (S1), and being an LTHET graduate are preferred.

Desired Skills and Attributes

Those seeking a position as the Combat Paramedic Branch chief or a CPP team chief must:

- possess superior communication skills and be able to quickly

establish rapport with and commitment from those both within and outside the organization;
- have exceptional technical competency and be able to plan, prepare, and execute training to a high degree of excellence;
- be comfortable leading and empowering advanced practice medical NCOs and civilians to identify problems, develop solutions, and implement plans to achieve resolutions; and
- be agile, adaptable, and willing to alter course to achieve desirable outcomes.

Conclusion

The Army's operational medicine training encompasses a wide swath of programs. Selected PAs who serve as leaders and instructors in these courses affect up to 9,000 medics, physicians, PAs, and nurses annually, across the spectrum of services. The experience and tactical and technical expertise of these PAs provide an excellent foundation of lifesaving skills and tactics to the operational force, and their importance to Army medicine at large cannot be overstated. Army PAs have served in an irreplaceable role in cutting-edge instruction and leadership for 7 decades, and by serving in the roles described here, will continue to lead in these capacities.

References

1. Committee on Tactical Combat Casualty Care. *Tactical Combat Casualty Care Guidelines 01 August 2019*. CoTCCC; 2019. Accessed August 10, 2020. https://deployedmedicine.com/

2. Defense Health Agency. Medical Education & Training Campus website. Accessed August 10, 2020. http://www.metc.mil/academics/DCMT/

3. Headquarters, Department of the Army. *Mandatory Pre-Deployment Trauma Training (PDTT) for Specified Medical Personnel*. HQDA; 2014. EXORD 096-09.

4. Brigade Combat Trauma Training Team Milbook website. Accessed August 10, 2020. https://www.milsuite.mil/book/groups/brigade-combat-team-trauma-training-bct3

5. The Prolonged Field Care Working Group. Prolongedfieldcare.org website. Accessed August 10, 2020. https://prolongedfieldcare.org/

6. US Department of Defense. Joint Trauma System website. Accessed August 10, 2020. https://jts.amedd.army.mil/

7. Army Training Requirements and Resources System website. Accessed August 10, 2020. https://www.atrrs.army.mil/atrrs2.aspx

8. US Congress. National Defense Authorization Act for Fiscal Year 2013. 2012. Accessed August 10, 2020. https://www.congress.gov/112/plaws/publ239/PLAW-112publ239.pdf

Chapter 19

ROLE OF THE CLINIC OFFICER-IN-CHARGE

Margie Deck, PA-C, MPAS; Paul V. Jacobson, APA-C, MPAS; Courtney D. Legendre, PA-C, MPAS; Patrick A. Sherman, APA-C, DSc, MHA; Erin Stibral, APA-C, MPAS; and Robert S. Heath, APA-C, MPAS

Introduction

This chapter discusses the job duties and responsibilities of a clinic officer-in-charge (OIC). Although each clinic OIC's exact duties and responsibilities will vary depending on the specific type and location of the clinic, there are certain standard functions of all OIC positions. Since most OIC positions are in primary care clinics, a section in this chapter is dedicated to the Army Medical Home (AMH) model, which encompasses some specifics of the Patient-Centered Medical Home (PCMH) and Soldier-Centered Medical Home (SCMH) models. These three models make up the Army's primary care system.[1] Taking a position as a clinic OIC is a challenging yet rewarding experience. For physician assistants (PAs), it provides an opportunity to expand their knowledge of the business of medicine, which is vital in both military and civilian health care systems. At the end of the chapter is a list of helpful resources.

Duties and Responsibilities

Army PAs selected as clinic OICs are responsible for the overall oversight and management of their assigned clinic. This oversight includes budgetary and personnel management, as well as ensuring clinic compliance with all clinic accreditation requirements. Fiscal duties involve overseeing the non-salary budget and ensuring that the clinic achieves productivity and receives maximum financial reimbursement. Personnel management duties include, but are not limited to, hiring actions, awards, counseling, evaluations, professional development, and disciplinary actions for both civilian and military personnel. The local troop command retains the Uniform Code of Military Justice and administrative authority over active duty staff. The management of civilian staff may be new to many PAs and involves working closely with the Labor/Management Employee Relations (L/MER) office and employee unions.

The OIC also oversees customer and patient services, strategic planning, business practices, and process improvement. The OIC is responsible for safety and compliance with requirements of the Joint Commission (a national organization that accredits more than 20,000 health care organizations and is considered a condition of licensure by the majority of state governments) and the Health Insurance Portability and Accountability Act (HIPAA). OICs must also update clinic standard operating procedures annually and develop appropriate memoranda of understanding between the local military medical treatment facility (MTF) and other units that work with the clinic. Also, the OICs are responsible for providing medical care to their assigned panel of patients.

Requirements

To serve in this position, a PA must:

- have experience as a PA and Army Medical Department officer,
- hold the rank of captain, major, or lieutenant colonel, and
- be a graduate of Intermediate Level Education or Captain's Career Course (recommended),
- be credentialed and privileged in the clinic they work in, and
- have access to and proficiency in the systems used in the clinic, such as Medical Protection System (MEDPROS), Automated Time and Assistance Production System (ATAAPS), Defense Medical Human Resource internet (DMHRSi), and the Armed Forces Health Longitudinal Technology Application (AHLTA)/Genesis, as well as additional systems required for a joint service clinic.

Desired Skills and Attributes

The following attributes are helpful:

- diverse operational experience including deployment experience, preferably in multiple roles of care;
- strong work ethic;

- ability to work well with both military and civilian organizations;
- interest in medical administration processes;
- excellent customer service skills;
- solid written and verbal communication skills;
- excellent rapport with the leadership of both the MTF and the supported unit; and
- the ability to balance the demands of multiple mission requirements while ensuring the staff are taken care of.

Training

Because PAs typically spend most of their company-grade (ranks of the second lieutenant to captain) time with Army units outside of MTFs, previous MTF experience, along with a period working with the outgoing OIC, is essential during the initial transition phase. Additional recommended training is listed below.

- **Basic Healthcare Administration Course**. This was a 1-week course that provided an introduction to the administrative side of health care, offering basic knowledge about data quality and productivity metrics for a better understanding of the medical business model and improved communication with administrators. As of publication, the Defense Health Agency (DHA), now owner of the Military Health System and the AMH model, will identify a course for defining levels of performance. For additional information, individuals should contact their respective regional health centers on the status of this course or its equivalent (Regional Health Command/Atlantic, Regional Health Command/Europe, Regional Health Command/Pacific, or Regional Health Command/Central).
- **Supervisor Development Course**. This course is essential in learning the requirements for managing civilian employees. It must be completed by all newly appointed supervisors within 1 year of appointment to the supervisory position. It is available through the Army Training Requirements and Resources System (ATRRS) online.[2]
- **Patient-Centered Medical Home Training**. This training provides students a good understanding of the PCMH/SCMH model, which is necessary to ensure the clinic meets all National Committee for Quality Assurance (NCQA) requirements.

- **Team Strategies and Tools to Enhance Performance and Patient Safety** (TeamSTEPPS; Health Research & Educational Trust, American Hospital Association). This system is the foundation for communication within the medical home.[3]
- **Lean Six Sigma**. This optional training is a continuous process improvement certification program used throughout the Army. Knowledge in this area will help in developing clinic process improvement plans.[4]
- **Army Medical Department Executive Skills Course**. This optional course is designed to prepare new and projected deputy commanders, command sergeants major, and other Army Medical Department leaders for executive medical positions within MEDCOM.[5] The course is part of the Joint Medical Executive Skills Program and focuses on teaching management and executive leadership skills.[6]

Key Facts

This position is typically a 2- to 3-year tour and is considered a broadening assignment, usually coded as an 05A (Army Medical Department immaterial officer) or 61H (Medical Corps officer in Family Medicine) position with no other additional skill identifier requirements. The exact position of the 65D PA within the organization varies depending on rank, the PA's experience, and openings available; however, it usually falls under the chief of the Department of Family Medicine or whichever department the clinic falls under. This is a leadership position and is primarily nonclinical, but the clinic OIC must maintain National Commission on Certification of Physician Assistant certification and MTF credentials, and perform the required patient workload or FTE requirements (which may vary but usually range between 0.25 and 0.7 FTE).

The rater is frequently the primary care chief, and the senior rater is the deputy commander for clinical services (DCCS), but this can vary from facility to facility. Alternatively, the OIC may be rated by the DCCS and senior-rated by the hospital commander. While the position is frequently a Medical Department activity position, some models operate under a memorandum of understanding (MOU) with the Forces Command (FORSCOM) unit providing the OIC.

Under this model, the rater is typically the unit executive officer, the intermediate rater is the primary care chief, and the senior rater is the unit commander.

The Army Medical Home Model

The SCMH, PCMH, and Community-Based Medical Home (CBMH) have been combined to make up the AMH. The use of the term AMH is designed to spread parity across the health care system and limit any perceived difference between the SCMH, PCMH, and CBMH. The implementation of the AMH is a top priority for DHA; if a clinic is not already an AMH, it is in the transition process of becoming one.[1]

The overall goal of an AMH is to "deliver care using the whole-person concept, coordinating and integrating evidence-based primary, specialty and wellness/preventive care in a comprehensive care plan process to customize care to the unique needs of each patient."[1] Health care is coordinated across the entire spectrum of care, including acute care, chronic care, preventive services, and care received outside of the facility. Doing this efficiently and effectively requires team organization and the understanding that it is a team effort. Each team member plays an integral and essential role in providing patient-centered health care.[3]

The AMH leadership team consists of the clinic OIC, medical director, practice manager/administrator, clinical nurse OIC, and clinic noncommissioned officer-in-charge (NCOIC). The leadership team deals with the day-to-day activities of running the AMH, ensuring that high-quality, evidence-based, friendly, and efficient patient care is provided at all times. The clinic OIC has overall responsibility for the supervision and management of the clinic. If the clinic OIC is a PA, there will also be a medical director, within either the clinic or the department, who is the senior clinical expert.[3]

The AMH is a business. It involves specific metrics that are reported to DHA through the accountable care organization (the MTF)[3] and the regional health command. The OIC serves as the commander's expert on the requirements for setting up an AMH and using the Healthcare Effectiveness Data and Information Set (HEDIS)—health care performance metrics used to determine and improve the overall health of the clinic's beneficiaries.[3,7] It is crucial that the OIC be well educated on the metrics and requirements of the NCQA.[8]

Tips for Success

These are the tips for success for the clinic OIC:

- Data quality and productivity measures are a crucial part of the job and are used to evaluate the success of the clinic. Coding is part of the data quality/productivity metrics used to assess the clinic's ability to be productive and adequately resourced.
- It is vital to have an excellent working knowledge of these data and ensure the clinic complies. The OIC must understand coding, apply it, and be able to articulate to subordinates and peers why it is vital to complete it correctly.
- The OIC should have monthly meetings with the division, corps, or senior command surgeon to optimize the use of division and corps assets (providers and medics) in the clinic. OICs should develop MOUs and installation support plans with the senior mission commander for the installation, which will help ensure that the AMH is primarily staffed with organic FORSCOM medical assets along with additional MEDCOM support. Having these documents in place and a good working relationship between MEDCOM and FORSCOM units is necessary for clinic success.
- Several operational order requirements involve having a specific number of specialties in the clinic. Specialties such as PharmD (Doctor of Pharmacy), registered dietician, physical therapist, behavioral health care provider, nurse case managers, public health nurse, and medical support assistant/administrative support will enhance the efficiency of the clinic.[3]
- The AMH model dictates a 3:1 ratio of support staff per provider, which is extremely important to ensure the proper flow of patients. This team includes licensed practical nurses, screening medics, team registered nurses, and medical support assistants.
- The MTF has a signed collective bargaining agreement with the employee union. It is essential to have a good working relationship with the L/MER specialist (an advisor to management in dealing with bargaining union employees concerning conditions of employment and personnel actions).[8] A good relationship will allow the organization to run smoothly, and buy-in from the union will make temporary changes easier.

- Stakeholder meetings with the active duty units supported by the clinic, including representatives from the unit family readiness group, will improve the working relationship between the clinic and patients and provide valuable feedback for clinic improvement. It is better to be proactive and meet beneficiaries outside of the clinic, where information on policies and procedures can be provided, than to meet them in the clinic after they have had a problem navigating the system or have filed a complaint.
- The OIC should handle patient concerns and complaints directly and quickly. They should develop an understanding of which concerns or complaints need their attention and which can be delegated to the medical director, administrator, or patient representative. Remember, there are three sides to every story (patient, staff, and correct). The effect of an OIC or key clinic leader speaking directly to a concerned patient, in person or via telephone, should not be underestimated.
- The OIC must have an understanding of the jobs and requirements of the administrator, clinic NCOIC, and medical director. OICs should not micromanage the staff, but should do spot checks and hold leadership accountable.
- The clinic will not run successfully if the OIC is behind the computer all day. It is imperative to walk through the clinic and engage staff and patients regularly. The OIC should also attend morning staff or team huddles and conduct routine checks to ensure standards are being met. Random visits should be made to the clinic during all hours of operation (morning sick call, regular duty hours, and evening clinics) to ensure standards are being met throughout the day.

Lessons Learned

These are lessons learned for the clinic OIC:

- Understanding the needs of the hospital and the supported units is critical for the OIC. If there is a robust training schedule for the supported units, the providers may not be available to meet all DHA metrics, and demand may vary based on training cycles.
- If several units fall under the clinic for support, the OIC should discuss and review the training calendars with unit providers. Anticipating absences well in advance will help reduce facility cancellations and allow time to adjust staffing.

- The OIC should attend required training as early into the tour as possible. The needs and rules of clinics are frequently interpreted because "it's the way we do it here." Learning the right way early will reduce these instances and improve the outcome when the Joint Commission visits.
- Leadership should be engaged early when problems arise. Some changes take several months to implement within the facilities, so the sooner leadership buys in, the more successful the OIC will be.
- The OIC should read and understand the installation health services plan and MOUs with any unit that falls within the clinic's footprint.
- The OIC, or a designated representative, should ensure that everyone working in the clinic knows how to input their DMHRSi timecards upon arrival to the clinic. Improper timecard entry may result in the loss of staff and support in the future.
- If the local hospital or clinic has established referral guidelines, the OIC should make sure new providers know how to find them. This will decrease unnecessary referrals and help maintain access for specialty providers.
- Documentation is still one of the most important things an OIC can do, even for civilian employees. Documenting good and poor performance will help everyone.

Conclusion

The clinic OIC position is an excellent opportunity for PAs to gain clinic leadership experience and implement changes that can transform the Military Health System, while learning the business of medicine. It is a challenging and rewarding position that is not afforded to all PAs. The OIC PA will learn the importance of supervising and rating civilian employees, coordinating with other departments in the facility, and balancing the demands of multiple entities within the footprint. Once the tour is complete, the PA will have a much greater knowledge of the role of the Military Health System and its impact on the medical readiness of Army soldiers and the PA profession.

References

1. US Army Medical Command. *Army Patient-Centered Medical Home*. MEDCOM; January 2011. Operation Order 11-20.

2. Civilian Human Resources Training Application System. Supervisor Development Course. Accessed June 15, 2020. https://usacac.army.mil/organizations/cace/amsc/supervisorDevelopment
3. Agency for Healthcare Quality and Research. Pocket Guide: Team STEPPS. Accessed June 15, 2020. https://www.ahrq.gov/teamstepps/instructor/essentials/pocketguide.html
4. MilBook Patient-Centered Medical Home resources. Accessed June 15, 2020. https://www. milsuite.mil/book/search.jspa?q=pcmh
5. Army Medical Command. *ARMY PCMH Implementation Manual: Leaders Guide to Army Patient-Centered Medical Home Transformation*. San Antonio, TX: USAMEDCOM; 2014. Accessed June 15, 2020. https://safe.menlosecurity.com/doc/docview/viewer/docN02BD308C545D6b439719afc118a00fb2eb7a80703bfe8556e58fc5d771ec0d564507ebcd1ebe
6. DHA. Leadership, Education, Analysis, Development, Sustainment. Accessed June 15, 2020. https://www.health.mil/About-MHS/OASDHA/Defense-Health-Agency/Education-and-Training/LEADS
7. Department of the Army. *Army Medical Department Officer Development and Career Management*. DA; 2007. Accessed June 15, 2020. DA Pamphlet 600-4. http://www.apd.army.mil/pdffiles/ p600_4.pdf
8. National Committee for Quality Assurance. HEDIS Measures and Technical resources. Accessed June 15, 2020. https://www.ncqa.org/hedis/measures/

Helpful Resources

- Standards and guidelines for the National Commission on Quality Assurance's Patient-Centered Medical Home (2014). Accessed June 15, 2020. http://www.ncqa.org/Programs/Recognition/Practices/PatientCenteredMedicalHomePCMH.aspx

- Army Patient-Centered Medical Home resource center. Accessed June 15, 2020. https://mitc.amedd.army.mil/sites/Communities/APCMHRC/Pages/default.aspx (special permissions required)
- Patient-Centered Medical Department Patient-Centered Medical Home training initiative. Accessed June 15, 2020. https://atn.army.mil/dsp_template.aspx?dpID=357
- Military Health System resources. Accessed June 15, 2020. https://health.mil/About-MHS
- American Federation of Government Employees website. Labor Relations Handbook for US Army Medical Command Supervisors and Managers. June 2012. Accessed June 15, 2020. https://www.afge. org/?documentID=4365
- Office of the Under Secretary of Defense for Personnel Readiness. *Medical Readiness Training (MRT)*. Department of Defense; 2018 (Effective March 16, 2018). DoDi 1322-24. Accessed June 15, 2020. https://jts.amedd.army.mil/assets/docs/policies/MRT-DoDI-1322-24.pdf
- Officer of the Under Secretary of Defense for Personnel Readiness. *Joint Trauma System (JTS)*. Department of Defense; 2016 (Change 1 effective August 5, 2018). DOD Instruction 6040.47. Accessed June 15, 2020. https://www.esd.whs.mil/Portals/54/Documents/DD/issuances/dodi/604047p.pdf?ver=2018-08-06-124902-047
- Defense Health Agency. The Joint Trauma System. Accessed June 15, 2020. https://jts.amedd.army.mil/

Chapter 20

ROLE OF THE ARMY PHYSICIAN ASSISTANT IN THE AIRBORNE AND RANGER TRAINING BRIGADE

Jon C. McBride, APA-C, MPAS

Introduction

The Airborne and Ranger Training Brigade (ARTB), headquartered at Fort Benning, Georgia, conducts the majority of high-risk, advanced skills training for the US Army Infantry School. It consists of the 4th, 5th, and 6th Ranger Training Battalions (RTBs), as well as the 1-507th Parachute Infantry Regiment. The ARTB conducts training to create and deliver combat-ready Rangers, paratroopers, jumpmasters, pathfinders, and reconnaissance leaders to the US Army and the Department of Defense in order to increase the leadership ability, tactical skill, and technical competence of the fighting forces of the United States.[1]

Ranger school is the Army's toughest course and the premier small-unit tactics and leadership school (Figure 20-1). The Ranger course is a mentally and physically challenging school that develops functional skills directly supporting units whose mission is to engage the enemy in close combat and direct fire battle. For 62 days, Ranger students train to exhaustion, pushing the limits of their minds and bodies. The course incorporates three phases (Benning, Mountain, and Swamp), each following the "crawl, walk, run" training methodology. After these three phases, Ranger students are proficient in leading squad and platoon dismounted operations around the clock in all climates and terrain. Rangers are trained to a higher level than most soldiers. Rangers are better trained, more capable, more resilient, and better prepared to serve and lead soldiers in their next duty position.[2]

The Reconnaissance and Surveillance Leaders Course (RSLC) is a 33-day program that teaches the fundamentals of dismounted

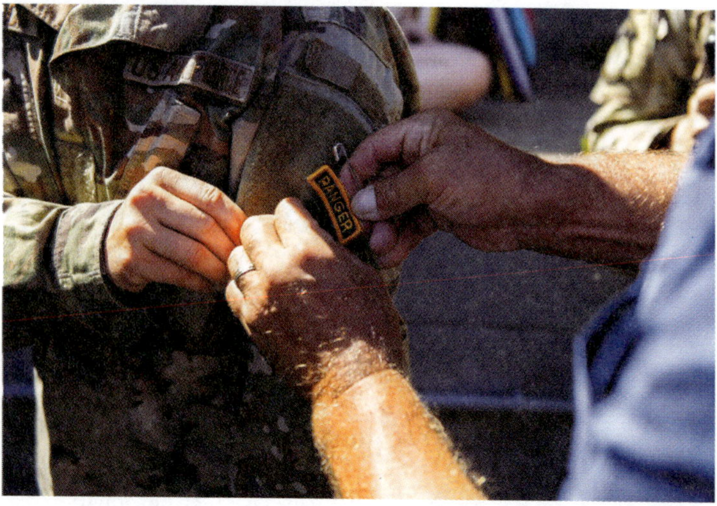

Figure 20-1. A Ranger student receives the coveted Ranger Tab during graduation at Hurley Hill, Fort Benning, Georgia. Photograph by Patrick Albright, Maneuver Center of Excellence, Fort Benning Public Affairs. Reproduced from: https://fortbenning.smugmug.com/Infantry-School/Airborne-Ranger-Training-Briga/Ranger-School/US-Army-Ranger-School/2019-08-30-Airborne-and-Ranger-Training-Brigade-Graduation/

reconnaissance, surveillance, and target acquisition to soldiers, noncommissioned officers, and officers. The RSLC physically and mentally challenges students, with each block of instruction building on previous blocks. It culminates in a multi-day, graded, field training exercise executed in both urban and woodland environments.[3]

The 1st Battalion, 507th Parachute Infantry Regiment, is responsible for training basic and advanced parachuting techniques, including pathfinder and jumpmaster training. These paratroopers from all services conduct airborne operations anywhere in support of the Department of Defense.[4]

Supervision

There are no authorizations for physicians within the ARTB, so there are no brigade or battalion surgeons. The medical director of the Department of Warrior Care at Fort Benning supervises PAs assigned to the ARTB. Battalion executive officers serve as raters for each Ranger Training Battalion (RTB) PA, battalion commanders serve as senior raters, and the medical director serves as intermediate rater. The brigade PA has a similar rating scheme, but is rated and senior-rated by the brigade executive officer and brigade commander.

Unit Structure

Each RTB is responsible for executing their respective phase of Ranger school in three geographic locations. The 4th RTB executes Benning Phase at Fort Benning. The 5th RTB executes Mountain Phase at Camp Merrill near Dahlonega, Georgia. The 6th RTB executes Swamp Phase at Camp Rudder, located on Eglin Air Force Base, Florida.

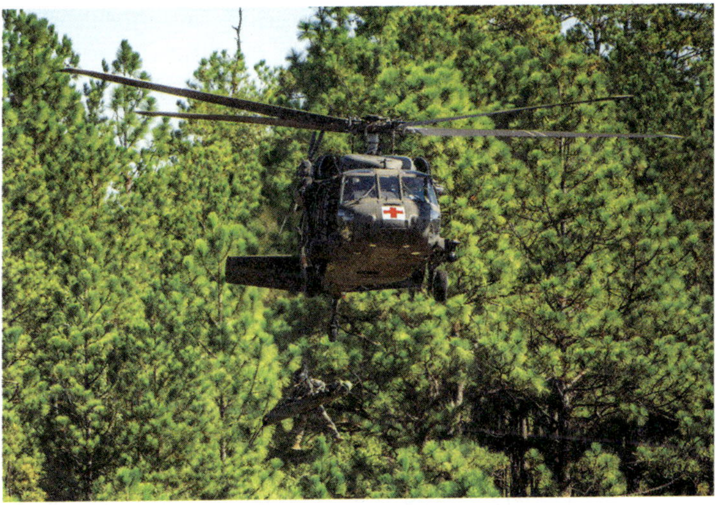

Figure 20-2. The 4th Ranger Training Battalion conducts hoist operations with an air ambulance detachment. Photograph by Patrick Albright, Maneuver Center of Excellence, Fort Benning Public Affairs.
Reproduced from https://fortbenning.smugmug.com/Infantry-School/Airborne-Ranger-Training-Briga/Ranger-School/US-Army-Ranger-School/2019-08-30-Airborne-and-Ranger-Training-Brigade-Graduation/

Each battalion has three line companies consisting of Ranger instructors who are responsible for all training and supervision of students. Each RTB has a Headquarters and Headquarters Company (HHC) element that executes normal staff functions, a medical platoon that provides 24/7 medical support, and an infantry platoon that acts as opposing forces during patrols. In addition to the standard task organization, the 4th RTB has an additional three companies. Echo Company, 4th RTB, executes RSLC. The air ambulance detachment provides medical evacuation coverage for the installation and surrounding areas, including Camp Merrill (Figure 20-2). Raven Flight Company conducts air movement, air assault, and other support to units on and around Fort Benning.

A PA, responsible for all medical functions within the battalion, is assigned to each RTB. The 4th RTB maintains two battalion aid stations that support the Benning Phase of Ranger school. Additionally, the 4th RTB PA and medical platoon cover all airborne operations conducted by the 1-507th Parachute Infantry Regiment. Both the 5th and 6th RTBs maintain a battalion aid station on their respective camps. Additionally, a troop medical clinic is located at both Camp Merrill and Camp Rudder. These serve RTB cadre and their families, as well as supplementing the medical care of Ranger students.

Roles and Responsibilities

PAs assigned to the ARTB are primarily responsible for the health and welfare of students attending Ranger school and RSLC. They conduct sick call and routine, urgent, and emergent care, as well as minor surgical procedures. PAs also provide recommendations to their commanders regarding the retention of ill or injured students. PAs are the only medical officers within the ARTB, so they shape all medical support and training within the unit. PAs also serve as advisors to their commanders on all student and cadre medical issues.

Each PA supervises a medical platoon that provides field medical support and maintains a battalion or forward aid station. Ranger students are subject to extreme physical conditions for 62 days, and generally present with more serious ailments than would be seen in a typical field or clinical setting. Therefore, PAs must have extensive clinical skills and be confident in an independent setting. Due to the austere settings, ARTB medics are also trained to a high level. RTB

PAs must maintain a high-functioning training program, and empower medics through standing orders and medical standing operating procedures.

The ARTB frequently conducts aviation and diving operations. In order to support these operations, PAs should be flight surgeon and hyperbaric and dive medical officer qualified. PAs that do not hold these qualifications must meet all prerequisites and volunteer for these courses as soon as possible.

Qualifications and Training Opportunities

Due to the unique training environment, the following qualifications are required (exceptions may be made for exceptional applicants):

- rank of captain,
- Ranger qualified, and
- airborne qualified.

Additional recommended training that may be provided while stationed at the ARTB:

- Advanced Life Support
- Tactical Combat Medical Care
- Delayed Evacuation Combat Management
- Rough Terrain Evacuation (Figure 20-3)
- Swift Water Rescue
- Wildlife Medicine

Qualified PAs who are interested in joining the ARTB should contact the ARTB senior PA to be considered for the position.

Lessons Learned

The intense conditions imposed on Ranger students create a difficult operating environment for the ARTB PA. PAs must be capable of making rapid decisions that will directly influence a student's ability to complete the course. Ranger students are not generally afforded a physical profile, which severely limits the PA's ability to rehabilitate the sick or injured. Therefore, PAs in the ARTB often

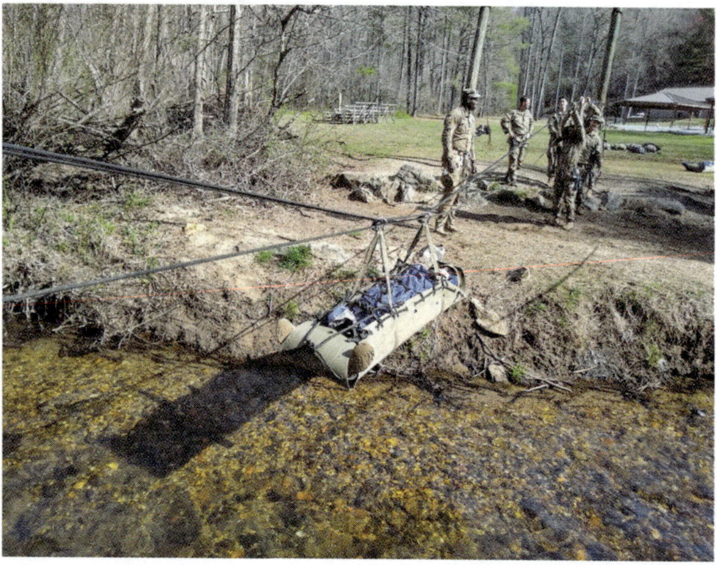

Figure 20-3. The 5th Ranger Training Battalion medical platoon moves a simulated casualty using a rope bridge in the Rough Terrain Evacuation Course. Photograph courtesy of Captain Andrew Nielsen, APA-C.

treat medical conditions more aggressively than is seen in a typical clinical setting for the purpose of returning students to training as rapidly as possible.

Reliable telemedicine is essential for an ARTB PA to be effective. ARTB PAs have limited diagnostic tools available due to the austere environment. Additionally, PAs will operate independently without direct support from other providers. In order to mitigate these limitations, PAs must maintain an extensive network of providers to call upon when assistance is needed.

The ARTB operates at a high operational tempo nearly year round. There is very little time available for training medics. PAs must maximize training opportunities during patient encounters as a means to ensure medics maintain both competence and confidence.

Conclusion

Serving as an ARTB PA is both extremely demanding and highly rewarding. PAs have a direct impact on the successful execution of the ARTB mission in many ways. In addition to providing expert medical care, PAs play a large role in shaping the methods used to train students, and in developing effective risk mitigation measures to protect students. In order to support the high-risk training, PAs will have multiple opportunities for additional training and certifications that are not commonly offered across the rest of the Army.

References

1. Fort Benning Airborne and Ranger Training Brigade (ARTB) website. Updated January 8, 2019. Accessed July 20, 2020. https://www.benning.army.mil/Infantry/ARTB/#
2. Fort Benning Ranger School website. Updated June 25, 2018. Accessed July 20, 2020. https://www.benning.army.mil/Infantry/ARTB/Student-Information/#
3. Fort Benning Reconnaissance and Surveillance Leaders Course website. Updated June 17, 2020. Accessed July 20, 2020. https://www.benning.army.mil/Infantry/ARTB/RSLC/#
4. Fort Benning 1-507th Parachute Infantry Regiment website. Updated May 28, 2019. Accessed July 20, 2020. https://www.benning.army.mil/Infantry/ARTB/1-507th/

Chapter 21

ROLE OF THE ARMY SERVICE COMPONENT COMMAND PHYSICIAN ASSISTANT AT US ARMY AFRICA

P. Jason E.E. Auchincloss, APA-C, MPAS, and Christopher R. Smith, PA-C, MPAS

Introduction

The US Army Africa (USARAF) physician assistant (PA) supports the USARAF command, which aligns under US Africa Command (USAFRICOM), the unified geographic combatant command. USARAF is an Army service component command currently headquartered in Vicenza, Italy. The assignment provides a unique opportunity for the PA to expand operational acumen and serve in a job that often bears both operational and strategic importance.

Unit Structure

USARAF, as an Army service component command, is typically a two-star command comprised of a headquarters and headquarters battalion (HHBn) with three companies (Figure 21-1). The companies are organized into two functional companies. The headquarters support company and the operations company form one large company with a single commanding officer and first sergeant. The intelligence and sustainment company creates the second company with its commander and first sergeant. The USARAF commander falls under the command group within the headquarters support company. The USARAF PA, along with the public affairs officer and chaplain, logically falls into the headquarters support company for administrative purposes, but is ultimately a member of the HHBn special staff.

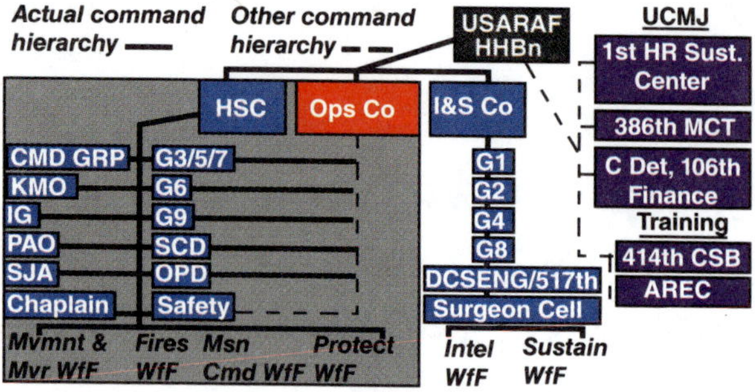

Figure 21-1. US Army Africa Headquarters and Headquarters Battalion organization diagram, presented in June 2018 as part of an inbrief for newly assigned personnel.
Diagram courtesy of Colonel Brett Medlin.
AREC: Army Reserve engagement cell; CSB: contracting support brigade; CMD: command; DCSENG: deputy chief of staff engineer; Det: detachment; GRP: group; HHBn: headquarters and headquarters battalion; HR: human resources; HSC: headquarters support company; I&S Co: intelligence and sustainment company; IG: inspector general; Intel: intelligence; MCT: movement control team; Msn: mission; Mvmnt: movement; OPD: Operational Protection Directorate; Ops Co: operations company; PAO: public affairs officer; SCD: Security Cooperation Division; SJA: staff judge advocate; Sust: sustainment; USARAF: US Army Africa; WfF: warfighting function

The HHBn medical team consists of the senior PA, a staff sergeant (E-6) combat medic (68W30) noncommissioned officer in charge, and one specialist (E-4) combat medic (68W10). The PA answers to the battalion commander, however, must be amenable to acting on medical guidance from the command surgeon (colonel/O-6) and USARAF commanding general (major general/O-8). The USARAF surgeon cell consists of the command surgeon and staff of Medical Service Corps officers, whose primary focus is planning.

Roles and Responsibilities

USARAF has only one PA authorized within the command. The USARAF command surgeon occupies the only other clinical position in the organization. The USARAF PA's primary role is to serve as special staff and medical advisor who supports the battalion commander, the command surgeon, and the regionally aligned force medical staff on the African continent. The latter is comprised of approximately seven physicians, nine PAs, seven nurses, and numerous combat medics. It is because of their oversight and input that the USARAF PA earns the moniker of "USARAF senior PA," despite no additional PAs or physicians assigned to the HHBn.

The USARAF senior PA advises the command team on all health, occupational, and environmental concerns while in garrison and when deployed. While in garrison, the USARAF senior PA provides routine and emergency medical care to USARAF and garrison personnel. Typically, the PA is also responsible for delivering health care to the two-star commander and executive staff. Additional clinical responsibilities may include daily urgent care visits, chronic care, and physical examinations. While not empaneled with the members of USARAF due to the additional special staff requirements, the PA does periodically operate in a borrowed manpower role at the US Army Health Clinic–Vicenza. The primary patient workload requirements range between 0.25 and 0.4 full-time equivalents.

Ultimately, the USARAF senior PA is responsible for battalion-level medical logistics, medical operations and plans, and the medical readiness of approximately 750 military and civilian employees. The PA is routinely assigned the management of day-to-day operations of the USARAF Travel Medicine Clinic at the Vicenza Health Clinic. The primary purpose of this clinic is to medically screen and medically clear personnel traveling to Africa in support of USARAF. The USARAF command surgeon is the waiver authority; however, the USARAF PA is delegated to assist with waiver adjudication for all US Army personnel with disqualifying medical conditions entering the AFRICOM theater.[1]

At all times, the USARAF senior PA is prepared to establish and staff a forward aid station in Africa for the USARAF contingency command post. In the forward aid station, the PA and USARAF medical team execute clinical medical support for select exercises in Africa hosted by USARAF. When directed, the USARAF senior PA serves as the medical officer in charge and the joint task force surgeon's clinical representative forward in the deployed setting.

As a special staff officer, the USARAF PA must balance the demands of the HHBn commander and staff, with those required by the USARAF commander, the executive team and directors, and the command surgeon and their directorate. It is during this daily fulfillment of obligations and requirements that USARAF PAs truly hone their skills in the art of diplomacy and the delivery of personalized care. While many will refrain from the term "executive medicine," one cannot overlook the timeless skill of providing "executive access to care."

Supervision and Evaluation

The USARAF PA is supervised by the HHBn commander, who serves as the PA's rater on the officer evaluation report. The PA's senior rater is the chief of staff, with the command surgeon providing medical input as the intermediate rater. However, a more traditional supervisory chain may exist based on rank (eg, the battalion executive officer as the rater, the command surgeon as the intermediate rater, and the battalion commander as the senior rater). Landstuhl Regional Medical Center (LRMC) in Germany processes credentialing and privileging for the USARAF PA.

Skills and Attributes

All candidates for the USARAF PA position must meet medical requirements to enter the Africa area of responsibilities.[2] In addition to medical eligibility, there are numerous desired skills and attributes of a PA in USARAF, including the following:

- current in all skills mandated by the individual critical task lists,
- operational experience,
- rank of senior captain or junior major,
- a graduate of the Captains Career Course, and
- outstanding written and oral communication skills.

The following attributes are also helpful for success as a USARAF PA:

- Mixed operational experience within multiple roles of care is preferred, with a minimum of Role I deploymentexperience.
- Knowledge and understanding of the joint and combined environments.
- The ability to work well with both military and civilian personnel and organizations, and excellent customer service skills. Having these skills will prove helpful when working in an environment

dominated by senior military and civilian leaders. A collegial working relationship must prevail at all times with the local health center and the surrounding units.

- An understanding and interest in the administrative aspects of managing a large medical equipment set that might be located in up to two or three countries simultaneously.
- The ability to work with multiple high-ranking African military leaders from the ranks of captain to a two-star general.
- Ability to understand, navigate, and execute the medical evacuation process using International SOS and the Theater Patient Movement Requirements Center–Europe.[2]

Training

The position requires no additional training outside of the credentials requirements.[3] However, the following additional training is highly recommended:

- **Brigade Surgeon Course.** This course prepares Medical Corps officers to function as brigade surgeons. It highlights the health and readiness issues that most often occur at the brigade or division task force levels. The course takes place at the Army Medical Center of Excellence.
- **Army Flight Surgeon Course**. This 6-week course teaches aviation and aviation survival, flight physiology, aviation operations, and mishaps and aviation medicine programs. It prepares graduates to implement an aviation medicine program at their home station and to address the medical needs of aviators. This course provides the Army service component command PA the ability to care for the aviators in the formation.
- **Joint Humanitarian Operations Course**. This is a 2-day course that highlights the relationship between the United States Agency for International Development, Office of Foreign Disaster Assistance and its partners.
- **Military Tropical Medicine Course**. This program of instruction offers enhanced training in tropical medicine to Army, Navy, and Air Force medical officers.[4] The course discusses a wide variety of topics to include environmental illnesses, pre- and post-travel medical evaluations, viral, bacterial, and parasitic infections, and

public health issues in the developing world. Any PA operating in the AFRICOM area of responsibility (AOR) must attend this course.

- **Tactical Combat Medical Care Course**. This course provides the clinician (physician, PA, nurse practitioner, and senior medics) with a practical working knowledge of how to deal with injured patients in a combat environment. The course provides training on the evaluation, resuscitation, stabilization, emergency surgical procedures, and the post-resuscitation management of the wounded soldier.

Recommended Certifications

- American Red Cross (ARC) Cardio Pulmonary Resuscitation (CPR) Instructor
- American Heart Association (AHA) Advanced Life Support (ALS)
- American Heart Association Pediatric Advanced Life Support (PALS)
- Advanced Trauma Life Support (ATLS)
- Advanced Burn Life Support (ABLS)

Basic Life Support, Advanced Cardiac Life Support, and Pediatric Advanced Life Support training are available through the Vicenza Health Clinic and Landstuhl Regional Medical Center.

Key Factors

The position is typically a 3-year assignment in Vicenza, Italy. The USARAF senior PA must be medically deployable to the very restrictive AFRICOM AOR.[5] The theater medical entry requirements reflect several factors including (1) the austere nature of the environment; (2) the size of the AOR (Figure 21-2); and (3) the medical infrastructure across the AOR.

Housing is available on base for families. The local housing office, staffed by English-speaking Italians, assists in finding appropriate accommodations for military and civilian personnel off-post. The Department of Defense Education Activity has an American elementary and high school for school-aged children.

Morale, welfare, and recreation (MWR) activities are plentiful in Europe. Outdoor recreation sponsors paid travel events to local Italian sites and other parts of Europe, providing a plethora of tourist

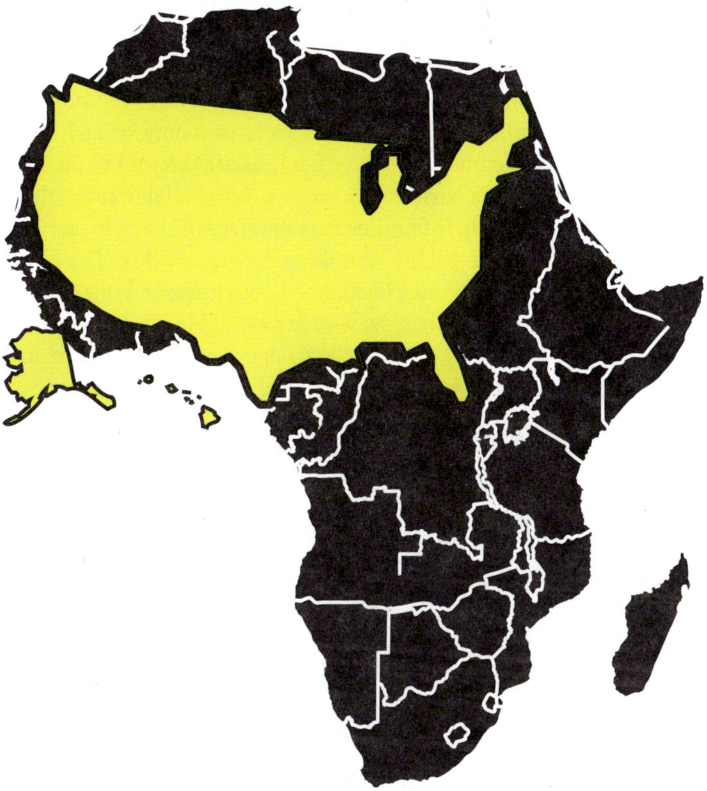

Figure 21-2. The true size of Africa—approximately 3.5 times the size of the continental United States. Medical evacuation and casualty evacuation movements frequently cover distances similar to moving a patient from Maine to Florida. There is NO "golden hour" in the US Africa Command area of responsibility.

experiences. Bike, ski, and kayak rentals are available. The local train network also offers an easy opportunity to travel. Venice Airport is located 45 minutes from Vicenza. Garrison provides a shuttle to and from the airport, with seating based on priority and availability. Preference is typically provided based on the following guidelines in order of precedence: emergency leave, permanent change of station travelers, temporary duty, and leave.

The Vicenza Health Clinic offers primary care for service members and their families. Additional services available include immunizations, hearing, optometry, behavior health, laboratory, radiography, pharmacy, physical therapy, and nurse case management. Services not provided at the clinic are either available on the local economy or at LRMC. Typically, service members and their families are referred to the local economy for imaging or basic health services not available at the clinic. Service members and their families may receive subspecialty services at LRMC. The Vicenza–LRMC shuttle runs twice weekly. The Italian San Bortolo Hospital provides local emergency care, and this hospital includes a staff of patient liaisons who are available 24/7 to assist the local military community with the language barrier. The nurse case managers at the Vicenza Health Clinic closely follow all inpatient care.

Opportunities and Experiences

The USARAF PA will travel to the Africa AOR frequently in support of exercises and real-world events (Figure 21-3). These activities gain notoriety from the international press and have high visibility at the strategic level. The USARAF PA is involved in the medical planning of exercises and forward operations, as a vital member of the staff.

The PA is often responsible for the medical care of senior commanders and leaders on the continent. Previous leaders and clients have included the chief of staff of the Army, the vice chief of staff of the Army, the AFRICOM and USARAF commanders, and many other senior government officials. The majority of this VIP medical coverage occurs annually during the African Land Forces Summit, which brings together chiefs of defense forces and senior military leaders from as many as 43 countries. This major event is vital to ensuring senior defense officials from across the continent can discuss regional and cross-regional challenges within the AFRICOM AOR.

In 2014 the USARAF PA was the primary clinical provider responsible for the health and welfare of the joint task force tasked to stop the spread of Ebola virus in Liberia, West Africa. The PA provided en-route and on-site medical coverage for the president of Liberia and other senior officials. At the same time, they visited the sites of the Ebola treatment units on a US Marine Corps V22 Osprey aircraft.

Later in 2015, the USARAF PA and a medic deployed to provide clinical oversight for the Special Purpose Marine Ground Task

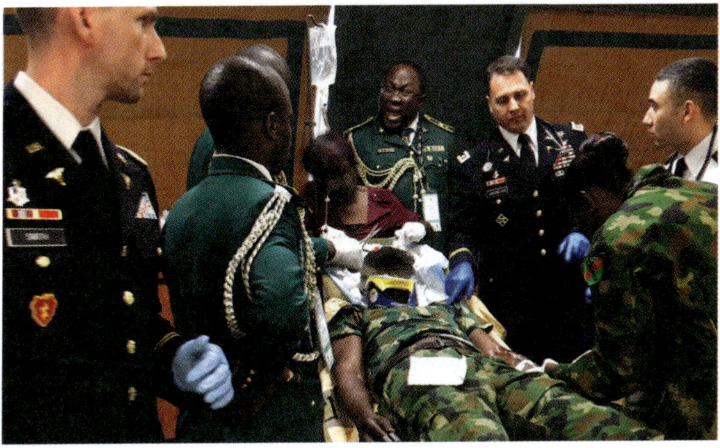

Figure 21-3. US Army Africa physician assistant and medics working alongside a Host Nation medical team to treat a patient injured during riots in West Africa. Photograph courtesy of Major Paul Auchincloss.

Force (SPMGTF) during their infiltration and establishment of a contingency location in Cameroon, West Africa. This deployment lasted approximately 3 months and was pivotal in the establishment of the AFRICOM policy regarding the use of antivenin by conventional forces on the continent.

Lessons Learned and Tips for Success

These are tips for success that will enable the future USARAF PA to succeed in their role:

- Attend command and staff meeting at least every other week. The command team and primary staff will appreciate involvement and input regarding the daily operations and medical readiness of the unit.
- Attend monthly meetings with the senior medical council members at the Vicenza Health Center.
- The USARAF PA will be extremely busy and on call most of the time. Developing an effective work–life balance is crucial to a successful assignment.

- Develop or maintain subject matter expertise regarding tropical diseases, and the threats service members of the command may be exposed to while forward on the continent.
- Step away from the office and circulate. Engage with the clinic staff and members of the command. Conducting weekly "rounds" to determine the health of the command team, staff, and directors is beneficial and appreciated. Everyone works extended hours, and individual health care is not always a priority for leaders.
- Attend morning staff or team huddles at least once a week at the health center. Doing so will solidify a relationship with the clinic staff and provide them an opportunity to discuss concerns regarding predeployment and travel requirements, as well as management of returning travelers who are ill.

Conclusion

US Army Africa offers a multitude of professional and international experiences not available at other duty stations. The position is unique due to the geographical and medical challenges associated with the Africa area of operation. As an assignment, it can provide a vital stepping stone to working in a joint environment.

References

1. US Africa Command website. AC form 43, USAFRICOM medical waiver request. Published January 15, 2019. Accessed May 14, 2020. https://www.africom.mil/media-room/document/32430/ac-form-43-africom-medical-waiver-request-form-15-jan-2019
2. Force Health Protection Requirements and Medical Guidance for Entry into the US Africa Command Theater. United States Africa Command. Published May 18, 2019. Accessed April 2, 2020. http://www.africom.mil/media-room/Document/32429/aci-4200-09a-force-health-protection-requirements-and-medical-guidance-for-the-africom-aor
3. DoD Instruction 1322.24, "Medical Readiness Training," October 6, 2011. Accessed May 28, 2020. https://jts.amedd.army.mil/assets/docs/policies/MRT-DoDI-1322-24.pdf

4. Military Tropical Medicine. Military Tropical Medicine. Accessed May 18, 2020. https://www.med.navy.mil/sites/nmpdc/courses/Pages/Military Tropical Medicine.aspx

5. US Africa Command website. AC form 42, USAFRICOM travel medical screening checklist. Published January 15, 2019. Accessed May 14, 2020. https://www.africom.mil/media-room/document/32432/ac-form-42-africom-travel-health-checklist-15-jan-2019

Chapter 22

ROLE OF THE THEATER SPECIAL OPERATIONS COMMAND PHYSICIAN ASSISTANT

P. Jason E.E. Auchincloss, APA-C, MPAS; F. Eddie Criss, APA-C, MPAS; Christopher Sacheli, APA-C, MPAS; and Geoffrey Washburn, APA-C, MPAS

Introduction

A Theater Special Operations Command (TSOC) is a one- or two-star subordinate, unified command of US Special Operations Command. TSOCs perform broad, continuous missions uniquely suited to special operations forces (SOF) and the capabilities they bring to the fight. The secretary of defense has assigned operational control of the TSOCs and their attached SOF tactical units to their respective geographic combatant commanders via the Global Force Management Implementation Guidance.[1]

While the geographic combatant command-aligned TSOCs vary widely in their task unit organization, and day-to-day operational activities, all TSOCs incorporate functional medical staffs designed to support and advise the commander on all aspects of health service support. The role of the physician assistant (PA) in the medical staff varies from senior primary care clinician, to deputy surgeon, to medical operations officer, or any combination thereof.

While there may be some slight variations in each TSOC (mainly due to manning, assigned forces, and geographic responsibility), the PA duties will be inherently similar. Filling a TSOC PA position is both rewarding and challenging. The assignment provides a unique joint force opportunity for the tactical PA to expand their operational acumen, and serve in a post that often bears both operational and strategic importance.

Unit Structure

Figure 22-1 shows an example of a TSOC organizational structure, although they vary. Each TSOC has a unique set of component commands, but the command relationship between the TSOC, US Special Operations Command, and the geographic combatant command remains the same (Figure 22-2).[2]

In some cases, the PA is assigned as the command surgeon, without a physician or additional deputy on staff (eg, Special Operations Command North). As the TSOC surgeon, the PA is medical advisor to the commander. The PA is also responsible for the entire medical directorate along with the previously stated responsibilities. The TSOC PA position is rewarding and career enhancing, unique within the PA (65D) career field. The TSOC PA for Special Operations Command Africa serves as the command PA and the deputy surgeon for clinical services and any other patient-related issues. Another medical officer, the operations deputy surgeon, is the lead medical planner.

For example, within Special Operations Command Africa, the command PA provides the "care there" clinical focus—honing in on clinical operations on the continent of Africa. A second PA (a US Army Reserve officer) works in the surgeon cell and focuses on "care here"—specifically in-garrison medicine and preservation of the force and family. This second PA position is not part of the baseline manning document and may not be filled. As a result, the command or TSOC PA must be familiar with all clinical duties, because they may have to assume both roles at any time.

Supervision

TSOC PAs traditionally practice medicine as general medical officers or within their trained specialties. The TSOC surgeon typically supervises these officers.[3–5] Depending on the unit's organizational structure, the TSOC PA may oversee other assigned or attached PAs, special operations medics, and additional medical and human performance enablers (eg, preventive medicine personnel and a preservation of the force and family team). Sometimes, the TSOC PA may be the senior medical staff member, requiring an intermediate

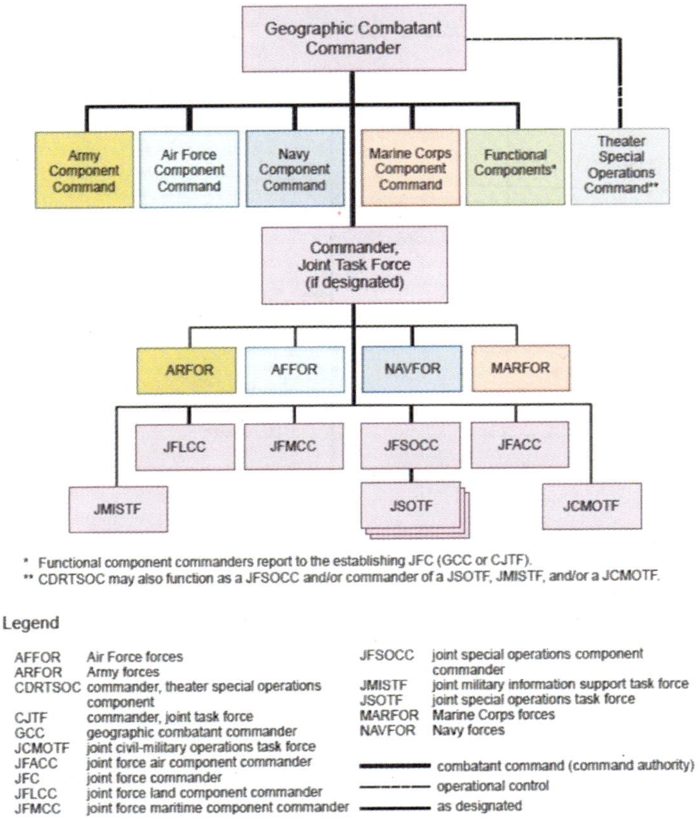

Figure 22-1. A notional organization chart that demonstrates the command structure and relationships of the different directorates in a Theater Special Operations Command. The surgeon falls under the personal staff (or special staff).
Reproduced from: US Department of Defense. *Special Operations.* DOD; 2014. Joint Publication 3-05, Figure III-2.

rater on official evaluations. In most TSOCs, the PA's rater will be the TSOC command surgeon, and the senior rater will be the TSOC chief of staff or TSOC commander.[2]

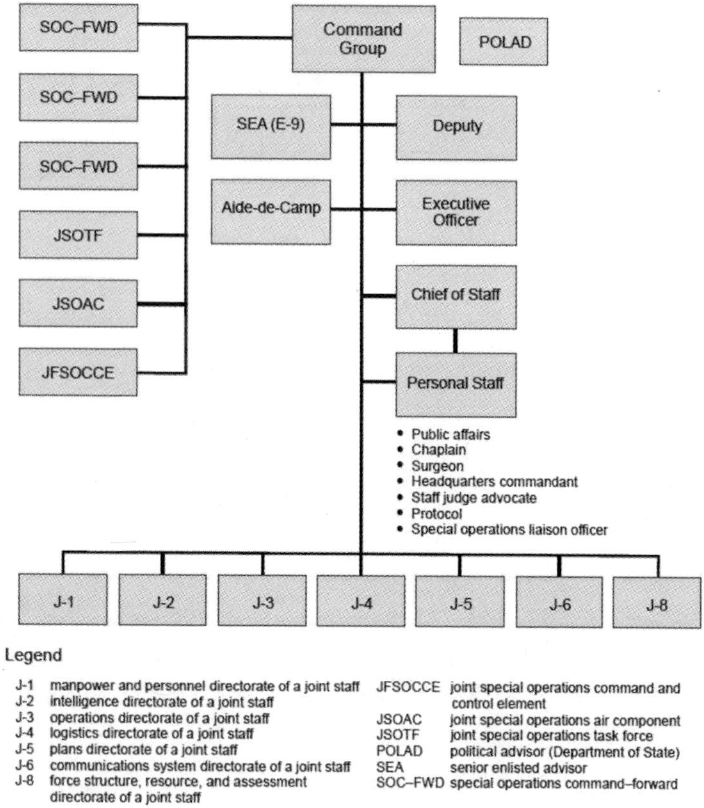

Figure 22-2. A notional organization chart that demonstrates the command relationships within a geographic combatant command. The geographic combatant commander has operational control over the Theater Special Operations Command.
Reproduced from: US Department of Defense. *Special Operations.* DOD; 2014. Joint Publication 3-05, Figure III-3.

Roles and Responsibilities

Primary Care Manager

The PA is responsible for the routine care of TSOC headquarters staff and their families. Duties may include functions such as facilitating completion of everyday medical readiness requirements and conducting routine physical examinations, sick call, and referral management. The PA often creates and maintains a deployable medical package (a modular, lightweight equipment set) for use in providing medical support for short-notice missions in their area of responsibility.

Deputy Command Surgeon

As the executive officer to the TSOC command surgeon, the PA is responsible for deputy director-level engagements and serves as a director in the surgeon's absence.

Human Performance Coordinator

The PA leads and facilitates the human performance team, which is made up of individuals in a variety of subspecialties, such as physical therapists, strength and conditioning coaches, athletic trainers, performance dietitians, and behavioral health specialists.

Medical Planner

The PA is the lead for health service support on operational planning teams, which develop operational and strategic policies and plans. In this role, the PA coordinates with higher and adjacent headquarters' medical staff. The PA also advises and reviews subordinate unit concepts of operation for both risks to mission and risk to forcc. Focus areas include medical support packages, the type of care available in the local hospitals, the level of care available on the mission, and the medical equipment needed.

Medical Exercise Planner/Scenario Controller

The PA serves as the lead medical exercise planner for joint and multinational special operations exercises. Duties include developing plans, determining resource requirements, and executing complex medical scenarios. At the end of each exercise, the PA provides relevant feedback to the training audience.

Requirements

The requirements to serve as a TSOC PA are the following:

- National certification and good standing with the National Commission on Certification of Physician Assistants.
- Eligible for credentials at a servicing military medical treatment facility.
- Current in all skills mandated by the individual critical task lists.
- Rank of major (recommended).
- Possess outstanding written and oral communication skills.

Desired Skills and Attributes

Desired skills and attributes of a TSOC PA include the following:

- Top secret-sensitive compartmentalized information security clearance.
- Graduate of Intermediate Level Education.
- Knowledge and experience in the training and scope of practice of special operations medics working throughout the joint force.
- Working understanding of the geographic area of responsibility, including relevant historical and current events, goals, opportunities, threats, military structures, and organizations.
- Working knowledge of US special operations core activities and the nuances of medical support to these operations.
- Understanding of the US Transportation Command and Defense Health Agency medical care, evacuation infrastructure, capabilities, and processes across the geographic area of responsibility.
- Knowledge of the capabilities, limitations, strengths, and weakness of joint force deployable medical treatment capabilities (eg, forward resuscitative surgical team, ground surgical team, emergency resuscitation surgical team, special operations surgical team, and special operations resuscitation team).
- Expertise in tactical combat casualty care.

- Working knowledge of the Joint Trauma System clinical practice guidelines, fundamentals of damage control resuscitation, and prolonged field care.

Training

- Joint Special Operations Medical Orientation Course
- NATO Special Operations Medical Planning and Support Course
- Flight surgeon and dive medical officer certifications
- Other recommendations by geographic area of responsibility
    - Operational Clinical Infectious Disease Course (3-day course)
    - Tropical Medicine Course (Special Operations Command Africa, either a 5-day or 1-month course)
    - Medical Management of Chemical and Biological Casualties Course and Medical Management of Radiologic Casualties Course (Special Operations Command North)

Recommended Certifications

- Cardiopulmonary Resuscitation Instructor
- Advanced Life Support
- Pediatric Advanced Life Support
- Advanced Trauma Life Support

Opportunities and Experiences

- Opportunity to engage, liaise, and learn from the whole US special operations joint force as well as partner and allied nation SOF.
- Broadening opportunity—working directly at the operational level and serving as a vital link between strategic policy and the "doers" at the tactical level.
- Geographic area of operations focus—opportunity to gain specific knowledge and expertise in the foreign policy goals, opportunities, and threats to a particular geographic area.

Lessons Learned

TSOC PA hours are often long, with many weekends spent on call as SOF continue their missions across the globe. TSOC PAs must be versatile and proficient in their clinical skills. They must be adept at communicating across multiple platforms, and with commanders and operators at all levels. The position will challenge TSOC PAs in the areas of casualty evacuation, medical evacuation, communication, and logistics. The mission seldom slows, so excellent time management skills that enable a reasonable family–work life balance are critical. If a TSOC PA knows something that may be important to the mission, they must speak up; if they do not know something, it is their duty to ask. Lives are often at stake, and as a professional, the PA must always place the soldier and the mission before personal pride.

Tips for Success

These tips for success can set up a rewarding tour:

- PAs should understand the operational environment and help the command team understand the medical risks. They should recommend risk reduction and mitigation activities that do not adversely affect the overall mission.
- Medical counterparts across the regionally aligned forces must be identified and integrated into each mission. If their supporting contributions are not planned and incorporated into the medical objectives they can hinder progress.
- Medical objectives must nest within command priorities. While seemingly obvious, medical lines of effort sometimes do not support directed priorities and threaten the credibility, resourcing, and relevance of the TSOC medical staff.
- PAs should always seek to expand and reinforce their medical knowledge at every opportunity.
- It is important to balance the requirement to provide primary medical care for patients with the operational and staff aspects of the TSOC PA job.

Conclusion

The TSOC PA is a very fast-paced and challenging position, albeit extremely rewarding. The position provides an excellent opportunity to straddle both the clinical and operational worlds of special operations. PAs will likely serve in both a health care delivery and primary trainer capacity, but also be heavily involved in operationalizing SOF medicine across the joint force. Special operations, under the TSOC proponent, have certain mission relevance as they are constantly engaged in all facets of special operations, across the full spectrum of military operations. The PA position offers a broadening opportunity, and a chance to serve in an operational-level joint headquarters, working alongside some of the finest officers and noncommissioned officers across both the joint SOF, and allied or partner nation SOF.

References

1. Joint Special Operations University. *Special Operations Forces Reference Manual.* 4th ed. JSOU Press; 2015:chap 2,2–13.
2. US Department of Defense. *Special Operations.* DOD; 2014. Joint Publication 3-05.
3. US Department of the Army. *Evaluation Reporting System.* DA; 2019. Army Regulation 623-3.
4. US Department of the Army. *Medical, Dental, and Veterinary Care.* DA; 2013. Army Regulation 40-3.
5. US Department of the Army. *Medical Services: Clinical Quality Management.* DA; 2004, Rapid action revision issue date: May 22, 2009. Army Regulation 40-68.

Chapter 23

ROLE OF THE BRIGADE SENIOR PHYSICIAN ASSISTANT

Stephanie Bocanegra, PA-C, MPAS

Introduction

The role of the brigade senior physician assistant (BDE PA) is arguably one of the best positions a physician assistant (PA) can be selected for in the Army. Why one of the best? Because in this position, a PA is no longer involved in the daily grind of balancing patient care with unit obligations, like a junior battalion PA (BN PA), and is not encumbered with the scope of responsibilities and complex planning duties of a division PA (DIV PA). A BDE PA works directly with BN PAs and medics and, while still involved with patient care, has the opportunity to provide more direct daily mentorship and shape policy within brigade medical operations. The BDE PA position bridges the middle ground between the BN PA and the DIV PA while working directly with the brigade surgeon (BDE SURG) to ensure that health service support and force health protection are executed appropriately. This chapter will provide a brief overview of both the clinical and the administrative duties and responsibilities of the BDE PA (refer to Chapter 12, Role of the Battalion PA, and to Chapter 25, Role of the Division PA, in this handbook for more in-depth details).

The BDE PA serves as the primary advisor to the BDE SURG on all clinical operations (CLINOPS), functions as the liaison between the local medical treatment facility (MTF) and division, and provides mentorship and career advice to all PAs within the brigade. The BDE PA plays an integral role in planning brigade garrison and deployment medical operations, developing mass casualty exercises, monitoring medical readiness, enforcing and coordinating medic military occupational specialty (MOS) sustainment training and continuing education for assigned providers, and performing oversight of daily CLINOPS in keeping with MTF quality management.[1]

Supervision

Supervision of the BDE PA is performed by the BDE SURG as outlined in Army regulations (ARs) 623-3, 40-3, and 40-68, and in the local MTF credential policies.[1–3] Traditionally, the BDE PA is rated by the BDE SURG and senior-rated by the brigade commander (BDE CDR). However, there can be a few variations, so a new BDE PA must ensure understanding of the rating scheme immediately (this is typically addressed in initial counseling by the supervisor or rater).

The Brigade Surgeon Section

The BDE SURG is responsible for the Army health system (AHS) support for the brigade combat team (BCT). In accordance with *Army Health Systems Support to Maneuver Forces* (Army Techniques Publication 4-02.3[4]), the BDE SURG is considered a:

> brigade-level special staff officer that coordinates AHS support activities with the brigade S-1 [personnel/administration officer] and other headquarters elements that affect AHS support in the brigade. The BDE SURG is responsible for the technical supervision of all medical activities in the command. The BDE SURG is part of the brigade commander's special staff, and as such, provides advice to the BDE CDR on all medical or medically related issues. The BDE SURG keeps the BDE CDR informed on the status of AHS support for the brigade and the health of the command.[4(p16)]

Per Army Techniques Publication 4-02.3,[4] the BDE SURG section does not include a BDE PA (although the BDE PA receives guidance from the section). The BDE SURG's staff consists of a field surgeon, a medical operations officer, and a health care noncommissioned officer who is battle staff-qualified. The section's three medical personnel are typically assigned to the headquarters company and are utilized as a sustainment warfighting component jointly with the S-4 (logistics) of an infantry BCT, armored BCT, or Stryker BCT. The sustainment element determines the type, amount, and the duration of support needed to meet command objectives. A BDE SURG section that is fully integrated in sustainment operations is responsible for planning, coordinating, and synchronizing the health service support mission for commanders and maneuver forces within the BCT's area of operations (Table 23-1).[4]

Table 23-1. Sustainment (S-4) medical staff.

Paragraph title	AOC/MOS	Grade	Title	Branch	Quantity
Sustainment–S/4 Medical	62B00	O-4	Field Surgeon	MC	1
	70H67	O-3	Medical Operations Officer	MS	1
	68W402S	E-7	Health Care NCO	NC	1

2S: battle staff operations
AOC: area of concentration
MC: Medical Corps
MOS: military occupational specialty
MS: Medical Service Corps
NC: noncommissioned
NCO: noncommissioned officer
S-4: logistics staff officer
Reproduced from: Department of the Army. *Army Health System Support to Maneuver Forces.* HQDA; 2014. Army Techniques Publication 4-02.3: Table 2-2.

The BDE PA is typically assigned to the medical company within the brigade support battalion. According to the modified table of organization and equipment (MTOE), the BDE PA is part of an area medical treatment squad, which provides basic primary care services and advanced trauma management to a supported area of operations within the brigade footprint. The treatment squad serves as the main source of medical care for the brigade support medical company's Role 2 treatment facility. The Role 2 consists of a medical treatment squad and other key elements that provide patient holding capabilities and multiple ancillary services, such as dental, laboratory, physical therapy, and radiology (Table 23-2).[4]

Job Duties and Responsibilities

Although the BDE PA does not align directly within the BDE SURG section, they function as the direct supporting element to the BDE SURG on all CLINOPS and PA matters. Typically, the BDE PA has been in the operational setting for several years. Therefore, their role is vital during garrison and deployment operations. The BDE PA's daily duties depend on the unit of assignment and the expectations of the BDE SURG and command team. Time is divided among meetings, staff work, training, and clinic. The BDE PA is often the first point of contact for incoming medical officers, so they will need to be heavily engaged

Table 23-2. The medical treatment squad (area).

Paragraph title	AOC/MOS	Grade	Title	Branch	Quantity
Medical Treatment Squad (Area)	62B00	O-4	Field Surgeon	MC	1
	65D00	O-4	Senior Physician Assistant	SP	1
	68W30	E-6	Health Care Sergeant	NC	1
	68W20	E-5	Health Care Sergeant	NC	2
	68W10	E-4	Health Care Specialist		1
	68W10	E-3	Health Care Specialist		2

AOC: area of concentration
MC: Medical Corps
MOS: military occupational specialty
NC: noncommissioned
SP: Medical Specialist Corps
Reproduced from: Department of the Army. *Army Health System Support to Maneuver Forces.* Washington, DC: HQDA; 2014. Army Techniques Publication 4-02.3: Table 2-14.

with sponsorship, communication, and streamlining credentialing and in-processing for these individuals.

Besides being heavily involved in day-to-day CLINOPS, the BDE PA should be significantly involved in the medical readiness training and associated professional development of all the medical personnel in the brigade. Teaching, coaching, and mentoring the approximately seven other PAs in the brigade, and support to the brigade nurse, physical therapist, dentist, and battalion surgeons are essential to the success of the brigade's overall medical mission. Fostering an environment of support and teamwork, while providing consistent communication and clear guidance on policies and systems that work, will ensure that all are moving forward together as a team. The BDE PA needs to actively encourage subordinate PAs to participate in medical and officer professional development opportunities in both the operational and clinical realms. They are also responsible for educating each BN PA to expand their technical and professional capabilities. These responsibilities include advising them through regular counseling (written and verbal) on how to write and review officer evaluation reports and officer record briefs, the importance of maintaining a current Army photo, and creating/updating their curriculum vitae. In some cases, the BDE PA may also serve as an intermediate rater for BN PAs.

Requirements

To serve in this position, a PA must:

- graduate from an accredited PA program, pass the Physician Assistant National Certifying Examination, and maintain certification with the Physician Assistant National Recertifying Exam through the National Commission on Certification of Physician Assistants[1];
- hold the appropriate rank;
- have completed the Captains Career Course;
- pass the current physical fitness test and be in compliance with height/weight standards of AR 600-9, *The Army Body Composition Program*[5,6];
- have current Basic Life Support certification at a minimum, and required Department of Defense Instruction (DODI) 1322.24 and service-directed medical readiness training[7];
- be credentialed at the local MTF;
- be a subject matter expert on readiness[7,8];
- know the entry criteria for warrior transition and soldier recovery units, and understand the Integrated Disability Evaluation System (IDES)[9–14]; and
- understand physical requirements of soldiers based on their MOS in accordance with DA Pamphlet 611-21, *Military Occupational Classification and Structure*.[15]

Desired Skills and Attributes

BDE PAs should:

- have an additional skill identifier of M2 (emergency medicine) per MTOE (this is not currently enforced due to personnel shortages);
- be able to operate in clinical, deployed, and field settings;
- be able to communicate effectively with their BDE SURG, command teams at the battalion and brigade levels, fellow health care providers and specialists, noncommissioned officers, soldiers, and patients;

- have deployment experience and be capable of worldwide deployment operations;
- be able to operate independently with little supervision or guidance;
- have solid written and oral communication skills;
- have current Tactical Combat Casualty Care foundational knowledge;
- have the knowledge and ability to train and supervise 68W combat medics and combat lifesavers, as well as other allied and ancillary health specialists;
- have a basic understanding of the individual critical task lists (ICTLs) for each medical area of concentration (AOC) for officers and military occupational specialty (MOS) for enlisted personnel under their purview[16]; and
- obtain access and understand the use of various software applications required for patient care and soldier readiness, including the electronic health record and key modules within the Medical Operational Data System (eg, the Medical Readiness Portal, Medical Protection System [MEDPROS], MEDPROS Web Data Entry, and Medical Health Assessment).

Intermediate Level Education is recommended but not required. BDE PAs are also encouraged to obtain and maintain Advanced Life Support (ALS).[1] Per AR 40-68, Advanced Trauma Life Support (ATLS), Medical Management of Chemical and Biological Casualties, and Tropical/Global Medicine are additional recommended courses.[1] However, ATLS and the Medical Management of Chemical and Biological Casualties are required courses on the 65D (PA) ICTL, along with ALS, Pediatric Advanced Life Support, Tactical Combat Casualty Care, and Medical Effects of Ionizing Radiation.

"Battle Rhythm"

Below are examples of the BDE PA's regular operations (this list is not all inclusive).

Daily

- Sick call (refer to "Sick Call Operations" in the Chapter 12, the BN PA).
- Clinic: BDE PAs are often primarily in charge of the day-to-day CLINOPS for their unit in both the garrison and field setting; this will

encompass the majority of their time. Managing provider schedules and medic coverage, ensuring algorithm-directed troop medical care[17] is incorporated into sick call and for acute walk-in patients, enforcing MTF safety protocols to prevent adverse outcomes, ensuring Health Insurance Portability and Accountability Act (HIPAA) compliance, and addressing patient satisfaction issues are just a few examples of a BDE PA's CLINOPS functions, in addition to overall unit readiness. BDE PAs are considered to fill an executive leadership role, and are therefore required to perform clinical care only to maintain their skills, proficiency, and credentialing (equating to 40 patient-contact hours per year, depending on MTF and unit leadership guidance). However, clinic time is often significantly more for involved BDE PAs, especially with recurrent PA shortages within the military.[1,3,4,7,9,13,14,17]

- Miscellaneous administrative duties and conference calls with various staff within the brigade, clinic, division, and MTF.

Weekly/Biweekly

- Command and staff meetings are typically twice monthly at the brigade level. BDE PAs should be present at both or at least one monthly (if splitting meetings with the BDE SURG), not only for situational awareness, but also to build rapport with unit leadership and staff.
- Regular clinic duties to maintain credentials and privileges of at least 40 hours of patient care and continuity of medical skill sets annually.
- Medical operations meetings outside the brigade to synchronize the AHS with higher headquarters.
- BDE SURG synchronization meetings with the other BN PAs and surgeons.
- Review of current operations orders (OPORDs) and fragmentation orders (FRAGOs) for clinically relevant material (be prepared to provide input and write OPORDs and FRAGOs to direct subordinate units as needed).

Monthly

- Monitoring the IDES management and non-deployable profile review boards at brigade and division levels for profiles that exceed 180 and 240 days, respectively.[10,11,13]

- Membership boards that involve key medical, behavioral, and legal subject matter experts who offer feedback on personnel identified by the command to be at a higher risk to themselves or others.
- Participation in warrior transition unit and soldier recovery unit entry boards.
- Division surgeon synchronization meetings.
- PA meetings, professional development, and team-building events.

Continuous/Ongoing

- Coaching, mentoring, and training new providers and medics.
- Professional development of self and others.
- Oversight of the first responder program and Combat Lifesaver training in accordance with the Tactical Combat Casualty Care guidelines.[7]
- Managing 68W sustainment training in close coordination with the installation medical simulation training centers, tracking certification status and ICTLs, and assisting units with the health care specialist management module of the medical operational data system web-based platform.
- Reviewing and updating standard operating procedures and continuity books.
- Open and effective communication with incoming providers and MTOE-assigned personnel.[18]
- Close coordination with clinic leadership and the local MTF concerning garrison health care issues, including borrowed military manpower personnel, clinic schedules, training, and deployment calendars.
- Ensuring sustainment and predeployment medical training requirements are conducted in accordance with Department of Defense Instruction 1322.24, AR 350-1, and AR 40-68, in close coordination with the MTF, the installation medical simulation training center, and the Medical Center of Excellence at Joint Base San Antonio–Fort Sam Houston, Texas.[1,5,7,16]

Lessons Learned and Tips for Success

For a BDE PA, the most important concept to understand is where they are in the hierarchy of leadership in relation to their battalion counterparts. Many PAs come into this position excited to have finally worked their way up to being in charge of a group of fellow professionals; however, being a BDE PA simply means they are the most senior and potentially the most experienced PA in their unit. The BDE PA is technically not in the BN PA or BN SURG chain of command; therefore, the BDE PA can provide guidance, input, and feedback on battalion-level daily operations and functions of the PAs and surgeons, but the unit will dictate their battle rhythm. Taskings must go through official operational channels for approval. While the BDE PA may be disheartened to limit themselves to what may seem "just an advisory role," they must understand that their BN PAs and surgeons still value their leadership position, mentorship, and advocacy on their part with their command teams.

The BDE PA position should be seen as an advocate for battalion providers, medics, and ancillary staff while also serving as a protective barrier against internal and external distractions that may hinder readiness and overall health service support operations. The BDE PA must take their role seriously as the most senior PA working with the health care professionals in their brigade; they are all focused on the same goals. If the BDE PA's subordinates know they are available to them, that they provide sound leadership and mentorship, and are a true team player while remaining flexible and resilient, they will together accomplish the mission in the most cohesive manner possible.

Conclusion

Filling a key leadership role that bridges the gap between the BN PA and DIV PA, the BDE PA plays a pivotal role in overall unit readiness, CLINOPS in the garrison and deployed setting, and sustained health service support and force health protection within the brigade area of operation. Daily, BDE PAs provide clear leadership, communication, and mentorship to their unit providers and staff while performing key advisory duties to the BDE SURG and BDE CDR. They also serve as liaison between the unit and the MTF, supporting readiness, health protection, and preventive care. Additionally, BDE PAs coordinate sustainment and continuing education training, clinical quality care, and professional development, ensuring their unit medical personnel are in keeping with the AMEDD motto, "to conserve the fighting strength."

References

1. Department of the Army. *Clinical Quality Management.* HQDA; 2009. Army Regulation 40-68.
2. Department of the Army. *Evaluation Reporting System*. HQDA; 2019. Army Regulation 623-3.
3. Department of the Army. *Medical, Dental, and Veterinary Care.* HQDA; 2013. Army Regulation 40-3.
4. Department of the Army. *Army Health Systems Support to Maneuver Forces*. HQDA; 2014. Army Techniques Publication 4-02.3.
5. Department of the Army. *Army Physical Readiness Training.* HQDA; 2012. Field Manual 7-22.
6. Department of the Army. *The Army Body Composition.* HQDA; 2019. Army Regulation 600-9.
7. Department of Defense. *Medical Readiness Training.* DOD; March 2018. DOD Instruction 1322.24.
8. Officer of the Under Secretary of Defense for Personnel Readiness. *Joint Trauma System (JTS)*. Department of Defense; 2016 (Change 1 effective August 5, 2018). DOD Instruction 6040.47. Accessed June 15, 2020. https://www.esd.whs.mil/Portals/54/Documents/DD/issuances/dodi/604047p.pdf?ver=2018-08-06-124902-047
9. Department of the Army. *Physical Evaluation for Retention, Retirement, or Separation*. HQDA; 2017. Army Regulation 635-40.
10. Department of the Army. *Medical Readiness Procedures*. HQDA; 2019. DA Pamphlet 40-502.
11. Department of the Army. *Standards of Medical Fitness*. HQDA; 2019. Army Regulation 40-501.
12. Department of the Army. *Warrior Care and Transition Program.* HQDA; 2015. AR 40-58.

13. Department of the Army. *Medical Readiness*. HQDA; 2019. Army Regulation 40-502.
14. Department of the Army. *Personnel Readiness Processing*. HQDA;2018. Army Regulation 600-8-101.
15. Department of the Army. *Military Occupational Classification and Structure*. HQDA; 2018. DA Pamphlet 611-21.
16. Department of the Army. *Medical Education and Demonstration of Individual Competence*. HQDA; 2015. Training Circular 8-800.
17. US Army Medical Command. *ADTMC: Algorithm-Directed Troop Medical Care (ADTMC)*. MEDCOM; November 13, 2019. MEDCOM Pamphlet 40-7-21.
18. Department of the Army. *Army Medical DepartmentProfessional Filler System*. HQDA; 2015. Army Regulation 601-14.

Chapter 24

ROLE OF THE PHYSICIAN ASSISTANT IN THE US ARMY TRAINING AND DOCTRINE COMMAND AND INITIAL MILITARY TRAINING

Sean M. Donohue, PA-C, MPAS, and Gail A. Evans, PA-C, MPAS

Introduction

The US Army Training and Doctrine Command (TRADOC), headquartered at Joint Base Langley-Eustis, Virginia, is the proponent for all Army training and doctrine. TRADOC works across the domains of doctrine, organization, training, materiel, leadership, personnel, facilities, and policy (DOTMLPF-P) to provide the structure and framework the Army operates within every day. TRADOC oversees 32 Army schools, organized under eight Centers of Excellence (CoE), each focused on a separate area of expertise within the Army (such as medical, maneuver, maneuver support, and signal). In total, these centers train over 500,000 soldiers, sailors, airman, marines, and international students worldwide each year.[1]

The US Army Center for Initial Military Training (CIMT), also located at Joint Base Langley-Eustis, was created by an act of Congress on September 24, 2009. CIMT is the core function lead under TRADOC for all initial military training (IMT). CIMT trains over 120,000 people annually, and the CIMT surgeon, an Army physician assistant (PA), is responsible for the health care oversight and policy affecting those trainees.

Training and Doctrine Command Unit Structure

TRADOC is commanded by a four-star general officer and has two core functional deputy commanding generals (DCGs): the DCG for

Combined Arms (Fort Leavenworth, KS), a lieutenant general (three-star) who oversees all CoEs, and the DCG for Initial Military Training (IMT), a major general (two-star) who oversees all IMT operations and the Army Training Center (Fort Jackson, SC). TRADOC also has oversight of the Army Recruiting Command, Army Cadet Command,

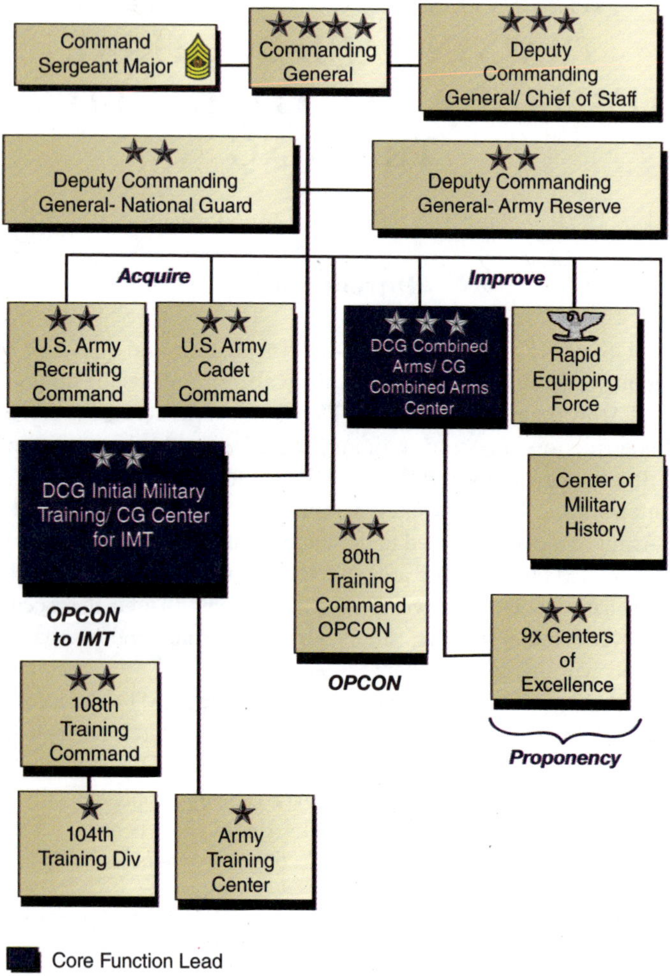

Figure 24-1. Training and Doctrine Command organizational chart (simplified).

Army Rapid Equipping Force, and Army Center of Military History. There are also DCGs (major generals) for the National Guard and Army Reserve components (Figure 24-1).

US Army Center for Initial Military Training Structure

CIMT oversees basic combat training (BCT), advanced individual training (AIT), one-station unit training (OSUT, where BCT and AIT are combined), the Basic Officer Leadership Course, and the Warrant Officer Basic Course. CIMT's Leader Training Brigade, located at Fort Jackson, educates, develops, and equips leaders with current, rigorous, and relevant curriculum in leadership, fitness, and resiliency. The brigade oversees three schools: the IMT Leadership School, Physical Fitness School, and Army Master Resiliency School. CIMT also oversees the Drill Sergeant Academy. These schools use a process that aligns the development of competencies (knowledge, skills, abilities, attributes) and behaviors so that civilian volunteers become soldiers who are physically ready, grounded in Army values, and competent in their skills. IMT includes developing baseline proficiency in warrior tasks, battle drills, and critical skills associated with the student's military occupational specialty or area of concentration. After completing IMT, graduates are prepared to contribute as leaders or members of a team upon arrival at their first unit of assignment.

CIMT is also the Army developer and proponent for the Army Expert Soldier Badge,[2] the *Soldier's Blue Book* (a guide to IMT),[3] the Army Combat Fitness Test (ACFT),[4] and the Holistic Health and Fitness (H2F) program.

Key Factors

The CIMT surgeon, an O-4 (major) PA (area of concentration [AOC] 65D), serves as the senior medical officer for the CIMT commanding general. Practically, the CIMT surgeon's role is to advise the commander on topics germane to the IMT training environment. These topics range from accessions and reception medical policy, the health care and wellness of recruits and soldiers in training at IMT courses, to evaluation and mitigation of attrition related to medical causes. Due to the proximity of CIMT to TRADOC, as well as the density of trainees in IMT, the CIMT surgeon also functions informally as the senior TRADOC PA. In the role of senior PA, the CIMT surgeon liaises with and advises the TRADOC command surgeon (an O-6 [colonel], AOC 60A, Operational Medicine Specialist) and serves as a coordinating or informal staff officer to the TRADOC surgeon. Because nearly all TRADOC surgeon initiatives and operations specifically affect the IMT population, the TRADOC surgeon staff and CIMT surgeon staff are inextricably linked.

TRADOC Surgeon Cell

TRADOC headquarters has a modest surgeon cell under the G1/4 (personnel and logistics staff section) at the headquarters element, principally consisting of the command surgeon and a deputy surgeon/environmental science officer (an O-5 [lieutenant colonel], AOC 72D), as well as three civilian positions: a medical operations officer, clinical operations officer, and executive assistant. The surgeon staff also includes a sergeant major (E-9), civilian command psychologist, and the civilian command ready and resilient integrator (CR2I).

CIMT Surgeon

The CIMT surgeon falls within the CIMT Research and Analysis Directorate. The directorate, under civilian leadership, also includes a senior medic (sergeant first class, military occupational specialty [MOS] 68W40, health care noncommissioned officer), command physical therapist (O-5, AOC 65B), command dietician (O-5, AOC 65C), and an occupational therapist (O-5, AOC 65A). Each position is intended for a traditional 3-year assignment and all positions serve as H2F action officers. The directorate also includes a variety of civilian analysts, doctrine writers, research physiologists, and the CR2I lead for Fort Eustis. The Research and Analysis Directorate areas of responsibility include:

- development and implementation of Army-level surveys, H2F doctrine, and pilots and tests for implementation of the ACFT;
- review of all proposed human subjects research involving trainees or cadre within IMT;
- tracking of attrition within IMT (including BCT, OSUT, and AIT); and
- developing policy, including Field Manual 7-22, *Army Physical Readiness Training*[5] (the name will soon become "Holistic Health and Fitness").

Additionally, the CIMT surgeon, dietician, and medical noncommissioned officer support the CIMT's Staff Assistance Visit (SAV) program to IMT sites (Figure 24-2) to evaluate compliance with applicable TRADOC regulations (TRs) and identify areas for support and improvement in the development of all initial training programs of instruction. The CIMT surgeon reviews and updates pertinent medical policy as it pertains to IMT, including the following TRs:

- TR 350-6, *Enlisted Initial Entry Training Policies and Administration*[6];
- TR 350-16, *Drill Sergeant Program*[7];
- TR 350-36, *Basic Officer Leader Training Policies and Administration*[8]; and
- TR 350-29, *Heat and Cold Casualties*.[9]

Other policy reviewed includes various Army regulations (ARs) as they pertain to CIMT:

- AR 40-501, *Standards of Medical Fitness*[10]; and
- AR 612-201, *Initial Entry/Prior Service Trainee Support*.[11]

Duties and Responsibilities

The daily duties of the CIMT surgeon are similar to those of other division or corps surgeon assets. Typical operations include enterprise-level observation of medical readiness, management of current and future operations, review and revision of policy guidance, generation of orders, contract preparation and execution, evaluation of studies and outcomes, evaluation of training programs for effectiveness and modification, and analysis of attrition. What truly makes the role of the CIMT surgeon unique, however, is the vast reach the position has across the DOTMLPF-P domain. In a typical day, the CIMT surgeon might address issues with the Military Entrance and Processing Command; review the program of instruction for Combat Lifesaver courses; evaluate the impact of community health threats on trainees and the greater population; participate in the planning, preparing, and budgeting and execution process; contribute to public affairs messaging; respond to congressional inquiries: present to various Army schools; meet with industry; and address problems with contracts. Because the CIMT surgeon's scope is so wide, it brings the incumbent into routine contact

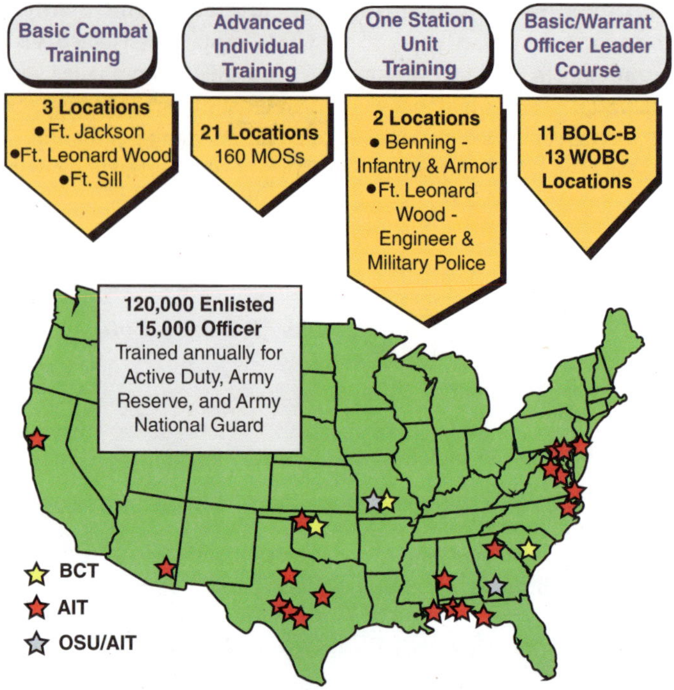

Daily Load				
BCT	OSUT	AIT	BOLC	Total
17,372	7,124	12,163	2,776	39,435

Annual Mission - FY 20	
Basic Combat Training	84,959
Advanced Individual Training	107,670
One-Station Unit Training	32,153
Basic Officer/Warrant Officer	15,002

Figure 24-2. Center for Initial Military Training map.
AIT: advanced individual training
BCT: basic combat training
BOLC-B: Basic Officer Leader Course
MOS: military occupational specialty
OSUT: one station unit training
WOBC: Warrant Officer Basic Course

with military medical treatment facility (MTF) commanders, CoE leadership, Office of the Surgeon General staff, and other Army senior leaders. Due to the sensitivities of representing IMT and TRADOC, whenever the CIMT surgeon travels on temporary duty, it is appropriate to notify the local MTF and senior commander staff.

The CIMT surgeon participates in human research study proposal review and approval, oversight of all medical trends and analysis, consultation and advice on accessions health policy and line-of-duty regulations, review of training deaths and significant injuries, and other topics of concern to the IMT commander. Recommendations for changes to regulations governing IMT outside of TRADOC are submitted directly to the proponent for the regulation (in many cases, Army Medical Command [MEDCOM]). It is CIMT's responsibility to identify and address any policy, extending across all Army components, that affects the initial military population, including international students.

The CIMT surgeon also performs other missions as assigned. As an H2F action officer, the CIMT surgeon serves as an integral member of the development of the Army concept on H2F, policy and doctrine development, and fielding to the Total Army. For the ACFT, the CIMT surgeon supports doctrine and policy development, fielding, and related research.

While the CIMT surgeon position is administrative rather than clinical in nature, it is imperative that the incumbent maintain clinical practice and relevant medical technology infrastructure access. Fort Eustis is home to McDonald Army Health Clinic (MCAHC), which operates one MTF, two troop clinics (one permanent party, one for trainees), and a community medical home for dependents in Williamsburg. The CIMT surgeon should maintain privileges with MCAHC and provide the MTF with semi-routine clinician support. Maintaining privileges supports the CIMT surgeon's clinical competency, and allows the surgeon to better understand the challenges of caring for trainees, observe firsthand the medical condition of trainees, observe the implications of TRADOC policy on trainee care decisions, and provide periodic health assessment and soldier readiness processing support for the small number of operational forces on the installation when needed. While observing medical and TRADOC leadership issues related to health care on an SAV is relevant, the impact of experiencing those same issues as a clinician brings better clarity for enterprise solutions.

As the TRADOC senior PA, the officer in this position provides routine operational and programmatic updates to the Army PA branch chief, the PA consultant to the surgeon general, and other senior medical staff across the Army, Navy, Air Force, MEDCOM, Joint Staff, and Department of Homeland Security elements. The CIMT surgeon also briefs the Medical Specialists (SP) Corps chief on a quarterly basis regarding TRADOC operations affecting the SP Corps writ large. The CIMT surgeon is also encouraged to conduct regular interactions and briefings internal and external to the SP Corps and the PA community. He or she routinely works with the CIMT public affairs officer to present ACFT and H2F topics to the media and groups with an interest in military training.

Because the CIMT commander also functions as the senior mission commander/senior commander of the Army element at Joint Base Langley-Eustis, the CIMT surgeon also functions as an interlocutor and liaison between the Installation Management Command commander, the MTF commander, and the commanding general. Similarly, in case of an emergency such as a pandemic or another situation requiring a unified incident command, the CIMT surgeon works to facilitate coordination of IMT organic and installation assets and resources in support of the senior mission commander.

Training and Desired Characteristics

The CIMT surgeon must have completed Command and General Staff College, and prior service on a corps or Army service component command staff is desirable. Some background in research or public health is beneficial, as is former service on the Army staff. There is no requirement for a background in doctrine development, capabilities development and integration, or contracting; however, a familiarity with these subjects is highly beneficial.

Individuals must be extremely diligent in time and workflow management. Executive-level operations require that numerous high-level missions be conducted concurrently and executed to the highest possible standard. Individuals must think critically and apply measured responses to high-intensity drivers for change. The CIMT surgeon must consider the impact that each decision could have across TRADOC and the IMT enterprise, and be prepared to present senior and command leadership with appropriate, relevant, and thoughtful guidance.

The direct leadership role of the CIMT surgeon is small, supervising one noncommissioned officer and one Army civilian. However, the indirect leadership role spans the entire Army, involving constant interaction with leaders inside and outside the Department of Defense. The CIMT surgeon must be succinct in presenting complex ideas, considerate of Defense and Army policy and guidance, and cognizant that their comments may be perceived as official policy guidance.

TRADOC Organic Medical Structure Initiative

As of the first quarter of fiscal year 2020, TRADOC has been approved to proceed with changes to the current organic medical structure. Historically, a very low number of medical officers and medical enlisted personnel have served in TRADOC to provide health care to trainees in IMT. The TRADOC Organic Medical Structure (TOMS) initiative will bring a brigade (BDE)/battalion (BN) surgeon cell capability, traditionally seen in Forces Command, to TRADOC. TRADOC BDE-level BCT and OSUT units will be resourced with one surgeon (O-4, AOC 65D or 62B, field surgeon), a behavioral health officer (O-3 [captain], AOC 66R, behavioral health nurse practitioner), a medic (68W40), and a behavioral health noncommissioned officer (staff sergeant, MOS 68X20, behavioral health noncommissioned officer). As of this writing, BN echelons will receive one surgeon (O-3, AOC 65D or 66P, nurse practitioner, or possibly a contract clinician) and two medics (MOA 68W, health care specialist).

The intent of the TOMS structure is to provide TRADOC units with the organic support they need to generate and sustain readiness. Eventually, AIT units and Army reception battalions will also receive a complement of medical personnel. The TOMS staff will also serve as part of the governance structure for H2F (described below). Conceptually, the BDE/BN providers will function much as they do in the Forces Command realm, as personal staff to the commander advising on medical issues and readiness. It will be imperative for these staff to be well versed in their core skill sets as providers, and to be willing to use great initiative to drive needed changes and support their units. The senior BDE positions will become CoE surgeons and have an informal linkage to the TRADOC surgeon via the TRADOC DCG for Combined Arms.

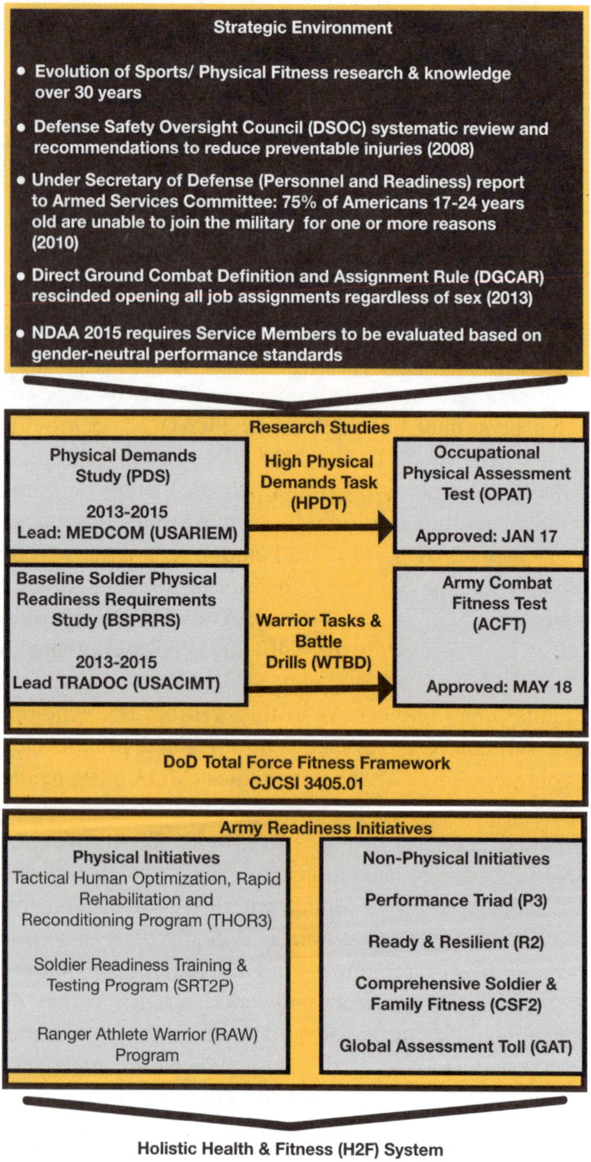

Figure 24-3. Holistic Health and Fitness (H2F) strategic environment. NDAA: National Defense Authorization Act

Holistic Health and Fitness

H2F is a comprehensive, integrated, and immersive health and fitness system that generates lethal soldiers who are physically, mentally, and spiritually ready to engage with and overmatch the enemy in multi-domain operations[12] (Figure 24-3). The system is composed of five elements—governance, programming, equipment, personnel, and leadership education—and spans five domains—physical, spiritual, mental, nutritional, and sleep. These elements, often absent or out of sync in legacy fitness programs, are essential to future Army readiness. As a system, the elements are aimed to comprehensively support all domains of soldier readiness.

The Army's continued investment in the human dimension will ensure soldiers are ready to deploy, fight, and win the nation's wars. From 2025 to 2030, physical and nonphysical performance training will continue to evolve as TRADOC, through IMT, develops plans for the integration of performance personnel into support brigades, Special Operations units, and training brigades. H2F personnel will expand to include cognitive enhancement and athletic trainer capabilities. In coordination with the Army Corps of Engineers and the Office of the Assistant Chief of Staff for Installation Management, TRADOC, through CIMT, will continue to develop the Soldier Performance Readiness Center training facility concept to provide a centralized location for unit-level physical and nonphysical performance training. Finally, TRADOC, through CIMT, will continue to align Army regulations and policies with the H2F doctrine, and begin systematic program assessment across units.

Army PAs must be prepared to support the H2F initiative as medical providers and medical readiness experts for their respective commanders. Army PAs must be integrated with the H2F leadership and staff to ensure continuity of care and conditioning for the entire command. While there are no formal leadership relationships between the BDE surgeon and the H2F staff, a preponderance of H2F staff are within the SP Corps, and include occupational therapists, physical therapists, and dieticians.

Lessons Learned and Tips for Success

Individuals considering service as the TRADOC CIMT PA should be prepared for a high-paced and rewarding position with a substantial impact on the generating force. Individuals must be willing to reach across the Army to accomplish a wide variety of missions and champion the health of the trainee. Understanding basic research and statistical analysis principles is helpful due to the wide variety of research and analysis conducted in the trainee realm. The CIMT PA should understand the generalizability of findings and be able to convey complex analysis in general terms. The position includes moderate amounts of travel.

Conclusion

Service as the TRADOC CIMT command surgeon is a rewarding position that provides the incumbent with the unique opportunity to affect the Army generating force. The scope of the position continues to grow as CIMT and TRADOC implement new Army-wide initiatives. The position allows the incumbent to leave a lasting and profoundly positive mark on the Army for years to come.

References

1. US Army Training and Doctrine Command website. Accessed April 14, 2020. http://www.tradoc.army.mil/
2. US Army Training and Doctrine Command. US Army Expert Soldier Badge. Accessed April 14, 2020. https://usacimt.tradoc.army.mil/ESB
3. US Army Training and Doctrine Command. *The Soldier's Blue Book.* TRADOC; 2019. TRADOC Pamphlet 600-4.
4. US Army. Army Combat Fitness Test. Accessed April 14, 2020. https://www.army.mil/acft/
5. Headquarters, Department of the Army. *Army Physical Readiness Training*. DA; 2019. Field Manual 7-22.
6. US Army Training and Doctrine Command. *Enlisted Initial Entry Training Policies and Administration*. TRADOC; 2019. TRADOC Regulation 350-6.
7. US Army Training and Doctrine Command. *Drill Sergeant Program*. TRADOC; 2018. TRADOC Regulation 350-16.

8. US Army Training and Doctrine Command. *Basic Officer Leader Training Policies and Administration*. TRADOC; 2017. TRADOC Regulation 350-36.
9. US Army Training and Doctrine Command. *Prevention of Heat and Cold Casualties*. TRADOC; 2016. TRADOC Regulation 350-29.
10. Headquarters, Department of the Army. *Standards of Medical Fitness*. DA; 2019. Army Regulation 40-501.
11. Headquarters, Department of the Army. *Initial Entry/Prior Service Trainee Support*. DA; 2017. Army Regulation 612-201.
12. US Army Training and Doctrine Command. *Holistic Health and Fitness Operating Concept Version 1-5.* TRADOC; 2020.

Section 4

Topics of Interest

Chapter 25

ROLE OF THE DIVISION PHYSICIAN ASSISTANT

Stephanie Bocanegra, PA-C, MPAS; David W. Broussard, PA-C, MPAS; Peter Carroll, PA-C, MPAS; Walter Engle, PA-C, MPAS; and Bradley Tibbetts, PA-C, MPAS

Introduction

The mission of the division physician assistant (DIV PA) is to serve as advisor to the division surgeon (DIV SURG) on clinical operations (CLINOPS), liaise with the local military medical treatment facility (MTF), and provide mentorship and career advice to all PAs within the division. With 10 active component divisions within the US Army, being selected to serve in one of these highly sought-after positions is not something to be taken lightly. The DIV PA serves as a medical subject matter expert under the sustainment warfighting function and is pivotal in helping create policy and synchronize health service support. Additionally, the DIV PA provides guidance, leadership, and mentorship to all medical personnel within the formation. DIV PAs have similar duties and functions as battalion or brigade PAs, but with differences in the level of complexity, scope of planning, and professional obligations affecting the Army health system. This chapter will provide information on both the clinical and administrative duties and responsibilities of the DIV PA.

Division Command Structure

The commanding general (CG) has clearly defined responsibilities and authorities for key leaders of the command group. Four principal assistants help the CG carry out their duties. They are the deputy commanding general for maneuver (DCG [M]), the deputy commanding general for support (DCG [S]), the chief of staff (CoS), and the division command sergeant major (DCSM). Each is delegated the authority to supervise execution of decisions and guidance policies, and to clarify these for subordinates as required.[1] The command group's medical responsibilities are as follows:

- The **DCG (M)** oversees brigade combat teams. Along with the DCSM, the DCG (M) also oversees expert field medical badge testing.
- The **DCG (S)** has responsibility for the combat aviation brigade, fires brigade, division headquarters, and headquarters battalion. Other areas of responsibility include force health protection, profile review boards, fatality review boards, and wounded warrior programs. The DCG (S) also oversees the division deployment and redeployment efforts, and the sexual harassment/assault response and prevention and suicide prevention programs.
- The **CoS** coordinates staff actions with the corps staff and brigade combat teams in support of policy and guidance from the CG and deputy CGs. The CoS supervises the general and special staffs, and every activity that occurs within the division is of special interest to the CoS. The DIV SURG staff works with other staff officers and reports through the CoS to the DCG (S) to ensure they are apprised of all matters related to medical support.
- The **DCSM** is the principal advisor to the CG on all matters pertaining to noncommissioned officers (NCOs), enlisted soldiers, and soldiers' family members. This includes being apprised of the health and welfare of the command. The DCSM oversees expert field medical badge testing in support of the DCG (M), all warrior tasks and drills, and individual training of soldiers, including medical training.

The Division Surgeon Section

The DIV SURG section (Table 25-1) is headed by the DIV SURG, who is a special staff officer to the CG and the senior medical advisor for the division. In accordance with Army Training Publication 4-02.3, the DIV SURG "…coordinates AHS [Army Health System] support under the sustainment warfighting function with the division assistant chief of staff, logistics, the division chief of staff, and other headquarters elements that affect AHS support in the division."[1(p20)] The DIV SURG

Table 25-1. Division Surgeon Section personnel.

Paragraph title	AOC/MOS	Grade	Title	Branch	Quantity
Division Surgeon Section	60A00	O5	Surgeon	MC	1
	70H67	O5	Medical Operations Officer	MS	1
	60W00	O4	Psychiatrist	MC	1
	65D00	O4	Physician Assistant	SP	1
	67J00	O4	Aeromedical Evacuation Officer	MS	1 1
	70E67	O4	Patient Administration Officer	MS	1
	70H67	O4	Medical Plans Officer	MS	1
	70K67	O4	Health Service Materiel Officer	MS	1
	72D67	O4	Environmental Science Officer	MS	1
	68Z50	E9	Chief Medical Noncommissioned Officer	NC	1
	68W50	E8	Operations Noncommissioned Officer	NC	1
	68W40	E7	Operations Sergeant	NC	1
	68J30	E6	Medical Logistics Sergeant	NC	1
	68W30	E6	Medical Noncommissioned Officer	NC	1

LEGEND:

AOC	area of concentration	MS	Medical Service Corps
MC	Medical Corps	NC	noncommissioned
MOS	military occupational specialty	SP	Army Medical Specialist Corps

Reproduced from: Headquarters, Department of the Army. *Army Health System Support to Maneuver Forces.* HQDA; 2014. Army Training Publication 4-02.3:20.

section is staffed differently in the Army's various divisions (airborne, cavalry, armor, air assault). The example in Table 25-1 is comprised of 14 soldiers, including 9 officers and 5 NCOs. When deployed, the DIV SURG section can also be augmented by additional personnel such as a preventive medicine officer, public health nurse, and pharmacist.

Besides the DIV SURG and the DIV PA, two additional key roles within this section are the chief medical NCO and the Deputy DIV SURG. The chief medical NCO, who works closely with the DIV SURG and is the senior enlisted leader for the section, typically holds the rank of sergeant major. The chief medical NCO is responsible for the same functions as the DCSM related to medical tasks and the assignments of NCOs and enlisted personnel, while working closely with Human Resources Command (HRC), division manpower and personnel (G1), and the DCSM. The deputy DIV SURG is typically the senior medical operations officer within the section. The deputy DIV SURG coordinates and supervises the work of the DIV SURG staff, tracks all internal and external tasks and projects that involve the section, and attends the CG's staff meetings, funneling information and guidance from the meetings to the separate sections within the DIV SURG office. In some cases, the DIV PA serves as the deputy DIV SURG and chief of CLINOPS (discussed in more detail below).

Supervision

Supervision of the DIV PA is performed by the DIV SURG as outlined in Army regulations (ARs) 623-3,[2] 40-3,[3] and 40-68,[4] and in the local MTF credential policies. The DIV PA is typically rated by the DIV SURG and senior-rated by the division CoS.

Requirements

Those seeking a position as a DIV PA must:

- be a certified PA with ability to maintain credentialed provider status and Basic Life Support certification at the installation MTF;
- have the rank of a senior major (Intermediate Level Education graduate preferred);
- be capable of deploying outside the continental United States;

- have a history of diverse assignments, including as battalion or squadron PA, brigade or regiment PA, or another table-of-organization-and-equipment unit staff position;
- have writing skills using the Army writing style;
- have knowledge of computer automation systems, including the Medical Readiness Portal and all modules within the Medical Operational Data System (MODS); and
- be familiar with orders production.

Duties and Responsibilities

The DIV PA functions as the advisor to the DIV SURG on all PA matters and CLINOPS. In the division, the DIV PA may also serve as the chief of CLINOPS and/or as the deputy DIV SURG, depending on mission and section manning. Primary functions of the position are divided into three main categories: CLINOPS, MTF liaison, and professional development of PAs.

Clinical Operations

The DIV PA is responsible for keeping the DIV SURG informed of all clinical aspects of the division. This responsibility covers both garrison and field operations, so clinical aspects of the garrison standard operating procedures and the medical annex to all operations orders (OPORDs) are his or her responsibility, when delegated. The DIV PA coordinates and provides guidance to the brigade surgeons and PAs on:

- predeployment readiness, the sustained readiness model, and redeployment preparation, in accordance with regulatory guidance and close coordination with the installation soldier readiness processing site or deployment readiness centers[5,6];
- battalion or brigade aid station operations and operations within the Soldier-Centered Medical Home clinics;
- the first responder program and combat lifesaver course in accordance with Tactical Combat Casualty Care guidelines and the Joint Trauma System[7];
- medical training and sustainment for medics (68W military occupational specialty)[8];
- clinical aspects of medical evacuation for air and ground in

coordination with the MTF, installation emergency medical services, and installation training area range control for daily operations and mass casualty management;
- profiles and the profile review board, including controlled substance profiling and reporting;
- management of the Integrated Disability Evaluation System;
- coordinate for clinical quality management[4]; and
- continuing medical education and individual critical task list (ICTL) training for credentialed providers in the division.[8]

Military Medical Treatment Facility Liaison

Close coordination between the units and the local MTF are crucial to medical support for soldiers. All garrison health care is the responsibility of the MTF commander. The way in which a DIV PA augments the MTF's mission directly impacts the support provided by the MTF for the division. The DIV PA can help foster this relationship by participating in the risk management program, or by contributing to root cause analyses after serious adverse events. Coordinating calendars for borrowed military medical personnel clinic schedules, training, or deployment with the MTF and Soldier-Centered Medical Home will support continuity of care.

Physician Assistant Professional Development

Teaching, coaching, and mentoring the division's approximately 40 PAs is essential to the success of the division's medical mission and the professional development of Army PAs. Fostering an environment of support and teamwork and providing guidance on policies and systems that work will ensure that no one fails the commander.

- The DIV PA should begin by educating the brigade PAs on the essential items in a professional officer's career: the officer evaluation report (OER), officer record brief (ORB), Army photo, and curriculum vitae. ORBs (including photos) should be reviewed during each routine counseling session and updated as necessary. ORBs are used not only by promotion boards, but also by the 65D (PA) consultant and the HRC branch representative to facilitate selections for special assignments. Recommendations for each PA's personal growth,

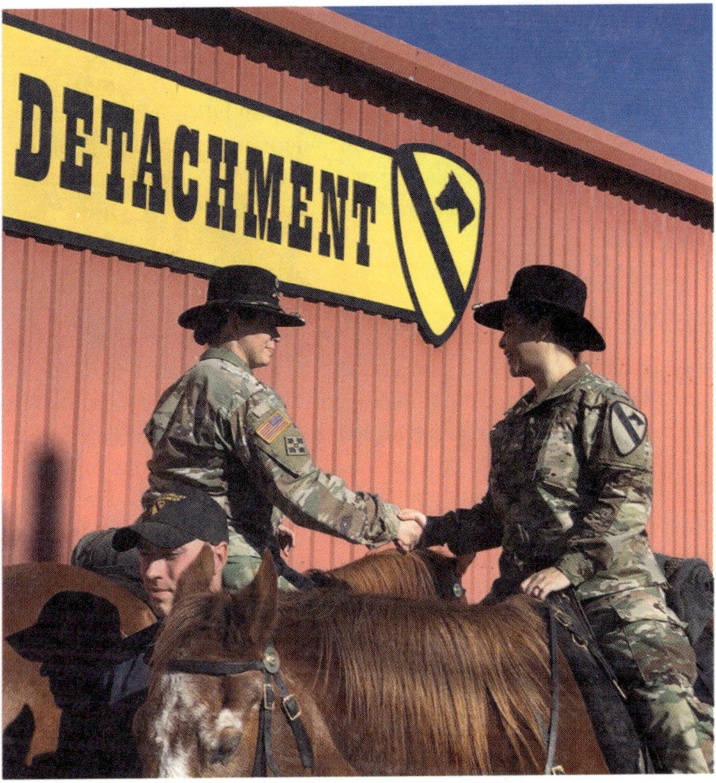

Figure 25-1. Major Stephanie M. Bocanegra (left), the 1st Cavalry Division physician assistant, dedicates time during a command post exercise to promote Captain Joelle I. Black (right) to major at the 1st Cavalry Division Horse Cavalry Detachment in December 2019. Photo courtesy of Major Stephanie Bocanegra.

military and civilian education, and assignments are also discussed during counseling sessions. Consideration should be given to attending appropriate military education and leadership schools, such as the flight surgeon, air assault, airborne, or expert field medical badge courses, and attaining skill sets and additional skill identifiers (ASIs) while accomplishing ICTL-required training.[8] Each brigade PA and the DIV PA can review all OERs and ORBs to assist brigade surgeons in their rating responsibilities and PA career progression.

- The DIV PA should seek counseling and mentorship for themself by pursuing a monthly telephone or in-person conference with the corps PA (III, XVIII, or I Corps) and the US Army-Europe PA to collaborate and share lessons learned by all DIV PAs.
- The DIV PA manages division personnel in special positions requiring ASIs or specific experience, such as serving in a combat aviation battalion or being aeromedically qualified (Figure 25-1).

Garrison Duties

The DIV PA has additional duties that can be categorized as garrison and deployment duties. Garrison duties are those that the DIV PA performs when they are not deployed. The DIV PA's garrison duties depend on the unit of assignment and the expectations of the DIV SURG. The deputy DIV SURG coordinates day-to-day operations of all DIV SURG staff personnel and their products. The DIV PA's time, unless otherwise directed, is divided among meetings, staff work, training, and clinic. A variety of meetings are attended on a weekly, monthly, or quarterly basis, such as the following (dependent on unit command, higher headquarters, and installation MTF timelines):

- clinic provider meeting (weekly),
- DIV SURG synchronization meeting (monthly),
- soldier recovery unit approval meeting (monthly),
- Suicide Engagement Response Team meeting (monthly),
- PA meeting (monthly),
- division and corps profile review board (monthly and quarterly respectively),
- medical evaluation board preparation meeting (quarterly),
- MTF risk management meeting (as needed), and
- MTF root cause analysis meeting (as needed).

The DIV PA should review all OPORDs and fragmentation orders for clinically relevant material. On occasion an order that is solely clinical in nature must be written by the CLINOPS section, with the DIV PA taking the lead. Reporting is limited to clinical information such as the disease and nonbattle injury report, narcotics inventory reports during field operations, and immunization reports. Time during the month must also be scheduled for providing health care. Because the DIV PA is a staff officer, command

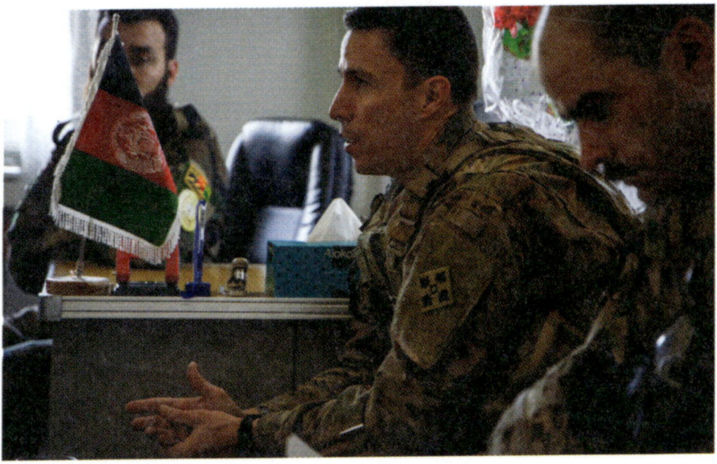

Figure 25-2. Major Christopher B. Cordova, the 4th Infantry Division physician assistant, conducts a medical advising engagement with the Afghan National Army, 203rd Corps, Medical School commandant, at Forward Operating Base Thunder in Gardez, Afghanistan, in February 2019. Photo credit Sergeant First Class Shana Hutchins.

group clinical support is not a primary responsibility, but it is essential for fostering the DIV PA's education and relations with colleagues.

The DIV SURG and DIV PA are responsible for the medical training conducted for division personnel. The DIV PA's ability to coordinate with the MTF, the installation medical simulation training center, and the Medical Center of Excellence at Joint Base San Antonio is vital to ensure that sustainment and predeployment preparedness medical training are conducted in accordance with Army Regulation (AR) 40-68,[4] Department of Defense Instruction 1322.24,[5] AR 350-1,[9] and Medical Command Pamphlet 40-7-21.[10]

Deployment Duties

During deployment operations, the DIV PA employs the training and preparation completed during garrison operations. Deployment is basically the capstone event, where the DIV PA's function will be tested. It is imperative to be up-to-date on medical regulatory guidance and tactics, techniques, and procedures (TTPs); to remain resilient and confident; and to be available to leadership as well as subordinate unit leadership as a subject matter expert. During deployment, the DIV PA normally supports the CLINOPS section of the DIV SURG staff, which has three additional personnel assigned:

- A preventive medicine officer (60C) physician, or environmental science officer (72D) non-physician, assigned to perform disease and nonbattle injury surveillance, advise the DIV SURG on matters relating to disease prevention, and inspect food and water sites and contracting personnel.
- A public health nurse (66B), who assists the preventive medicine officer with surveillance, immunization tracking, rabies treatment monitoring, positive results on blood donation screening, and other assignments.
- A pharmacist (67E), who assists with narcotics inventory reports, adverse drug reactions, cold chain monitoring, and special drug requests (Figure 25-2).

Battlefield Circulation

One of the most important deployment functions of the DIV PA, as the chief of CLINOPS, is battlefield circulation. Battlefield circulation requires the DIV PA to move across the division footprint into brigade battlespaces to assess the different roles of care. This is not only a morale function, but will also address shortfalls, test new TTPs, and capture lessons learned from the overall experience. A regular rotation of visits to battalion aid stations throughout the operational environment can provide a wealth of experience and guidance to new providers and medics needing assistance. During battlefield circulation, information is gained that no amount of reporting can achieve.

As part of their battlefield duties, the DIV PA assists in preparations for Purple Heart presentations. The CG, DCSM, and a State Department senior civilian representative present Purple Heart medals at Role 3 MTFs to soldiers within their command. The DIV PA reviews the medical records for pertinent information to answer command group inquiries on the patient's condition prior to the presentation. The DIV SURG is responsible for briefing the CG, and may also be involved in briefing State Department officials prior to the presentation.

Personnel Recovery Coordination Cell Medical Advisor

The DIV PA is also the personnel recovery coordination cell (PRCC) medical advisor. The division is responsible if a soldier, sailor, airman, or marine becomes isolated due to capture, aviation mishap, or dislocation. During phase 1 reintegration of a formerly isolated returnee, the primary focus is the medical and psychological care of the returnee and the tactical debriefing.[11] The PRCC varies according to unit size and need, but contains at a minimum a chief; assistant chief; medical advisor; survival, evasion, resistance, and escape psychiatrist; and debriefer. As the medical advisor, the DIV PA advises the PRCC chief on the medical condition of the recovered personnel and the options for a timely debrief should the availability exist. Personnel recovery training is provided prior to deployment by the Joint Personnel Recovery Agency.[11,12]

Lessons Learned and Tips for Success

Good expectation management is essential when entering this position. Intending to take the position and change the PA world overnight will result in a great deal of frustration. In a time when PA shortages are significant, DIV PAs will fill different roles within subordinate units in order to assist with their mission. It is important to remain flexible, empower junior PAs to figure things out on their own, and try to "be the change you want to see."

Conclusion

The DIV PA plays an integral role in the overall Army health system, affecting division readiness and CLINOPS in both garrison and deployed settings. The DIV PA is a leader and subject matter expert who works hand-in-hand with the DIV SURG in key advisory and operational roles while synchronizing health service support across division activities. DIV PAs serve as a bridge between the unit and the MTF, promoting readiness, health protection, and preventive care while also coordinating sustainment warfighter functions, continuing education training, clinical quality care, and professional development. To serve as a US Army DIV PA is an incredible honor and a credit to those selected.

References

1. Headquarters, Department of the Army. *Army Health System Support to Maneuver Forces*. HQDA; 2014. Army Training Publication 4-02.3.
2. Headquarters, Department of the Army. *Evaluation Reporting System*. HQDA; 2019. Army Regulation 623-3.
3. Headquarters, Department of the Army. *Medical, Dental, and Veterinary Care*. HQDA; 2013. Army Regulation 40-3.
4. Headquarters, Department of the Army. *Clinical Quality Management*. HQDA; 2009. Army Regulation 40-68.
5. Department of Defense. *Medical Readiness Training*. DOD; March 2018. DOD Instruction 1322.24.
6. Headquarters, Department of the Army. *Standards of Medical Fitness*. HQDA; June 2019. Army Regulation 40-501.
7. Officer of the Under Secretary of Defense for Personnel Readiness. *Joint Trauma System (JTS)*. Department of Defense; 2016 (Change 1 effective August 5, 2018). DOD Instruction 6040.47. Accessed June 15, 2020. https://www.esd.whs.mil/Portals/54/Documents/DD/issuances/dodi/604047p.pdf?ver=2018-08-06-124902-047.
8. Headquarters, Department of the Army. *Medical Education and Demonstration of Individual Competence*. HQDA; October 2015. Training Circular 8-800.
9. Headquarters, Department of the Army. *Army Training and Leader Development*. HQDA; 2017. Army Regulation 350-1.
10. US Army Medical Command. *Algorithm Directed Troop Medical Care*. June 2006. Army Medical Command Pamphlet 40-7-21.
11. Headquarters, Department of the Army. *Army Personnel Recovery*. HQDA; 2014. Field Manual 3-50.
12. US Department of Defense. *Personnel Recovery*. DOD; 2011. Joint Publication 3-50.

Chapter 26

ROLE OF THE PHYSICIAN ASSISTANT AS THE CONGRESSIONAL LEGISLATIVE LIAISON

Sean M. Donohue, PA-C, MPAS, and Maureen Giorio, PA-C, MPAS, MHA

"The Congress shall have the power to . . . raise and support Armies, but no Appropriation of Money to that use shall be for a longer term than two years."

—*Article I, Section 8, Clause 12 of the US Constitution*

Introduction

The mission of the Office of the Chief, Legislative Liaison (OCLL), is to provide effective liaison between the US Army and Congress to gain congressional trust and support. This is a strategic mission that involves the participation of legislative subject matter experts from across the Army. The chief of legislative liaison (CLL) is directly responsible to the secretary of the Army (SECARMY) regarding legislative affairs, including formulating, coordinating, supervising, and executing the Army's congressional policy and strategy. The CLL ensures the overall integration of the Army's efforts with Congress, develops comprehensive congressional engagement strategies for Army senior leaders (ASLs), and disseminates critical information on all significant congressional activities.[1]

Army congressional fellows, other Army officers, senior noncommissioned officers (typically sergeants major), and Army civilians comprise the staff of OCLL. These individuals represent various interests and portfolios to members of Congress (MoCs) and their personal and professional staff. Numerous Army civilians, including two in Senior Executive Service positions, manage daily operations, strategic planning, and routine correspondence to MoCs and congressional staff who serve on committees of authorization (primarily the House Armed Services Committee, and Senate Armed Services Committee, and associated subcommittees). The assistant secretary of the Army for financial management, budget liaison (SAFM-BUL), accomplishes much of the same functions as the OCLL; however, the SAFM-BUL deals specifically with MoCs responsible for congressional appropriations (eg, the House Committee on Appropriations–Defense).

Army Medicine Within the Legislative Community

Army medicine maintains two positions within the legislative liaison community. The first position is an 05A (area-of-concentration-immaterial Medical Portfolio Lead) within the OCLL Programs division, which has been occupied by officers from the varying medical branches of the Army Medical Department (Army Nurse Corps, Medical Specialist Corps, Medical Corps, Medical Service Corps). This position is assigned to the Army Medical Command (MEDCOM) with duty in the Pentagon under the personnel services directorate. The position covers all topics germane to Army health care and is focused on defense authorizers with oversight interests in the Army health system, as well as committees within their jurisdiction, including the House and Senate armed services committees. Typically, the officer is a senior major and a Command and General Staff College graduate who is selected by the Office of the Surgeon General (OTSG) in consultation with MEDCOM.

The second position, coded for a 70C (Medical Comptroller), is assigned to OTSG with duty at SAFM-BUL, also located at the Pentagon. The SAFM-BUL position focuses exclusively on congressional appropriation committees. The OCLL and SAFM-BUL medical portfolio liaisons work closely with the MEDCOM congressional affairs contact officer (CACO) and senior OTSG/MEDCOM leaders to craft Army medicine messages, develop a congressional engagement strategy to socialize and explain Army medical policies to relevant MoCs and committees, escort Army medical leaders to meetings and hearings on Capitol Hill, and escort MoCs and their staff to Army health care entities worldwide.

A third position was established within the OCLL House Liaison Division (HLD) by Lieutenant General Patricia Horoho, the 43rd Army surgeon general, to increase the Army medicine presence on Capitol Hill and perform critical functions as a forward medical liaison. As liaison to the House, this person serves the preponderance of the congressional community. Responsibilities of this position are primarily those of a legislative liaison and include planning, supporting, and executing Army events on Capitol Hill; rapidly responding to questions about medical policy and operations; supporting ASL meetings and engagements with MoCs and their staff; and supporting congressional travel when requested. As a MEDCOM asset, the position provides an unparalleled opportunity to support Army medical leadership engagements on Capitol Hill.

Unit Structure

The OCLL falls under the Secretariat of the Army (Figure 26-1) and is led by a major general who reports directly to the under secretary of the Army and the SECARMY (both of whom are nominated by the president and confirmed by the Senate). Within OCLL are seven subdirectorates (Figure 26-2), each led by a colonel (or GS-15 civilian): the House, Senate, Operations, Inquiry, Programs, Investigations and Legislation, and Management and Support divisions.[2] The Senate division functions much like the House division, but with a smaller staff. The Operations division manages OCLL plans, training, and strategy. The Inquiry division tracks, researches, and replies to inquiries originating from MoCs and their staff. The Programs division contains subdivisions that manage various portfolios, including medical, munitions, tracked vehicles, rotary-wing aircraft, cyber, missile defense, personnel, and many other subjects. Investigations and Legislation manages all operations involving legal review and prepares political appointees and general officers for confirmation hearings. The Management and Support office conducts the daily management of OCLL and supports congressional travel operations. The medical legislative liaison is typically rated by the division deputy chief (a GS-14 civilian) and senior-rated by the division chief, usually a colonel or equivalent (O-6 or GS-15).[2] A liaison who is a practicing medical provider may choose to have an intermediate rating by their supervising physician if applicable under the provisions of Army Regulation (AR) 623-3, *Evaluation Reporting System*.[3]

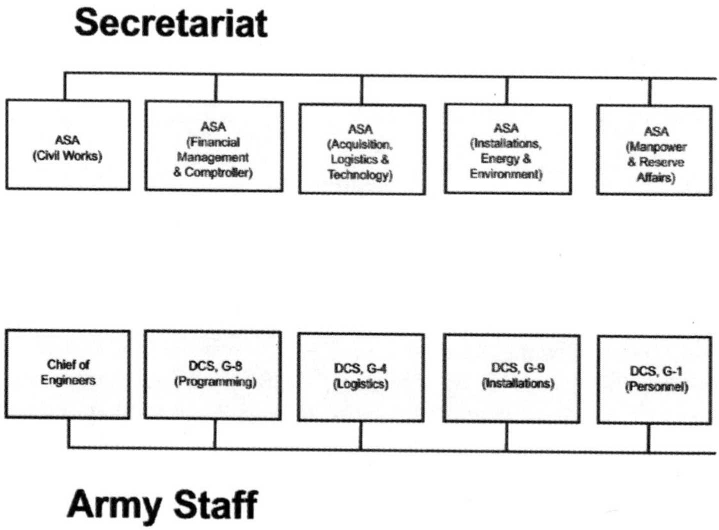

Figure 26-1. Structure of the Headquarters, Department of the Army.
ASA: Assistant Secretary of the Army
CSA: Chief of Staff of the Army
DCS: Deputy Chief of Staff
SECARMY: Secretary of the Army
USA: Under Secretary of the Army
VCSA: Vice Chief of Staff of the Army

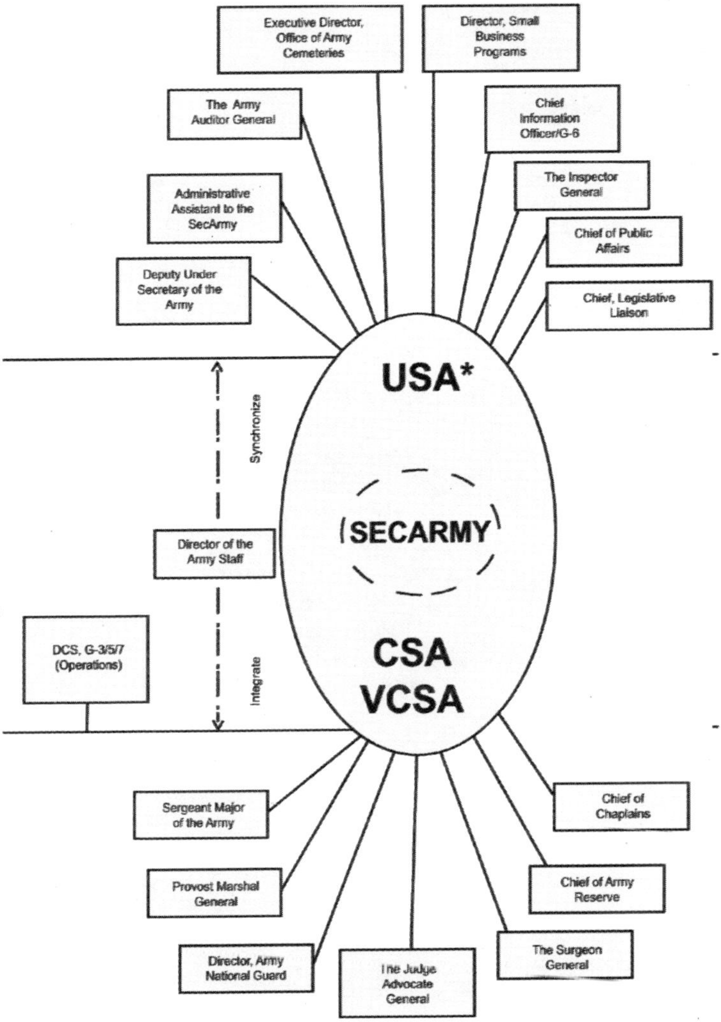
Executive Director, Office of Army Cemeteries
Director, Small Business Programs
The Army Auditor General
Chief Information Officer/G-6
Administrative Assistant to the SecArmy
The Inspector General
Chief of Public Affairs
Deputy Under Secretary of the Army
Chief, Legislative Liaison
USA*
Synchronize
SECARMY
Director of the Army Staff
DCS, G-3/5/7 (Operations)
Integrate
CSA
VCSA
Sergeant Major of the Army
Chief of Chaplains
Provost Marshal General
Chief of Army Reserve
Director, Army National Guard
The Judge Advocate General
The Surgeon General

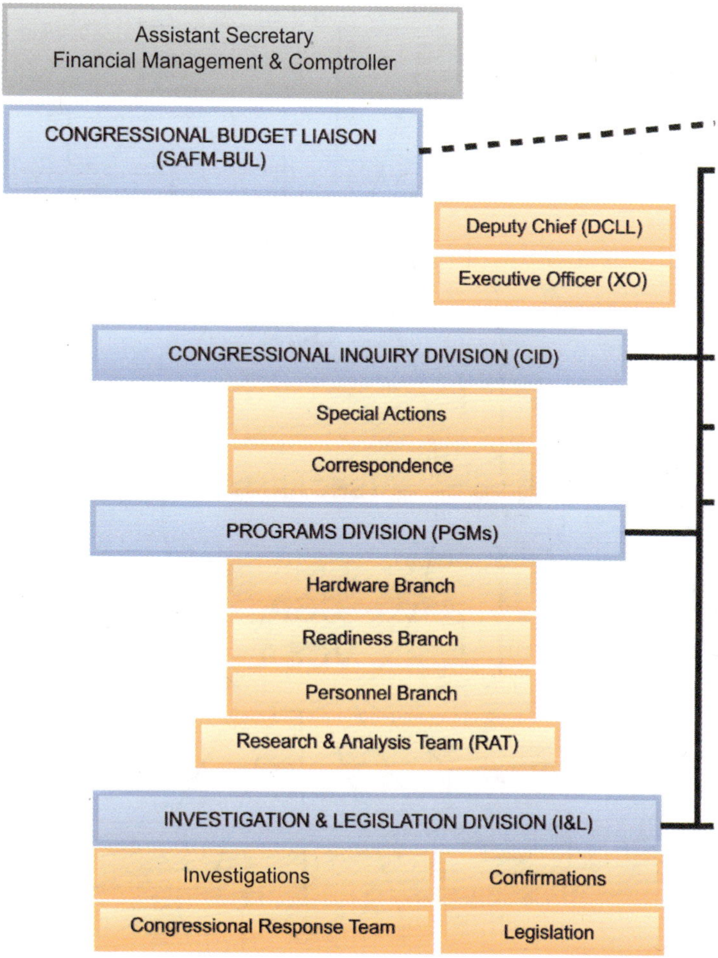

Figure 26-2. Office of the Chief, Legislative Liaison, organization chart.
ACOM: Army command
ARSTAFF: Army staff
ASCC: Army service component command
DRU: direct reporting unit
SAFM-BUL: Secretary of the Army, Financial Management–Budget Liaison

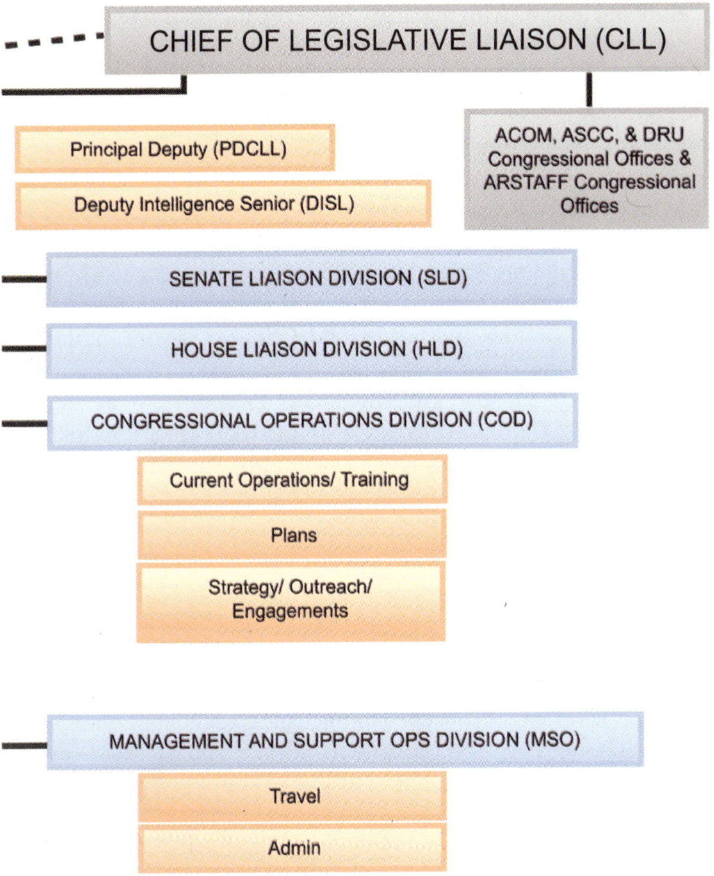
CHIEF OF LEGISLATIVE LIAISON (CLL)
Principal Deputy (PDCLL)
Deputy Intelligence Senior (DISL)
ACOM, ASCC, & DRU Congressional Offices & ARSTAFF Congressional Offices
SENATE LIAISON DIVISION (SLD)
HOUSE LIAISON DIVISION (HLD)
CONGRESSIONAL OPERATIONS DIVISION (COD)
Current Operations/ Training
Plans
Strategy/ Outreach/ Engagements
MANAGEMENT AND SUPPORT OPS DIVISION (MSO)
Travel
Admin

Legislative Liaison as a Clinician

The legislative liaison position is not wholly consistent with the execution of routine clinical duties due to the OCLL's high operational tempo. With planning, however, the position is amenable to maintaining at least the minimum clinical requirements called for in policy: title 37 USC § 335, Pay and Allowances of the Uniformed Services[4]; Department of Defense Instruction (DoDI) 6000.13, *Accession and Retention Policies, Programs, and Incentives for Military Health Professions Officers*[5]; and AR 40-68, *Clinical Quality Management.*[6]

Options for credentialing in the national capital region (NCR) are numerous, including Walter Reed National Military Medical Center, the Fort Meade Army Medical Activity, and Fort Belvoir Community Hospital. DiLorenzo Troop Medical Clinic (DTMC), under the oversight of Fort Belvoir, is located in the Pentagon (8th corridor) and may provide the most appropriate option for guest providers due to its proximity to Capitol Hill and the OCLL-HLD offices. Individuals can easily utilize the Washington DC Metro, Pentagon shuttles, or a personal vehicle (parking is available at the Pentagon). The Fort McNair Army Health Clinic, under the oversight of Fort Meade, and Radar Health Clinic, at Joint Base Myer-Henderson Hall, also offer guest provider options, with dedicated parking and quick access to the Waterfront Metro Station. The DTMC serves a preponderance of the 26,000 people working in the Pentagon and consistently needs support in the acute, primary, or executive care clinics. Credentials and privileges at DTMC are obtained through the credentialing coordinator at Fort Belvoir. It is also possible to work at other regional clinics within the NCR, including Fort Myers, Joint Base Anacostia–Bolling, and Andrews Air Force Base.

Numerous MoCs and their staff are members of the Army National Guard or Reserve and routinely contact OCLL for various support functions. When OCLL-HLD is occupied by a credentialed and privileged provider, the position is capable of supporting basic Army medical readiness requirements, such as periodic health assessments and vision screenings, for these individuals; additional support can be provided as appropriate. Providers assigned to OCLL do not function as the primary care provider or medical operations officer for MoCs or the OCLL and should maintain caution and boundaries as appropriate. Health care for MoCs and congressional staff with congressional health insurance is provided by the Office of the Attending Physician or through the individuals' insurance provider.

Daily Operations

Liaisons who work exclusively on Capitol Hill usually wear formal business attire (business suits that are dark in color, white or blue shirt with a conservative tie, or similar attire for men, and commensurate business attire for women). When Congress is not in session, more relaxed business casual attire is appropriate (eg, open-collar shirts or Army-related polo-style shirts). There is no uniform allowance for officers assigned to OCLL. When working at the Pentagon, liaisons may wear the Army Combat Uniform (ACU) within the building, but must wear formal business attire (or Army Service Uniform with cap or Army Green Uniform with cap) when conducting business on Capitol Hill. At no time should soldiers wear the ACU on Capitol Hill. When escorting ASLs, liaisons commonly wear business attire. When traveling in support of congressional delegations or congressional staff delegations, liaisons should anticipate wearing both business attire and business casual attire throughout; liaisons will not wear military uniforms or carry weapons (Figure 26-3).

Beyond daily interaction with military legislative staff, liaisons provide a critical role in supporting and shaping congressional oversight travel. MoCs and their staff routinely execute oversight visits to military treatment facilities (MTFs) and other medical facilities to ensure that the Department of Defense (DOD) and Army Medical Department (AMEDD) are responsible stewards of appropriated funds and in compliance with legislative changes and policy implementation. Congressional travel may be investigative in nature (causing elevated concern), or purely informational (Figure 26-4). In conjunction with various CACOs, liaisons help develop delegation itineraries that include presentations, demonstrations, tours, and activities of interest to the MoC or their staff. Coordinating for travel includes planning for all aspects, including but not limited to arranging air and ground transportation; coordinating with government, nongovernment, and possibly foreign agencies to conduct requested meetings; managing all baggage and support supplies for travel, planning events, and meals; and managing and disbursing per diems. The OCLL Management Support Operations office supports liaisons in these efforts.

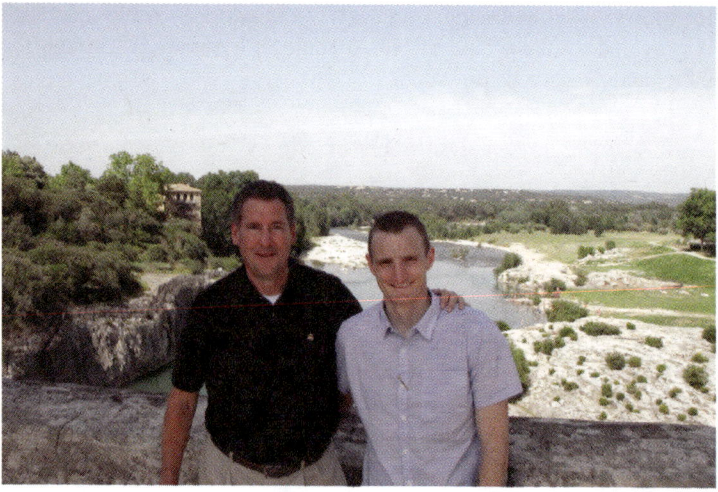

Figure 26-3. Major Sean Donohue and Representative Greg Harper of Mississippi's 3rd Congressional District, in Provence, France, on a congressional delegation addressing national museums, digitizing national archive content, and cybersecurity for national museum operations; May 2019.

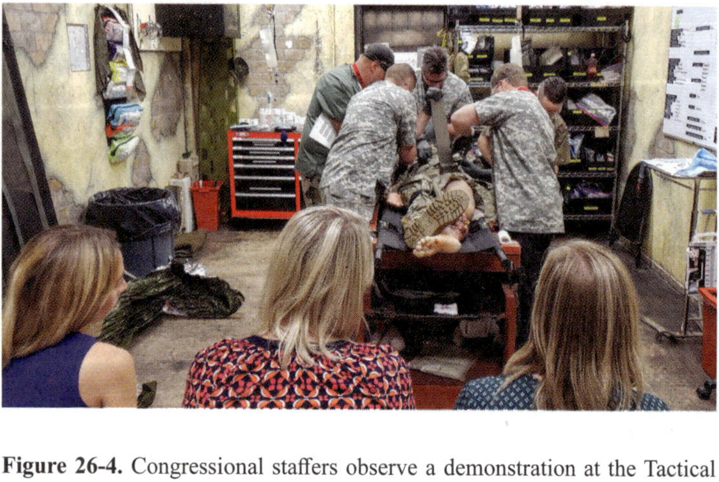

Figure 26-4. Congressional staffers observe a demonstration at the Tactical Combat Medicine Course, Joint Base San Antonio, Texas, September 2018.

Liaisons may also be tasked with coordinating and executing Army briefings in the US Capitol complex. This includes advertising the events, contracting for catering, and providing a room and audio-visual support. Liaisons may also plan for and execute large-scale events such as the Army Birthday Congressional Cake Cutting ceremony (Figure 26-5), the Joint Service Congressional Social, and other Army and Defense Secretariat-level congressional receptions. Liaisons may also be called on to support other defense and NCR missions such as state funerals, the State of the Union address, and the presidential inauguration.

Medical Recruiting Liaison

The legislative liaison positions also serve as a liaison between Army medical recruiting and Congress. Historically, the OCLL-HLD liaison has assisted in the recruitment of MoCs into the Army Reserve Medical

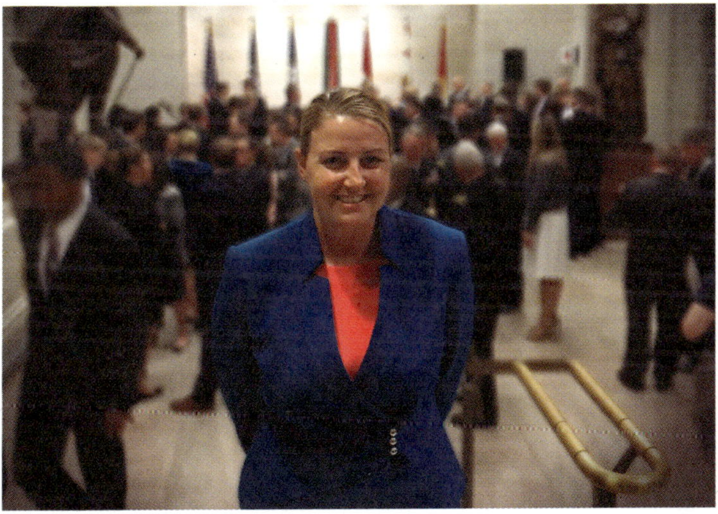

Figure 26-5. Lieutenant Colonel Maureen (Mo) Giorio stands in the US Capitol Congressional Atrium during the Army Birthday Congressional Reception, June 2016. The Congressional Cake Cutting ceremony recognizes the connection the Army has with Congress and the establishment of the Continental Army by congressional resolution in 1776.

Corps, assisted staff with enlisting in the Army, recruited civilians visiting the office, and helped congressional offices assist constituents who join the AMEDD through their local medical recruiting office.

Army Congressional Fellowship Program

Those wishing to complete the Army Congressional Fellowship Program should reference AR 1-202, *Army Congressional Fellowship Program.*[7] The fellowship program provides outstanding commissioned officers, noncommissioned officers, and Army civilians with firsthand experience and understanding of the strategic relationships between the Army and Congress, and allows fellows to learn about the Army as an institution through contact with Army personnel working in their office. Officers wishing to apply for the fellowship should be in the grade of captain or major (O-3 or O-4), with at least 6 years of active federal commissioned service, and have graduated from the Captains Career Course. Upon selection by the annual liaison selection board, students will conduct a permanent change of station move to the NCR, with an assignment to the Army Student Detachment at Fort Jackson, South Carolina. Fellows will complete a Masters in Legislative Affairs at George Washington University and work as a legislative fellow within the office of a MoC (typically a member of the House Armed Services Committee). Upon completing the fellowship, the officer will execute a 2-year utilization tour and concurrent active duty service obligation with OCLL or SAFM-BUL. (Selection for the fellowship as an Army medical officer does not mean that the officer will serve their utilization as the medical liaison.)

Medical Command Congressional Affairs Contact Officer

The MEDCOM CACO is a colonel (O-6) position serving as a personal staff officer to the surgeon general. The CACO's staff includes two major (O-4) positions, one senior enlisted, and two civilians (Figure 26-6). The MEDCOM CACO is the proponent for all Army medicine-related issues involving Congress, supporting AMEDD and OTSG efforts such as congressional testimony, and supporting the OCLL Programs medical lead. The MEDCOM CACO also interviews and recommends officers for proponency positions within OCLL when appropriate. It is also worth

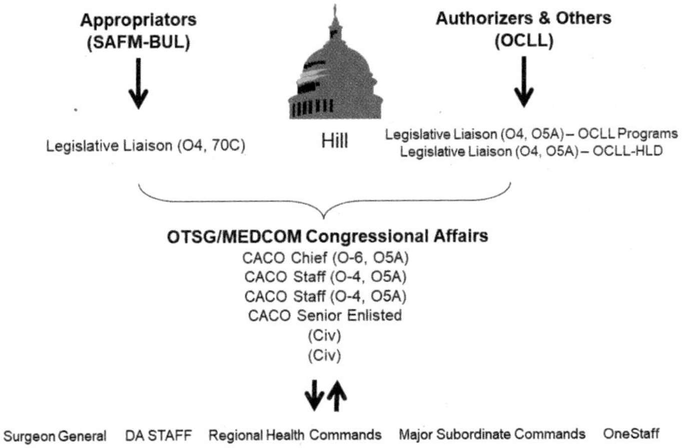

Figure 26-6. Legislative relationships and structure.
CACO: Congressional Affairs Contact Office
CIV: civilian
HLD: House Liaison Division
OCLL: Office of the Chief, Legislative Liaison
SAFM-BUL: Secretary of the Army, Financial Management–Budget Liaison

noting that most Army garrisons and division elements and above have a formal or informal CACO responsible for congressional interactions, often combined with the political advisor position. Historically, the O-4 staff positions have been filled by a Medical Service Corps officer, one of whom concentrates on appropriations (budgeting) and the other on authorizations (programmatic). In 2016, a 65D (Army Physician Assistant [PA]) served in the appropriation position (therefore, precedence exists for future consideration of PAs). A clinician working as a CACO must be prepared for an increased operational tempo; however, guest privileges can be obtained for biweekly or monthly clinic time for skills maintenance (see Legislative Liaison as a Clinician, above).

While the CACO position is largely a deviation from clinical practices, it rewards the clinician with a greater understanding of medical policy and the delicate balance of the finite medical resources required to achieve readiness across the Army, MTFs, and other military services. A clinician as CACO also has a unique opportunity to see and learn from best practices across clinical service lines, MTFs, Centers of Excellence, and operational units—and how to avoid common clinical leadership issues and pitfalls. Moreover, there is ample mentorship opportunity and face-time with ASLs. Skills gained in the CACO position set up the PA clinician for future broadening and leadership opportunities.

The CACO's staff communicate daily with the legislative liaison to support and enhance the overall congressional engagement strategy. As liaisons plan and organize staff and congressional delegations, the CACO's staff works in parallel to prepare medical leaders and MTF commanders for visits. Delegation preparation includes a thorough analysis of current political optics, MoC interests, past congressional visits, and any relevant activities to highlight. Delegations are *strategic opportunities* for ASLs to communicate success, needs, and challenges to legislators. Military services are unable to lobby; therefore, the liaison, CACO, and ASLs must synergize efforts to ensure that timely information is delivered via the right platform to successfully influence future legislation or policy implementation.

CACO staff also prepare official responses to congressional inquiries, compose oral and written testimony for the surgeon general, and prepare witnesses (ASLs) for congressional hearings. Testimony writing and preparation is a sensitive and time-consuming process that can be stressful when a hearing is called on short notice or in response to a negative issue.

The CACO, OTSG staff, legislative liaison, and senior leaders work closely to ensure delivery of consistent themes, messages, and talking points, and to articulate best practices and relevant concerns across MTFs and other medical equities. Of recent interest, the military health system reform first prescribed in the 2017 National Defense Authorization Act (NDAA) has dominated ASL attention and the AMEDD's congressional interactions. Changes set in motion by this groundbreaking legislation have caused both concerns and opportunities for care delivery. The CACO and legislative liaisons serve as the AMEDD's front line to form and maintain beneficial relationships and facilitate key leader meetings to communicate concerns, affected entities, and projected outcomes associated with the NDAA and related policy implementation.

Desired Skills and Attributes

Those considering service with OCLL, as CACO, or as a congressional fellow should have solid and advanced organizational, writing, and briefing skills; maintain good fiscal habits; and be comfortable with public speaking. A history in government policy or politics is not required but can be helpful. Because liaisons are routinely trusted with sensitive national military strategic messaging priorities, sensitive social military topics, and large sums of money, a solid ethical and moral footing is paramount to success. To be successful, individuals serving in the OCLL must be sound time managers, as well as proving themselves accountable, efficient, and dutiful.

Lessons Learned

Army PAs thinking of serving within the congressional community should consider several issues before undertaking such a position, primarily the impact on family. Living in the NCR can be fun and exciting, with the proximity to museums, sports, and outdoor activities, but the area is also notorious for traffic problems. Housing becomes more affordable the further it is from the Pentagon or the Capitol, but even a mile outside the beltway can significantly increase commute times. However, joint-basing has improved options for those who desire to live closer to the city and are willing to make some trade-offs. Joint Base Anacostia-Bolling is on the southeast side of Washington and within an easy commute of the Capitol or the Pentagon by car or commuter bus. Because liaisons must often work hours outside the typical 0800 to 1700 workday, and there is consistent travel (typically flying from Dulles or Reagan National airports, and occasionally from Andrews Air Force Base), choosing where to live is important.

Inconsistent schedules also make it difficult to maintain personal fitness. Legislative liaisons working at the Capitol can join the congressional staff gym for a nominal fee; those working at the Pentagon or MEDCOM headquarters also have gyms within their respective footprints.

Liaisons working in the congressional realm must be responsive and tactful. Any engagement, from email to casual conversation, may include topics of national interest and defense policy. Liaisons must understand that their every word may be circulated well outside their immediate realm of influence and be seen and heard by numerous general officers and elected officials. It is crucial to understand that a liaison's role is to stick to talking points while remaining approachable and forthright in conversation. Although it is best to maintain conduct as though every conversation is "on the record," there are still many opportunities to forge personal relationships with congressional staff and MoCs. Liaisons must not forget they are specially selected representatives of the Army and DOD.

Tips for Success

Legislative liaisons must be highly organized and detail-oriented; have solid grammar and editing skills; and be proficient in Microsoft Office software. To guide the approach of ASLs to MoCs and their staff, it is imperative that liaisons and CACOs track the MoCs' personal preferences, committee assignments, and constituent interests. Liaisons must maintain close working contacts across congressional offices to understand the mood and opinions on Capitol Hill. These relationships are forged with hard work and consistent contact; they subsequently help inform ASLs about congressional opinions of Army efforts and programs. Coordinating correspondence and requests for information

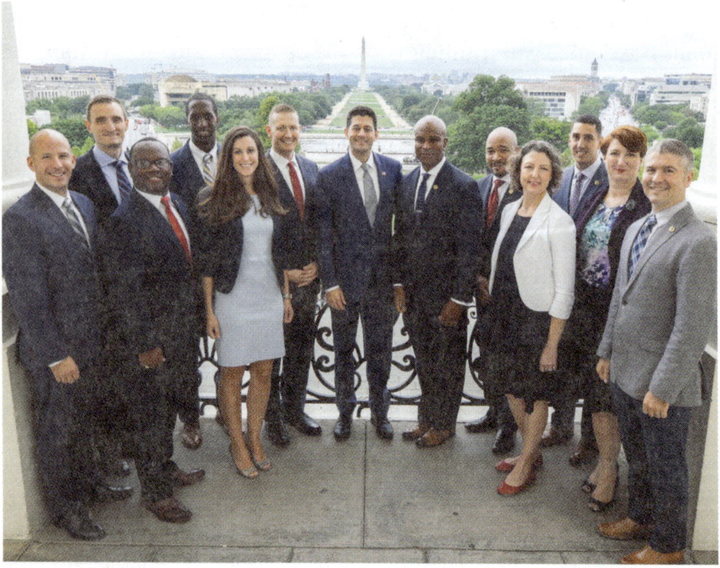

Figure 26-7. Major Sean Donohue (second from the left) with members of the Army House Liaison Division staff and the 54th Speaker of the House, Paul Ryan, during the 115th Congress.

are essential to daily liaison operations, who must ensure that each question is answered to the satisfaction of the office requesting the information (Figure 26-7).

Conclusion

Service as a legislative liaison or a CACO is a highly competitive and rewarding broadening opportunity that brings selected individuals into daily contact with senior DOD and elected government leadership. These assignments will provide participants a high-level, behind-the-scenes understanding of the legislative branch of government and Army operations.

References

1. US Army Office of the Chief Legislative Liaison. *2019 Congressional Actions Responsibilities Standing Operating Procedures (CARSOP)*. OCLL; 2019.
2. US Department of the Army. *Legislative Liaison*. USDA; 2013. Army Regulation 1-20.
3. US Department of the Army. *Evaluation Reporting System*. USDA; 2019. Army Regulation 623-3.
4. Pay and Allowances of the Uniformed Services of 2006, 37 USC § 335 (2011).
5. US Department of Defense. *Accession and Retention Policies, Programs, and Incentives for Military Health Professions Officers (HPOs)*. DOD; 2016. DOD Instruction 6000.13.
6. US Department of the Army. *Clinical Quality Management*. USDA; 2019. Army Regulation 40-68.
7. US Department of the Army. *Army Congressional Fellowship Program*. USDA; 2017. Army Regulation 1-202.

Chapter 27

ROLE OF THE PHYSICIAN ASSISTANT IN A JOINT ENVIRONMENT

Cleve Sylvester, PA-C, DSc, MPAS, and Colin Frament, APA-C, MPAS

The Joint Chiefs of Staff, in view of their global responsibilities and their perspective with respect to the worldwide strategic situation, are in a better position than any single theater commander to assess the risk of general war. Moreover, the Joint Chiefs of Staff are best able to judge our own military resources with which to meet that risk.

—Chairman of the Joint Chiefs of Staff Gen. Omar N. Bradley to the Senate Foreign Relations Committee, 1951[1]

The Army physician assistant (PA) serving at the Office of the Joint Staff Surgeon (OJSS), Joint Staff, Pentagon, must have a firm set of clinical and operational skills with significant planning acumen. It is important to begin the tour of duty with basic knowledge of joint operations and understand that the joint environment transcends all services, specialties, and combatant commands (CCMDs).The PA must have or be prepared to develop a strategic mindset, with the ability to conduct analyses, develop processes, generate solutions, articulate risks to senior leaders at the three-star and four-star levels, and occasionally convey the Department of Defense (DOD) position on applicable subject areas to congressional leaders and other government agencies. The Army PA is the most well-rounded medical officer in the DOD, and as a Joint Staff officer, must always be prepared to offer subject matter expertise on demand. This expertise may range from individual medical readiness to operational medicine or even hospital operations. The PA experience is instrumental in providing crucial insight that may shape care for the warfighter across the joint force.

Strategic Environment

The PA must be prepared to interface and coordinate with both military and civilian senior leaders, including general/flag officers, congressmen, department secretaries, and foreign representatives. Senior leaders expect good staff officers to have well-developed communication and technology skills, including conducting basic research, using productivity software, and performing general analyses. Additionally, the staff officer must acquire working knowledge of other capabilities such as the Joint Staff tasking management system, the Joint Staff action process (JSAP), and other joint systems and tools such as the Joint Operations Planning and Execution System (JOPES); the Joint Capabilities Integration and Development Systems (JCIDS); the Joint Training Information Management System (JTIMS); and the integrated priority list process.

All Joint Staff officers, including the PA, must have a firm understanding of national strategies as well as the roles, duties, and responsibilities of the chairman of the Joint Chiefs of Staff (CJCS) and the Joint Staff; the PA must also focus on the roles and responsibilities of the Joint Staff surgeon. This perspective is extremely important when framing responses and corresponding across the joint force. Arriving on the Joint Staff with some basic knowledge may significantly ease transition and potentially decrease the learning curve—slightly. For starters, awareness of national strategy, joint doctrine, and the function and priorities of the OJSS may be very helpful. The following major national strategy documents drive all military operations and are required knowledge for all Joint Staff officers.

- **The National Security Strategy (NSS)** informs the National Defense Strategy (NDS), which, in turn, informs the National Military Strategy (NMS). The NSS is written by the White House (executive branch) and presented to the American public and Congress during the president's State of the Union address. The document is grounded in the Goldwater Nichols Act of 1986 and outlines the president's assessment of the capabilities necessary to mitigate threats to the nation. The administration presents both a classified and unclassified version of the report.[2]
- **The National Defense Strategy (NDS),** written by the secretary of defense, is informed by the NSS. The NDS outlines the threats to the

complex global security environment and the risks and challenges posed by great power competition. The 2018 NDS states, "The central challenge to US prosperity and security is the reemergence of long-term, strategic competition by what the National Security Strategy classifies as revisionist powers."[3] As such, the three lines of effort outlined in the strategy are (1) rebuilding military readiness through a more lethal joint force; (2) strengthening alliances and partners; and (3) reforming the DOD's business practices for higher performance and affordability.

- **The National Military Strategy** (NMS), written by the Joint Chiefs of Staff and signed by the CJCS, is informed by the NDS. It is issued to the secretary of defense and outlines the strategic aims of the armed services. The 2018 NMS provides an integrated approach composed of three national military objectives: (1) to deter, deny, and defeat state adversaries; (2) to disrupt, degrade, and defeat violent extremist organizations; and (3) to strengthen the global network of US allies and partners.[4] The NMS also includes the overlapping concept of the "continuum of strategic direction": "Force employment (how the Joint Force will meet the challenges of the current strategic environment); Force development (adaptation of the existing Joint Force to do what it does better; and Force design (innovation to enable the Joint Force to do what it does differently in a fundamentally disruptive way)."[5]

The Joint Staff

The PA may have the opportunity to directly engage the CJCS and executive staff (vice chairman, director of the Joint Staff, vice director of the Joint Staff), as well as other military and civilian leaders. Therefore, it is important to understand the Joint Staff and its functions (Figure 27-1). The Joint Chiefs of Staff consist of the CJCS, the vice chairman of the Joint Chiefs of Staff, the chief of staff of the Army, the chief of naval operations, the chief of staff of the Air Force, the commandant of the Marine Corps, and the chief of the National Guard Bureau.[6] The CJCS is the senior ranking member of the Joint Chiefs of Staff. *The Joint Staff supports the* CJCS *in meeting the congressional* intent to provide "(1) for the unified strategic direction of the combatant forces; (2) for their operation

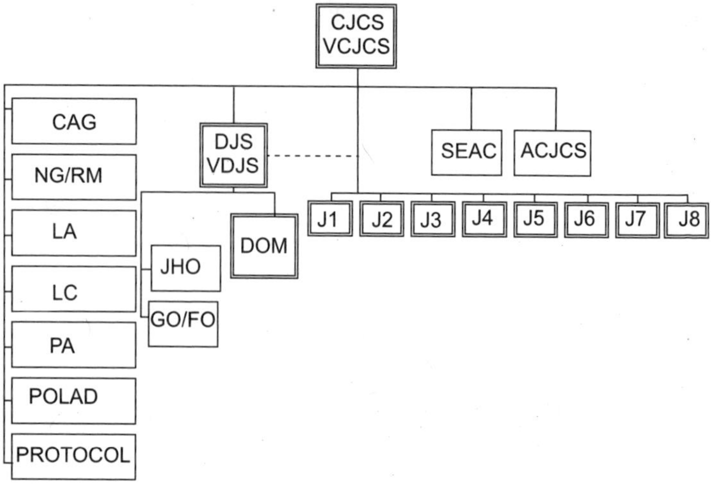

Figure 27-1. The Joint Staff organizational structure.
ACJCS: Assistant to the Chairman, Joint Chiefs of Staff; CAG: Chairman's Advisory Group; CJCS: Chairman, Joint Chiefs of Staff; DJS: Director, Joint Staff; DOM: Directorates of Management; GO/FO: General Office/Flag Officer; JHO: Joint History Office; LA: Legislative Affairs; LC: Legal Counsel; NG/RM: National Guard and Reserve Matters; PA: Public Affairs; POLAD: Policy Advisor; SEAC: Senior Enlisted Advisor to the Chairman; VCJCS: Vice Chairman, Joint Chiefs of Staff; VDJS: Vice Director, Joint Staff

under unified command; and (3) for their integration into an efficient team of land, naval, and air forces."[7] Responsibilities as members of the Joint Chiefs of Staff take precedence over duties as the chiefs of military services.[6] The CJCS is the global integrator and exercises Title 10 responsibilities that include comprehensive joint readiness, strategic direction and planning, global military integration, joint capability, and joint force development.[8] In the role of global force integrator, the CJCS has the responsibility of advising the secretary of defense on the risks to the mission and risks to the force involved in the transfer and allocation of forces across geographic commands. Staff sections, called joint directorates, that support the CJCS in their duties are as follows[9]:

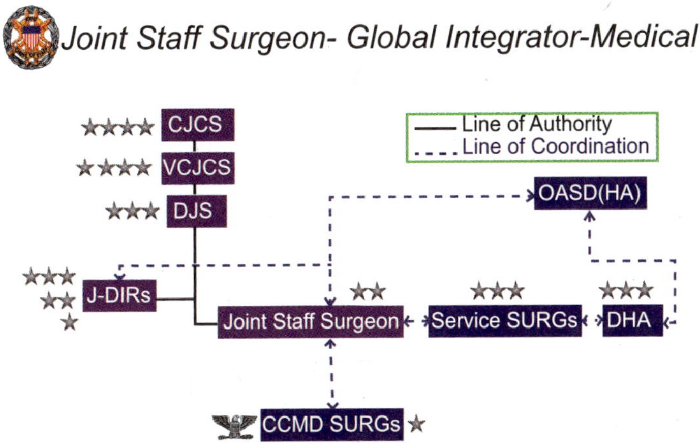

Figure 27-2. Joint Staff global medical integration. The Joint Staff surgeon maintains robust lines of coordination across the Department of Defense. CCMD SURG: Combatant Command Surgeon; DHA-Defense Health Agency; J-Dir: Joint Directorate; OASD(HA): Office of the Assistant Secretary of Defense for Health Affairs

DOM: Directorates of Management
J1: Manpower and Personnel
J2: Intelligence
J3: Operations
J4: Logistics
J5: Strategy, Plans, and Policy
J6: Command, Control, Communications, and Computers/Cyber
J7: Joint Force Development
J8: Force Structure, Resources, and Assessment

The OJSS, originally under J4, is now under DOM (see Figure 27-1).

Office of the Joint Staff Surgeon

The Joint Staff surgeon is the global medical integrator for the Joint Staff and synchronizes health services to enable globally integrated operations across the joint force (Figure 27-2). In this capacity, the Joint Staff surgeon provides medical advice to the CJCS; oversees medical requirements and capabilities; manages education, evaluations, and assessments; synchronizes CCMD and service efforts; and maintains a full sphere of influence through strong coordination relationships with other government agencies, the CCMDS, and the services. The OJSS is responsible for several strategic documents that shape medical operations across the DOD, two of which are Joint Publication (JP) 4-02, *Joint Health Services*,[10] and the *Joint Concept for Health Services (JCHS)*.[11]

- JP 4-02 is the doctrine for health services support across the joint force, and provides guidance for the exercise of authority by the CCMDs and other joint force commanders regarding force health protection, health service support operations, and health service support planning.[10] The PA must fully understand the scope and purpose of JP 4-02 and may be a key player in its interpretation and ultimately its revision.
- The JCHS, released by the CJCS in 2015, presents a comprehensive set of medical capabilities that enable joint, integrated, and optimized health services across the continuum of care. The JCHS is informed by several strategic documents,[11] including the *MHS Strategic Plan: A Roadmap for Medical Transformation*, 2008; *The Joint Operating Environment*, 2010; *Health Readiness Concept of Operations*, 2010; the Navy Medicine Strategy Map FY15,[12] and the *2018 Army Medicine Campaign Plan*.[13]

Unit Structure

Currently there are eight permanent positions on the OJSS manning document. The other 13 personnel on staff are a mix of contractors, liaison officers, and detailed personnel from the services. The OJSS is a two-star billet, with a civilian deputy (GS-15) and a uniformed deputy (O-7 [general or flag officer] or O-6 [colonel or captain]). The rest of the staff include specialists in plans, operations/logistics, clinical operations, force health protection, and strategic management. This composition may change based on availability of personnel.

Knowledge, Skills, and Attributes

The PA's experience and prior assignments on the Joint Staff will impact their effectiveness and efficiency. Previous assignments at the Army Medical Command and or a CCMD will assist them in understanding the roles and responsibilities of the Joint Staff surgeon. The PA's expertise and clinical experience become important during meetings, working groups, and capability-based assessments. The PA is a clinical subject matter expert on readiness and care of the warfighter. The operational experience a PA has from supporting "the line" can be instrumental in providing perspective during discussions that will impact the future of the joint medical force and how care is provided to service members. Concise written and verbal communication skills are important to being a successful staff officer, and the PA's ability to write and brief effectively will continue to be developed during a Joint Staff assignment.

Duties and Responsibilities

The primary duties and responsibilities of the PA are to assist the Joint Staff surgeon in providing the CJCS with the best medical advice on time, every time. A PA assigned to the OJSS should be the rank of lieutenant colonel or major (promotable) and have completed the requisite professional military education. Prior assignment as a Joint Staff intern, an Army staff officer, or CCMD staff officer may enhance understanding of the strategic environment and better facilitate strategic planning and resourcing at the OJSS.

Daily Routine

The OJSS has a very dynamic "battle rhythm." The typical day begins with the morning meeting, nicknamed the "Jolt," in which the staff provides an internal update and attempts to synchronize and crosswalk priorities, actions, tasks, and deliverables. Generally, the Monday Jolt includes an update to the Joint Staff surgeon, and the Tuesday Jolt includes a session on professional development. The rest of the day is spent performing staff work, coordinating, planning, performing action officer (AO) taskings, and attending meetings. A significant portion of the day is spent coordinating and generating correspondence. This

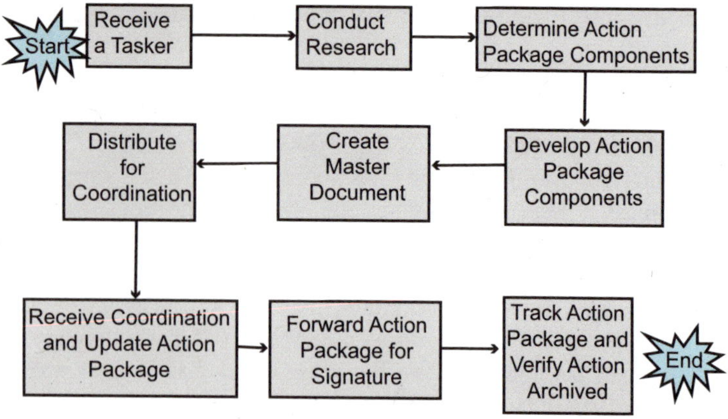

Figure 27-3. Joint Staff action package process flowchart.

includes a lot of research, reading, and writing action and information memoranda, information papers, position (decision) papers, and talking points. Other correspondence includes fact sheets, memoranda for the record, background papers, and coordination papers (summary sheets, letters, messages, and estimates).[14]

The PA will become integrated into the team that steers the joint force into the future while simultaneously receiving a high level of professional military education as outlined in *Developing Today's Joint Officers for Tomorrow's Ways of War: The Joint Chiefs of Staff Vision and Guidance for Professional Military Education & Talent Management*.[15] The PA generates products that will influence decisions at the level of the secretary of defense and, on occasion, assist Congress and the White House in shaping national policies. The OJSS is the Joint Staff's repository for all things medical, and the PA supports the Joint Staff surgeon in providing the best available military medical advice to the CJCS. The PA must be mentally agile and flexible, and must be prepared to respond to inquiries at the speed of strategic relevance. A tardy but accurate answer (in some cases, minutes late) may no longer be needed because the discussion has already progressed or the decision has already been made. Requests for information may come to the OJSS via phone calls, email, office visits, or formally through the JSAP.

Joint Staff Action Process

The JSAP system (Figure 27-3) is the tasking process of the Joint Staff used to formally request information, direct action, coordinate responses, or disseminate information across the DOD. A prime responsibility of Joint Staff officers is to work action packages using the JSAP system. The DOM funnels all tasks that require medical responses to the OJSS, and the JSAP manager within the office assigns each task an AO. Working a task as an AO is perhaps one of the most important, time-consuming actions at the OJSS, with potential high visibility and high impact. The JSAP task instructions may direct the AO to consolidate information and responses from other organizations, prepare packets for senior leader approval/signature, or disseminate information across the joint force. Additionally, AOs may develop executive summaries, letters, memoranda, and other documents, or coordinate actions among directorates, services, CCMDs, and other government agencies. The AO working a JSAP must ensure that the response meets the intent of the tasker and that the packet is completed by its suspense date. Late JSAPs are reported to the level of the director of the Joint Chiefs of Staff.[16]

Other aspects of the PA's portfolio are integrated into the daily routine and mainly include areas within clinical operations that require medical or clinical expertise. The PA may also perform duties related to JCIDS, global health engagement, research and development, or science and technology.

Joint Capabilities Integration and Development System

The PA must understand the intricacies of the JCIDS and be able to articulate and explain the process to those seeking clarification and guidance from the OJSS. The CCMDs and services use the JCIDS process to identify, develop, and validate requirements; identify and match capabilities to those requirements; identify capability gaps; and develop sourcing solutions. The Joint Requirements Oversight Council owns the JCIDS process and is chartered to conduct JCIDS activities and validate capability requirements, unless independent validation authority is identified.[17] The purpose of the JCIDS process is to support and enable the council in executing the CJCS's responsibilities in identifying, assessing, validating, and prioritizing joint military capability requirements.[18]

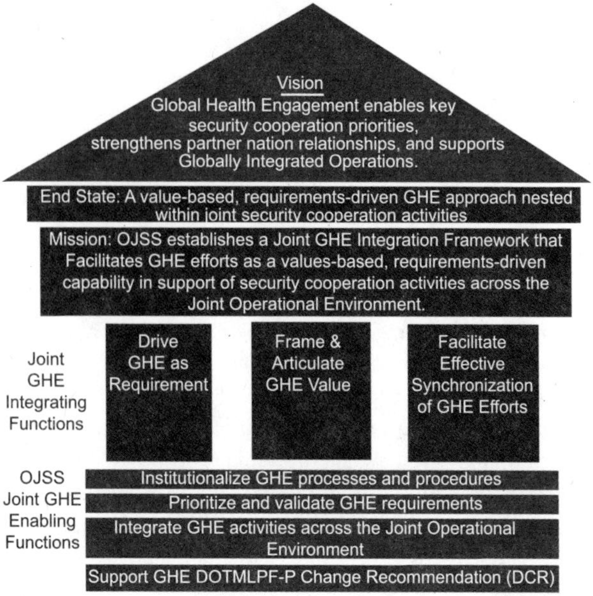

Figure 27-4. Joint Global Health Engagement Integration Framework facilitates global health efforts as a values-based, requirements-driven capability in support of security cooperation activities across the joint operational environment.

Non-materiel solutions proposed from capabilities-based assessments result in doctrine, organization, training, materiel, leadership, personnel, facilities, and policy (DOTMLPF-P) change recommendations (DCRs). The DCR is part of the JCIDS process and provides a format for considering solutions for each DOTMLPF-P domain.[19] The OJSS chairs the Health Services Working Group, which serves as a gateway and validation authority for capabilities-based assessment outputs as well as tasks assigned within a DCR. Current DCRs with enduring requirements include:

- The **Defense Trauma Enterprise** DCR identifies gaps in DOD's ability to deliver and manage trauma care from the point of injury to Role 4.
- The **Forward Resuscitative Care** DCR identifies gaps in DOD's ability to provide and manage resuscitative care during operations in austere and remote environments.

- The **Medical Readiness Skills Sustainment During Deployed Operations** DCR identifies capability requirements for preserving the highly perishable mission-essential medical skills of deployed medical personnel involved in patient treatment in support of the joint force.
- The **Global Health Engagements** DCR identifies global health engagement shortfalls across the joint force that limit practical and useful support to the combatant commander's theater objectives.

Global Health Engagement

The PA must have a working knowledge of global health engagement and understand how it is informed by strategic documents and executed at the CCMD level (Figure 27-4). Global health engagement is nested within security cooperation and is an interdepartmental collaborative of DOD global health engagement, the Joint Staff, the Uniformed Services University Center for Global Health Engagement,[20] services, and CCMDs, as well as other governmental agencies such as the Defense Threat Reduction Agency, Centers for Disease Control and Prevention, and US Agency for International Development.

Current Operations

Activities within current operations range from the Defense support for civil authorities during disaster response (southern border operations, hurricane and other natural disaster support, infectious diseases, epidemic and pandemic support) to CCMD activities. The PA may be the subject matter expert with the requisite experience and knowledge to appropriately respond to requests for assistance from other government agencies or to validate requests for forces from the CCMD.

Lessons Learned

The following are lessons learned from service at the OJSS:

- A few courses that are not required but will be helpful are How the Army Runs, Joint Medical Officer's Course (JMOC) Basic and JMOC-Advanced, and the Joint Senior Medical Leaders Course.

- Balance is important. Being an AO for the Joint Staff surgeon requires self-discipline and balance between work and home. The office's high operational tempo can be daunting; being mindful of life outside the Pentagon walls is very important.
- An assignment on the Joint Staff is an opportunity to understand the role of the OJSS and its influence on how health care is provided to the joint warfighter. The challenge is to adjust focus from an Army-centric view to a joint view. Army PAs assigned to the Joint Staff must understand they are AOs whose mission is to develop joint solutions that nest with the Joint Staff surgeon's priorities.
- Movement, action, and decision-making at the strategic level can be slow and deliberate. Exercising tactical patience is rewarding. Conversely, impatience and ignorance can lead to frustration, especially during the first 6 months.
- Learning to navigate the Pentagon is essential. Many meetings require physical attendance, so understanding the Pentagon's layout makes coordination and daily tasks less daunting. The Pentagon is composed of five floors, five interconnected rings with ten interlinked corridors, several internal hallways, and an open courtyard in the center of the building. It is easiest to identify a corridor or office by going through the center courtyard. Walking along the rings is generally ill-advised if time is of the essence; the outmost ring (E-ring) is almost 1 mile long.

Tips for Success

Along with lessons learned, the following tips will help future Joint Staff PAs succeed:

- The Joint Staff PA should allow at least 90 days for orientation and onboarding. A good sponsor will ensure a smooth transition and in-processing. This time affords the Joint Staff PA an opportunity to put things into context.
- Joint Staff PAs must be prepared to live outside their comfort zone. Being called on to respond to unfamiliar things is a way of life at the Pentagon. The PA should project confidence, ask for help, ask if they do not know something, and never refuse help when offered.

- "There is no casual conversation; every discussion is an evaluation." The Joint Staff PA should know that media is present throughout the building, and always assume someone is watching or listening.
- The Joint Staff PA must put conversations into context. Conversations taken out of context, discussions that are unintentionally expanded beyond intended audiences, or emails circulated inadvertently and inappropriately can have devastating consequences. Office discussions, often intended to frame and support internal tasks and actions, can pose unintended consequences when discussed with persons outside the group.
- "Words have meaning." The Joint Staff PA's discussions with senior leaders and fellow Joint Staff officers must be as accurate, brief, and concise as necessary.
- The Joint Staff PA must not forward general officer/flag officer emails.
- The Joint Staff PA must listen and learn. No matter how much a PA thinks they know, there is much more that they do not.
- The Joint Staff is about joint solutions. Service-specific solutions that do not support CCMD interests or conflict with the CJCS's priorities are of less interest to the Joint Staff. A PA who cannot move beyond Army-specific issues will certainly struggle.

Conclusion

An assignment to the OJSS is an excellent opportunity for field-grade officers to further develop their strategic acumen. Service on the Joint Staff affords the opportunity to interact with service medical leadership, Defense Health Agency staff, CCMD surgeons, and senior leaders from other government agencies. These engagements will not only build career-long relationships but also set the stage for future operational and strategic assignments for PAs as future Army leaders.

References

1. The Joint Chiefs of Staff. Global integration: what is it? Accessed September 10, 2020. https://www.jcs.mil/About/Global-Integration/

2. The White House. *The National Security Strategy of the United States of America December 2017*. Accessed September 10, 2020. https://www.whitehouse.gov/wp-content/uploads/2017/12/NSS-Final-12-18-2017-0905.pdf
3. Department of Defense. *Summary of the 2018 National Defense Strategy of the United States of America*. Accessed September 10, 2020. https://dod.defense.gov/Portals/1/Documents/pubs/2018-National-Defense-Strategy-Summary.pdf
4. The Joint Chiefs of Staff. *Description of the National Military Strategy 2018*. Accessed September 10, 2020. https://www.jcs.mil/Portals/36/Documents/Publications/UNCLASS_2018_National_Military_Strategy_Description.pdf
5. Garamone J. National Military Strategy addresses changing the character of war. Department of Defense website. Published July 12, 2012. Accessed September 10, 2020. https://www.defense.gov/explore/story/Article/1903478/national-military-strategy-addresses-changing-character-of-war/
6. The Joint Chiefs of Staff. About. Accessed September 10, 2020. https://www.jcs.mil/About
7. Joint Staff, 10 USC §155. Accessed September 10, 2020. https://uscode.house.gov/view.xhtml?req=granuleid:USC-prelim-title10-section155&num=0&edition=prelim
8. Department of Defense. *Functions of the Department of Defense and Its Major Components*. DOD; December 21, 2010. DOD Directive 5100.01. Accessed September 10, https//cmo.defense.gov/Portals/47/Documents/PDSD/510001p2.pdf
9. The Joint Chiefs of Staff. Directorates. Accessed September 10, 2020. https://www.jcs.mil/
10. The Joint Chiefs of Staff. *Joint Health Services*. JCS; December 11, 2017 (Incorporating Change 1, September 28, 2018). Joint Publication 4-02. Accessed September 10, 2020. https://www.jcs.mil/Portals/36/Documents/Doctrine/pubs/jp4_02ch1.pdf
11. The Joint Chiefs of Staff. *Joint Concept for Health Services (JCHS)*. JCS; August 31, 2015. Accessed September 10, 2020. https://www.jcs.mil/Portals/36/Documents/Doctrine/concepts/joint_concept_health_services.pdf?ver=2017-12-28-162027-633

12. Navy Medicine. Navy Medicine Strategy Map FY15. Accessed September 14, 2020. https://www.med.navy.mil/Pages/StrategicMap.aspx

13. US Army Public Health Command. *2018 Army Medicine Campaign Plan*. Accessed September 10, 2020. https://armymedicine.health.mil/~/media/78E0C20AB5D74DEDAB0A31F912999261.ashx

14. The Joint Chiefs of Staff. *Joint Officer Handbook Staffing and Action Guide*. 3rd ed. JCS; August 2012. Accessed September 13, 2020. https://www.pacom.mil/Portals/55/Documents/pdf/newcomers-Joint-Staff-Officer-Handbook-2012.pdf

15. The Joint Chiefs of Staff. *Developing Today's Joint Officers for Tomorrow's Ways of War: The Joint Chiefs of Staff Vision and Guidance for Professional Military Education & Talent Management*. JCS; May 1, 2020. Accessed September 10, 2020. https://www.jcs.mil/Portals/36/Documents/Doctrine/education/jcs_pme_tm_vision.pdf?ver=2020-05-15-102429-817

16. The Joint Chiefs of Staff. *Policy on Action Processing*. JCS; September 10, 2010. Chairman of the Joint Chiefs of Staff Instruction 5711.01C. Accessed September 10, 2020. https://www.jcs.mil/Portals/36/Documents/Library/Instructions/5711_01.pdf?ver=2016-02-05-175047-203

17. The Joint Chiefs of Staff. *Manual for the Operation of the Joint Capabilities Integration and Development System*. JCS; August 31, 2018. Accessed September 10, 2020. https://www.acq.osd.mil/jrac/docs/2018-JCIDS.pdf

18. The Joint Chiefs of Staff. *Charter of the Joint Requirements Oversight Council (JROC) and Implementation of the Joint Capabilities Integration and Development System (JCIDS)*. Joint Staff; August 31, 2018. CJCSI 5123.01H. Accessed September 10, 2020. https://www.jcs.mil/Portals/36/Documents/Library/Instructions/CJCSI%205123.01H.pdf?ver=2018-10-26-163922-137

19. Rausch J. Joint Capability Integration & Development System overview. Accessed September 10, 2020. https://www.acq.osd.mil/log/MR/.PSM_workshop.html/2019_Files/Day_One/3_New_JCIDS_Instruction_Guidebook_Rausch.pdf

20. Uniformed Services University of the Health Sciences. Research. Accessed September 10, 2020. https://www.usuhs.edu/cghe/research

Additional Sources

- Department of Defense. *DoD Manual for Written Material: Correspondence Management*. DOD; October 26, 2010. DOD Manual 5110.04-M-V1. Accessed September 10, 2020. https://execsec.defense.gov/Portals/34/Documents/511004m_v1.pdf
- The Joint Chiefs of Staff. *Guidance for Developing and Implementing Joint Concepts*. JCS; August 16, 2018. Chairman of the Joint Chiefs of Staff Instruction 3010.02E. Accessed September 10, 2020. https://www.jcs.mil/Portals/36/Documents/Library/Instructions/CJCSI%203010.02E.pdf?ver=2017-02-08-173223-657
- The Joint Chiefs of Staff. *Planner's Handbook for Operational Design*. JCS; October 7, 2011. Accessed September 10, 2020. https://www.jcs.mil/Portals/36/Documents/Doctrine/pams_hands/opdesign_hbk.pdf#:~:text=The%20handbook%20is%20not%20approved%20doctrine%2C%20but%20it,of%20using%20this%20information%20in%20actual%20operations.%205
- The Joint Chiefs of Staff. *Joint Planning*. JCS; June 16, 2017. Joint Publication JP 5-0. Accessed September 10, 2020. https://www.jcs.mil/Portals/36/Documents/Doctrine/pubs/jp5_0_20171606.pdf

Chapter 28

ROLE OF THE CHIEF OF THE READY AND RESILIENT INTEGRATION BRANCH AT HEADQUARTERS, INSTALLATION MANAGEMENT COMMAND

Amelia M. Duran-Stanton, PA-C, PhD, DSc, MPAS; Donna Clouse, MS, CEAP; Derek Ferrell, MSM, MHA; Frances Measells, DSW, LCSW, CEAP; Paul Smith, MBA, MA; and Pamela Budda, BSW, MEd

Introduction

The physician assistant (PA) assigned as the chief of the Ready and Resilient (R2) Integration (R2I) branch and deputy surgeon at Headquarters, Installation Management Command (HQ IMCOM), provides recommendations to IMCOM staff, the deputy commanding general, and the commanding general, as subject matter expert for all aspects of the Army's strategy for maintaining a ready and resilient force, including sexual harassment/assault response and prevention (SHARP), risk reduction, and suicide prevention programs. To provide a comprehensive awareness of the chief, R2I, role, this chapter will also provide information on the IMCOM and R2/Alcohol Substance Abuse Program (ASAP) Division.

Supervision

The chief of the R2I branch is a branch immaterial (O1A) position aligned under the HQ IMCOM G1 (Personnel) R2/ASAP Division. It is rated by the R2/ASAP division chief and is senior-rated by the HQ IMCOM G1 deputy director.

Roles and Duties

The position requires assisting in the execution of health care policies pertaining to soldiers, families, and civilians at 64 garrisons worldwide. Primary duties include coordinating and contributing health care expertise across the Installation Management Command leadership worldwide to execute a comprehensive plan to communicate and address immediate and enduring R2 programs for soldiers, families, and communities. The position unifies efforts across all services, as well as external civilian agencies, to coordinate multidisciplinary teams to implement Army readiness programs and initiatives. If the incumbent is a clinician, they can also fill the role of the IMCOM deputy surgeon, who advises and acts as a medical liaison between Army service component command surgeons, the US Army Medical Command, Training and Doctrine Command, Office of the Surgeon General, Defense Health Agency, and support staff.

Desired Knowledge, Skills, and Attributes

Knowledge

- Knowledge of Army culture and organizations, systems, policies, and processes.
- Understanding of military medicine and the business of health care.
- Experience with writing and updating policies.
- Good understanding of joint, Army, IMCOM, and Army Medical Command cultures.
- Competence in using Microsoft Office, MilSuite, and SharePoint applications.

Skills

- Strategic thinking.
- Exceptional written and oral communication skills.
- Unwavering military bearing and tact with senior leadership.
- Strong interpersonal skills; consensus-building across a variety of stakeholders and agencies; persuasion/negotiation skills and tactics; team-building.
- Attention to detail and exceptional organizational skills are an absolute must.

- Proficiency in editing military and civilian correspondence and other documents.
- Strong leadership skills; the ability to coach, teach, and mentor civilian employees.

Attributes

- Critical thinking and problem-solving skills.
- Self-starter; able to see a need and begin action in response.
- Systems thinker; able to connect dots and see the big picture.
- Ability to effectively handle pressure, remaining calm and rational.
- Ability to effectively multi-task.
- Willingness to do any task required for mission success.
- Assertive; able to tactfully enforce requirements with senior staff.
- Good at planning; able to anticipate needs and develop options.

Training

Systems training required for managing civilian employees includes the Automated Time and Attendance Production System (ATAAPS) and

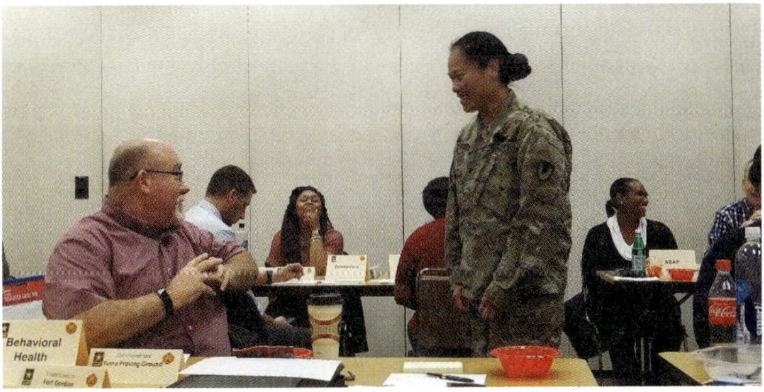

Figure 28-1. Lieutenant Colonel Amelia Duran-Stanton engages with a program manager during a scenario-based discussion at the Army Substance Abuse Program Manager Course.
Photo courtesy of Ms. Leslie Sweeney.

Defense Performance Management and Appraisal Program (DPMAP). There is also the opportunity to attend the training conducted by the staff, such as the Suicide Prevention Program Manager, Risk Reduction Program Manager, and Army Substance Abuse Program Manager Courses (Figure 28-1). Table 28-1 lists courses offered by the R2/ASAP Division. When the incumbent is a clinician and fills the role of a deputy surgeon, there are training recommendations that will be outlined in the IMCOM surgeon chapter (Chapter 47).

Key Factors

This position is typically a 2-year tour and is coded for 01A (branch immaterial) lieutenant colonel (O-5) with no additional skill identifier requirement. The position is primarily nonclinical but utilizes clinical regulatory knowledge learned throughout a clinician's career, which enhances the ability to make sound and timely decisions in managing the programs and civilian staff. PAs in the position must maintain their credentials and perform at least 40 hours annually of the clinical duties they are privileged and credentialed for at the local medical treatment facility.

Installation Management Command

A three-star-level command currently located at Joint Base San Antonio–Fort Sam Houston, Texas, IMCOM integrates and delivers base support for all assigned installations to enable readiness for a globally responsive Army. IMCOM is committed to providing base operations support in accordance with established standards to accomplish the mission. It is also invested in providing appropriate programs and services at the right time and place for soldiers and their families. IMCOM's tagline is "We are the Army's Home" (Figure 28-2).

Ready and Resilient/Army Substance Abuse Program Division

The HQ IMCOM G1 R2/ASAP Division is comprised of two branches: the Prevention Services Branch and the R2I Branch (Figure 28-3). Each branch has a chief and is aligned with specific programs, discussed in detail below. The division's **vision** is to establish integrated community

Table 28-1. Courses offered by the Ready and Resilient/Alcohol and Substance Abuse Program Division.

Course	Target Audience
Drug Testing Coordinator Recertification Course	Drug testing coordinators
Suicide Prevention Program Managers Course	Suicide prevention program managers
Community Ready and Resilient Integrator Course	Community R2 integrators who are IMCOM employees
Drug Testing Coordinator Full Course	Drug testing coordinators
Prevention Coordinators Course	Prevention branch chiefs and prevention coordinators
Army Substance Abuse Program Manager Course	Army substance abuse managers
Commander's Risk Reduction Dashboard/Risk Reduction Coordinators Course	Risk reduction prevention coordinators
Prime for Life	Prevention coordinators
Employee Assistance Program Coordinator Course	Employee Assistance Program coordinators

IMCOM: Installation Management Command; R2: Ready and Resilient

resources that enhance readiness and resiliency. Its **mission** is to strengthen readiness and support the resilience of the Army's most valuable resource: people. The R2/ASAP Division operates along three lines of effort: to deter, to prevent, and to assist.

- To **deter** risky behaviors involves setting conditions to help individuals to make the right choice. The goal of deterrence is to discourage high-risk behaviors by clearly identifying consequences of negative choices (eg, drug use, drinking and driving, sexual harassment, and assault).
- To **prevent** risky behaviors includes efforts that increase knowledge, skills, or experience as the desired outcome. Educational/motivational programs focus on the adverse effects and consequences of alcohol and other drug abuse. These efforts create and foster conditions that promote mission readiness by preventing high-risk behaviors.

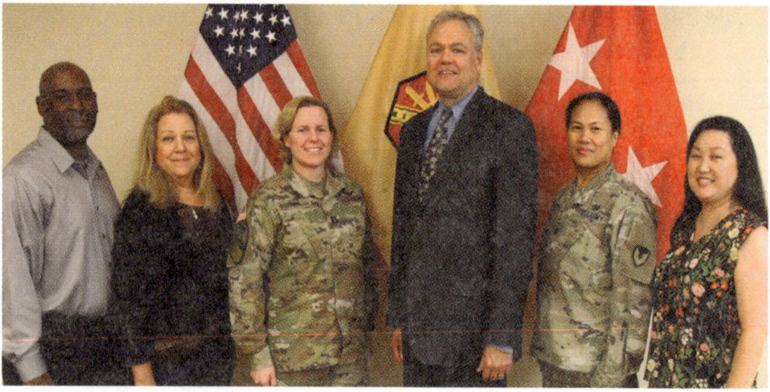

Figure 28-2. Staff of Headquarters, Installation Management Command (IMCOM), left to right: Derek Ferrell (Suicide Prevention/Risk Reduction program manager), Leslie Sweeney (Ready and Resilient integrator), Captain Cynthia Stephenson (aide-de-camp to the IMCOM commanding general), J. Randall Robinson (executive deputy to the IMCOM commanding general), Lieutenant Colonel Amelia Duran-Stanton, Rhonda DeVries (assistant to the IMCOM chief of staff).
Photo courtesy of Installation Management Command Public Affairs Office.

- To **assist** means intervening early to lessen the impact of risky behaviors and to help individuals return to full functioning and full duty.

Prevention Services Branch

This branch provides the following services: drug testing, budget assistance, prevention and education, and employee assistance.

Drug Testing

Drug abuse is inconsistent with Army values and readiness. Drug testing is governed by Army Regulation (AR) 600-85, The Army Substance Abuse Program.[1] Program staff perform the following services:

- Provide professionals at garrisons the tools necessary to deter soldiers from abusing drugs (including illegal drugs, other illicit substances, and prescribed medication).

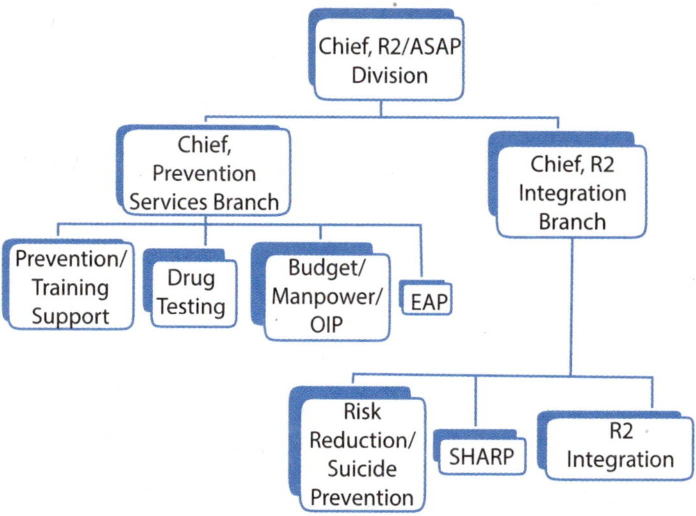

Figure 28-3. Ready and Resilient/Alcohol and Substance Abuse Program (R2/ASAP) Division organizational chart.
EAP: Employee Assistance Program; OIP: Organizational Inspection Program; SHARP: Sexual Harassment/Assault Response and Prevention Program

- Provide information for garrison ASAP staff to facilitate early detection of drug abuse.
- Enable commanders to assess the security, military fitness, and good order and discipline of their units, and to use information obtained to take appropriate disciplinary or other administrative actions.
- Collect data on the prevalence of drug abuse within the Army.
- Track aggregate garrison drug testing collection numbers across IMCOM to ensure compliance with AR 600-85.[1]
- Promote the Army Drug-Free Federal Workplace Drug Testing Program as directed by the Executive Order 12564, dated September 15, 1986, and establish the goal of a drug-free federal workplace.[2]
- Provide certification courses to garrison ASAP staff (namely, drug testing coordinators and drug testing technicians) or any other staff members who carry out drug testing functions to maintain forensically sound drug testing collection points at each garrison.

- Advocate for a workplace that is free from illegal use, possession, or distribution of controlled substances by its civilian workforce and that is safe, healthful, productive, and secure.

Budget Assistance

- Assist garrisons with budget requirements and spend plans.
- Partner with IMCOM G8 (budgeting) in carrying out workforce studies for ASAP coaches and mentors, and assist garrison drug testing coordinators in service delivery.

Prevention Services

- Promote ASAP services using marketing, networking, and consulting strategies.
- Ensure garrisons comply with regulatory requirements and support the Army's priorities.
- Analyze prevention data for trends in service delivery as well as completed alcohol and drug abuse prevention training.
- Provide training and other services to assist organizations in ensuring all military and civilian personnel are provided prevention education training.
- Provide an array of professional development opportunities for ASAP professionals.
- Design and develop community-targeted, group-oriented alcohol and other drug interventions in coordination with the ASAP staff and other installation prevention professionals.

Employee Assistance

- Coach, mentor, and assist the garrison Employee Assistance Program (EAP) coordinators in service delivery.
- Provide working groups to create EAP client satisfaction surveys and other data-gathering resources.
- Provide screening, assessment, short-term counseling (one to four sessions), and referral for problems that may affect work performance.
- Provide guidance, advice, mediation, and prevention education on topics that promote the well-being of civilian employees.
- Services are not limited to worksite-related problems.
- Provide supervisory consultation to supervisors.

- Eligibility for EAP services: Army civilians, civilian and military family members, military retirees, and family members of military retirees.

The Ready and Resilient Integration Branch

The R2I Branch is comprised of four programs: Risk Reduction, Suicide Prevention, Ready and Resilient Integration, and SHARP.

Risk Reduction Program

The Risk Reduction Program uses a database to collect and report on risk factors, using an interface called the Commander's Risk Reduction Toolkit.

- Designed to remove the burden of multiple meetings for commanders and leaders.
- Initially collected data on 20 Army-defined risk factors.
- Currently reports on 14 of those factors to installation commanders and leaders.
- Has flexibility and capability to obtain and report on risk factors not identified by the Army but deemed necessary to installation leadership.
- Collects data on active duty Army personnel only.
- Able to report on geographically dispersed units.

Suicide Prevention

The Army's efforts to prevent suicide are executed in three phases; (1) prevention; (2) intervention (education with "ACE" [Ask, Care, and Escort] and "ACE-SI" [Ask, Care, and Escort—Suicide Intervention] courses); and (3) "post-vention" (follow-up support services and care). The installation's suicide prevention program manager (SPPM) is the subject matter expert for the senior commander and installation leaders on all suicide prevention matters.

- The SPPM is aligned under and works for the ASAP manager in most cases.
- The SPPM provides data and trend analysis and advises and assists the community R2 integrator on all suicide prevention matters pertaining to the Community Ready and Resilient Council (CR2C).

- The SPPM is responsible for tracking all ACE-SI and Applied Suicide Intervention Skills Training trainers.[3]
- The SPPM is required to submit a monthly report to HQ IMCOM.

The Ready and Resilient Integrator

The HQ IMCOM R2 integrators synchronize and provide support for garrison-level community R2 integrators. The information below provides background information on the R2 Council and integrators at the garrison level.

- **Community R2 Councils** integrate and synchronize the Army's multiple efforts and programs designed to improve readiness and resilience.[4] The process integrates garrison, medical, and mission efforts in support of the synchronization of health promotion, risk reduction, and suicide prevention programs. At the installation level, the council is chaired by the senior commander. It includes the garrison commander, medical treatment facility commander, brigade commanders, tenant unit representation, and appropriate subject matter experts across the installation. AR 600-63[5] specifies the objectives of the health promotion program to enhance the quality of life, resiliency, and wellness for all soldiers, family members, civilians, and retirees and to optimize and coordinate organizational efficiencies related to health promotion.[4,5]

- **Community R2 integrators** are responsible for coordinating, planning, organizing, and implementing comprehensive health promotion and well-being processes based on initiatives to enhance readiness and resilience for the total Army.[4] The Suicide Prevention Task Force, the Installation Prevention Team, and five other workgroups support the resiliency pillars that support the senior commander's priorities. Community R2 integrators are also responsible for the Community Resource Guide, an app-based resource that provides information for all the local communities.

Sexual Harassment/Assault Response and Prevention Program

The IMCOM HQ SHARP program manager standardizes processes with multiple organizational alignments at the garrison level, coordinating with over 50 other program managers to support the senior mission commander (there is no cookie-cutter approach). They provide guidance on policy, track client caseloads, manage training, and collate required annual reports.

Some sexual assault response coordinators/victim advocates (SARCs/VAs) fall under different chains of command depending on the installation. Based on experience, the IMCOM SHARP Manager recommends including the garrison commander or deputy/command sergeant major in the rating scheme. The garrison SHARP office manages about 80% installation cases and about 20% garrison cases.

- Per Army Directive 2018-23, only face-to-face SHARP refresher training is mandatory (the online version is not required, but still available to use).[6]
- SHARP personnel must be certified or recertified every 2 years, and have background checks every 3 years.
- The Army G1 SHARP Program Improvement Forum is a national forum where senior SHARP personnel discuss policies and procedures for the program. Breakout workshops are conducted to brainstorm issues and challenges.
- SHARP staff participate in a National Organization for Victim Assistance (NOVA) annual training event. NOVA is a DOD-endorsed credentialing program.[7]

Lessons Learned

These lessons learned may help PAs assigned to IMCOM as well as in other assignments. The PA should:

- gain an understanding of the IMCOM leadership vision and mission, and how the organization fits into the bigger scheme of the Army as a large organization;
- maintain a network of liaisons established from previous organizations, and gain new ones;
- manage competing priorities and seek guidance when necessary;
- attend, and get credit for, all the courses conducted by the R2/ASAP team as early as possible (these courses may lead to future opportunities);

- manage their calendar wisely and ensure internal team members have access to it;
- know the functions of the IMCOM directorates in garrisons worldwide;
- learn how to write civilian evaluations before coming to IMCOM, and hone skills while at IMCOM;
- manage regulatory guidance updates and be familiar with both previous and current policies;
- create a continuity mechanism to share experience and lessons learned with the next team; and
- empower subordinates in creating standard operating procedures.

Tips for Success

Along with lessons learned, these tips for success will enable PAs to maximize the opportunity afforded to them at IMCOM. The PA should:

- maintain ties with the medical community (it is a value-added network of professionals that IMCOM will benefit from);
- maintain a routine battle rhythm but be prepared for ad hoc meetings and events;
- collaborate locally with civilian entities in all R2-related programs;
- maintain clinical credentials and privileges;
- manage leave wisely and ensure the team does the same;
- stay humble and learn from everyone they contact (the IMCOM team is a highly functional group of professionals, and each individual will add value to the PA's experience at IMCOM and beyond);
- seek opportunities to improve personal health and fitness, and fit them into their schedule routinely;
- continue to be involved in the Army Medical Specialist (SP) Corps and the Medical Center of Excellence by taking every opportunity as schedule permits to meet with SP Corps leaders who are stationed or on temporary duty at Joint Base San Antonio (JBSA);
- remain flexible and keep the team informed of any schedule or event changes as needed; and
- take full advantage of local courses at JBSA as schedule permits.

Conclusion

An assignment with IMCOM is a unique and broadening experience that will provide PAs an opportunity to build on their previous skills and also to develop new ones. A unique leadership experience that requires management of multiple, high-visibility programs and portfolios, this position will enable PAs to develop and display their strengths in clinical, administrative, management, and leadership abilities.

References

1. Department of the Army. *The Army Substance Abuse Program*. DA; July 23, 2020. Army Regulation 600-85. Accessed July 31, 2020. https://armypubs.army.mil/epubs/DR_pubs/DR_a/ARN30064-AR_600-85-000-WEB-1.pdf
2. Reagan R. Executive Order 12564—Drug-free Federal workplace. Published September 15, 1986. Accessed July 7, 2020. https://www.archives.gov/federal-register/codification/executive-order/12564.html
3. Suicide Prevention Resource Center. Army ACE Suicide Intervention Program. Accessed July 8, 2020. http://www.sprc.org/resources-programs/army-ace-suicide-intervention-program
4. Department of the Army. Community readiness and resiliency integrators. Stand-To! The Official Focus of the US Army. Published May 17, 2017. Accessed July 8, 2020. https://www.army.mil/standto/archive_2017-05-17
5. Department of the Army. *Army Health Promotion*. DA; April 14, 2015. Army Regulation 600-63. Accessed July 8, 2020. https://armypubs.army.mil/epubs/DR_pubs/DR_a/pdf/web/ARN15595_R600_63_admin_FINAL.pdf
6. Esper MT. *Army Directive 2018-23 (Improving the Effectiveness of Essential and Important Army Programs: Sexual Harassment/Assault Response and Prevention, Equal Opportunity, Suicide Prevention, Alcohol and Drug Abuse Prevention, and Resilience)*. Secretary of the Army; November 8, 2018. Accessed July 8, 2020. https://armypubs.army.mil/epubs/DR_pubs/DR_a/pdf/web/ARN14010_AD2018-23_Web_Final.pdf

7. National Organization for Victim Assistance website. Accessed July 7, 2020. http://www.try-nova.org/

Chapter 29

WHAT ARMY PHYSICIAN ASSISTANTS NEED TO KNOW ABOUT ELIMINATING POTENTIALLY SURVIVABLE DEATHS ON THE BATTLEFIELD

Christopher B. Cordova, PA-C, DSc, MPAS; Mitchell R. Andreas, PA-C, MPAS; Brandon M. Carius, PA-C, DSc, MPAS; Gonzalo de Taboada, PA-C, DSc, MPAS; Alixandra M. Mackey, PA-C, DMSc, MPAS; Mandy L. Pears, PA-C, MPAS; Tiffany L. Pittman, PA-C, MPAS; Adam R. Sahlberg, APA-C, MPAS; Megan L. Smith, PA-C, MPAS; and Andrew D. Fisher, MD, PA-C, MPAS, LP

Introduction

The diversity of the physician assistant (PA) profession in the armed forces offers opportunities for PAs to lead the way in eliminating preventable deaths on the battlefield. Army PAs are subject matter experts in the application of Tactical Combat Casualty Care (TCCC) for their assigned units, which places them in a position to impact combat medic training and the development of TCCC guidelines. During the Iraq and Afghanistan conflicts, combat casualty care evolved to dramatically improve delivery of life-saving measures to service members at the point of injury and beyond. Data collection from battlefield casualties has led to paradigm shifts in many types of battlefield care, with the ultimate goal of eliminating preventable deaths on the battlefield. The evolution and implementation of TCCC principles continues to change the definition of preventable deaths.

In a 2011 article, "Eliminating Preventable Death on the Battlefield,"[1] Kotwal et al reported the 75th Ranger Regiment's casualty survival rate from October 2001 to March 2010, which was higher than the rate for the Department of Defense as a whole. The article described the concepts the unit implemented to achieve their superior casualty survival rate: tactical leader prioritization of TCCC medical training for all unit members, tactical leader ownership of the casualty response system, and using feedback from the trauma registry to drive medical treatment protocols in the prehospital setting. This model should be thoroughly understood by all PAs, communicated to the unit leadership for implementation, and embraced by all deploying units.

Emerging capabilities in damage control resuscitation (DCR) and advanced resuscitative care (ARC), coupled with forward delivery of these interventions, are changing the definition of a potentially survivable death on the battlefield. The ability to deliver DCR and ARC interventions demonstrates great potential to improve battlefield survivability. This chapter will describe how the Army PA can continue to lead Army medicine by taking a key role in the development and execution of the use of fresh whole blood (FWB), resuscitative endovascular balloon occlusion of the aorta (REBOA), ARC, and prolonged field care (PFC).

Background of Tactical Combat Casualty Care and the Committee on Tactical Combat Casualty Care

In the final years of the 20th century, battlefield medicine was driven by advanced trauma life support (ATLS) principles.[2] While ATLS remains the standard of emergency department trauma care, it was not designed to address the most common causes of potentially preventable death on the battlefield.[3] The TCCC guidelines resulted from a 2-year study by the US Special Operations Command,[2] and the groundwork for their early adoption took place in the special operations community. Although TCCC is still evolving, the current guidelines embody the core principles of battlefield medicine as it is practiced today. In 2001, the Committee on Tactical Combat Casualty Care (CoTCCC) was formed.[4] As of 2019, the CoTCCC falls under the Joint Trauma System (JTS), has 42 members, meets biannually, and provides several updates per year. The JTS TCCC Guidelines for Medical Personnel Clinical Practice Guideline (CPG), listed in the Resources section of this chapter, provides the current TCCC recommendations.

Tactical Combat Casualty Care Phases

According to Butler et al, the goals of TCCC are to treat the casualty, prevent additional casualties, and complete the mission.[4] To accomplish these goals, there are several factors specific to TCCC and the distinct phases that must be considered, which include[4]:

1. The care team and the patient may be receiving accurate fire while care is being rendered. This requires that treatment be performed selectively at appropriate times and in a focused, deliberate, and timely manner.
2. Interventions should be focused on the leading causes of preventable death in combat: limb hemorrhage, airway obstruction, tension pneumothorax, junctional hemorrhage, and noncompressible torso hemorrhage (NCTH).
3. Evacuation times may be much longer than what is commonplace in civilian hospital systems.
4. Multiple casualties may be sustained in a single incident.
5. TCCC practitioners must often plan for and care for injuries in austere environments under adverse weather conditions.

Basic knowledge of TCCC begins with understanding the TCCC phases, defined as follows:

- **Care under fire.** Care that occurs at or close to the point of injury while the injured person and the care provider are under effective hostile fire. Equipment is generally limited to what can be carried by the medical provider. Care is limited to limb tourniquet application.[3]
- **Tactical field care.** Similar to care under fire, but there is no effective hostile fire. Medical equipment is limited to that which was brought on the mission.[3]
- **Tactical evacuation care.** Describes the care provided in both casualty evacuation (CASEVAC) and medical evacuation (MEDEVAC) scenarios. It begins with staging a casualty for evacuation and ends with delivering the casualty to the next level of care, with continual reassessment of previous interventions. Medical capability is augmented by both pre-staged equipment and personnel or dedicated medical evacuation assets and personnel.[3]

In order to understand the "why" behind the TCCC guidelines, it is important to know the data that drives the guidelines. The driving data point is the leading cause of preventable death on the battlefield.

Leading Causes of Preventable Death on the Battlefield

The leading causes of death on the battlefield as identified by Butler et al at the inception of TCCC were extremity hemorrhage, airway compromise, and tension pneumothorax.[2] More recent studies comparing data from before and after the widespread institution of TCCC training and interventions highlight a steep reduction in preventable deaths on the battlefield.[5,6] With the widespread issuance of ceramic hard plate body armor and Kevlar (DuPont) helmets and vests, injury patterns in Operation Iraqi Freedom and Operation Enduring Freedom shifted to include more extremity injuries and fewer head and torso injuries.[7] Widespread issuance of and training on tourniquets, nasopharyngeal airway adjuncts, and chest seals have served to equip battlefield first responders with the tools to address aspects of all three leading causes of preventable battlefield death.[8] Additionally, empowering 68W combat medics with the ability and training to conduct more advanced interventions, such as supraglottic airways, needle chest decompression, and in some cases cricothyrotomy, has affected causes of death far forward from even the battalion aid station.[9–11]

A further innovation has been treatment of both junctional hemorrhage and NCTH. The military has introduced junctional tourniquets and hemostatic impregnated gauze in an attempt to improve battlefield survivability of junctional hemorrhage. Unfortunately, treatment for NCTH remains difficult at Role 1. While an extended focused assessment with sonography for trauma (e-FAST) exam can assist in the decision to transport a casualty to definitive management, and tranexamic acid (TXA) and FWB can address coagulopathy and hemostasis, the mainstay of treatment for NCTH is rapid transport to surgical management.[12]

Fresh Whole Blood

The next innovation in advancing medical capabilities beyond the TCCC phases at the point of injury and Role 1 was administration of FWB (Figure 29-1). FWB entails blood recently acquired from local

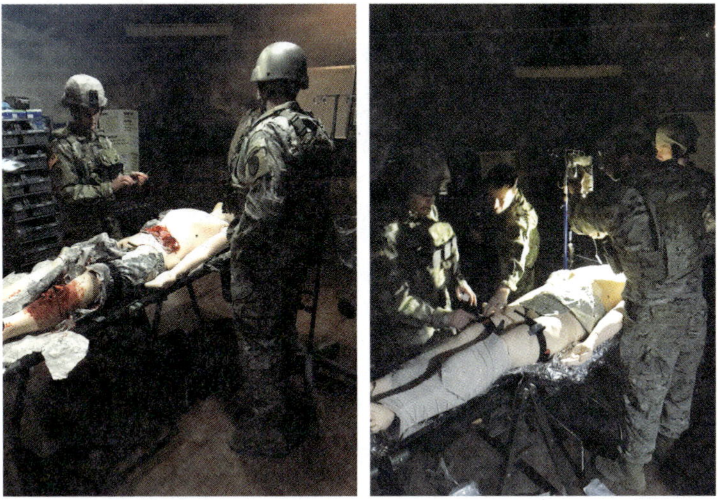

Figure 29-1. Major Christopher Cordova, PA-C, conducts trauma training scenarios, incorporating TCCC principles and fresh whole blood transfusion capability, to PA students (Captain Alixandra Mackey, Lieutenant Mitchell Andreas, and Lieutenant Benjamin Williams) at the Fort Carson Medical Simulation Training Center in January 2018.
Photographs courtesy of Captain Tiffany Pittman.

volunteer donors, generally through the use of walking blood banks, in which volunteers are called en masse to donate blood for patients in hemorrhagic shock. Although cold stored whole blood is preferred over FWB because it has been prescreened and transfusions can be started immediately, it may not be available in all forward deployed locations. Army PAs are commonly deployed to remote locations without the logistical support to store whole blood or blood component products, so FWB collection from donors is likely the only blood product available in most scenarios. The blood collected through this method does not go through regulated testing; therefore, the resulting product is not approved by the Food and Drug Administration (FDA). In order to implement a successful FWB program, planning should occur well before the execution of this capability.

Use of FWB is an important capability available to frontline medical providers with the potential to prolong survivability of critically injured patients.[13] However, FWB must be employed in conjunction with other DCR principles.[14] The implementation of FWB transfusion protocols must be guided by the recommendations of Strandenes, Fisher, and JTS CPGs.[15–19] Army PAs deployed or preparing to deploy should thoroughly review these protocols. The protocols must be adapted to individual trauma teams of forward deployed units, and the tailored protocols must be repeatedly trained and implemented by the provider-led trauma team, well before the unit is deployed to a combat environment.

Implementation

FWB transfusion is currently widely implemented at most Role 1 facilities and executed at the point of injury and during air medical evacuation in combat theaters. The JTS Whole Blood Transfusion and Damage Control Resuscitation CPG, listed in the Resources section of this chapter, provides the most recent recommendations for implementation. Planning is paramount! The implementation and execution of a successful FWB protocol must be integrated well before the combat training center rotation and combat deployment. Through proper coordination, the Armed Services Blood Program (ASBP) can screen soldiers for transfusion-transmitted diseases (TTDs) and anti-A/anti-B titer less than 1:256 (low-titer group O whole blood [LTOWB]). The ASPB documents screening results in the Theater Medical Data Store (TMDS) blood module. This critical predeployment action enables faster administration of FWB at the time of need because it eliminates point-of-care (POC) blood typing for the donor and recipient.

Equipment

Upon completion of screening, the next focus is acquisition of equipment required to execute the transfusion. Blood transfusion kits or sets are available for purchase through a variety of medical companies. These products contain the items required for performing an FWB transfusion, such as blood type test kits (if blood was not prescreened), like the EldonCard (Eldon Biologicals) to test recipients and donors; blood collection bags; intravenous (IV) tubing with a filtered chamber; and typical items used to obtain IV access. PAs must also ensure possession of Standard Form 518, Blood or Blood Component Transfusion Medical Record, to properly document the medical intervention.

Blood collection bags differ from other standard IV fluid bags in their additives and anticoagulants that allow for preservation of donated blood. Each bag contains either citrate phosphate dextrose (CPD) or citrate phosphate dextrose adenine-1 (CPDA-1), which prevent blood clot formation by binding calcium in the donor's blood and thus inhibiting the coagulation pathway. CPD allows for 21 days of refrigerated storage in case an FWB donation is not utilized immediately, while CPDA-1 allows for up to 35 days of refrigerated storage.

The use of proper IV tubing, containing a micron filter, is essential to further mitigate the risk of blood clots. These administration sets filter blood and any clots that may be formed and, combined with the use of blood collection bags containing CPD or CPDA-1, significantly reduce the likelihood of clot formation and transfusion into the recipient.

Storage of blood should be avoided but is possible at room temperature up to 6 hours, after which it must be refrigerated. However, it is still considered FWB up to 48 hours after donation.[17] Blood storage devices can extend capabilities in combat missions. Portable storage devices like the Golden Minute Container and Golden Hour Medic Thermal Blood Transfer Container (both manufactured by Pelican BioThermal) are available. Storage options requiring a constant power supply may be obtained for a fixed military medical treatment facility (MTF).

Importance of Training

All medical capabilities should be rehearsed repeatedly, utilizing the most realistic scenarios possible, in order to execute the capability during a high-stress trauma situation. Executing an FWB transfusion should not be taken lightly. This capability should be rehearsed thoroughly with critical focus on the administrative details in order to avoid incorrect administration of type-specific blood.

As the primary trainers of medical skills to unit medics, Army PAs should be deeply involved in the implementation and execution of an FWB training program. Mastery of military and medical skills requires effective initial training, and continued training is required to maintain proficiency. While most procedures involved with FWB transfusion, such as initiating an IV, are baseline skills for combat medics and medical providers, regular training must be conducted to maintain confidence in equipment and personnel. To ensure optimal blood matching and avoid unnecessary hemolytic reactions for training purposes, autologous transfusions (self-to-self) are used for FWB transfusion training. This process involves drawing blood from one location of the body (such as the left antecubital fossa) and "donating" it into another location (such as the right antecubital fossa).

Training Risks and Mitigation

All training, including FWB transfusion, involves risks that should be mitigated to the fullest extent. Despite the use of autologous transfusions, risks remain. As the medical subject matter expert in their unit, the Army PA should understand and acknowledge all risks while making every effort to effectively mitigate them. The Army PA should conduct a formal risk assessment with approval of the accepted risk by the unit commander.

The most common side effect with blood donation is the onset of a vasovagal reaction (VVR).[20] In a recent military study by Donham et al, VVR occurred in less than 0.5% of participants.[20] As with most regular donor protocols, VVR can be mitigated by ensuring participants eat and drink regularly prior to donation and lie flat on a stable surface during the donation event. If a reaction occurs, the donor's legs should be lifted above the level of their heart to optimize venous return.

A study of over 3,400 US military autologous transfusions found that besides VVR, ocular blood exposure and a minor allergic reaction (urticaria) occurred only twice and once, respectively.[20] There were no reports of anaphylaxis or major hemolytic transfusion reactions.[20]

Clinical Indication for Fresh Whole Blood Transfusion

Once population screening and equipment acquisition is complete, the Army PA is fully prepared to execute the FWB transfusion when encountering a casualty meeting the clinical indication. The clinical signs of hemorrhagic shock (decreased mentation, pulse > 120 beats per minute, absent or weak radial pulse, systolic blood pressure < 90 mm Hg), along with a mechanism of injury suggesting significant blood loss (eg, limb amputation, penetrating chest or abdominal injury) are the indications for initiation of the DCR protocol[17]: hemostasis through tourniquet use in junctional and peripheral penetrating wounds, administration of TXA within 3 hours of injury, and early blood product resuscitation.[14]

Fresh Whole Blood Tips for Success

The following are tips for success for the Army PA regarding fresh whole blood.

1. The PA must review and understand the FWB CPG produced by the JTS.[19]
2. The PA must conduct unit screening for LTOWB and TTDs 3 to 6 months prior to deployment through the ASPB or local MTF. The roster should be verified through the TMDS blood module.
3. The PA must procure necessary equipment from installation supply channels or through vendor purchase 3 to 6 months prior to deployment to perform FWB and store FWB or cold stored whole blood in austere environments as the mission conditions dictate (eg, FWB kits, Golden Minute Container or Golden Hour Medic Thermal Blood Transfer Container).
4. The PA must rehearse protocols routinely with dedicated medical staff in collective unit training exercises and in the deployed MTF. Training should include:
   a. identification of FWB transfusion indications in notion casualties;
   b. notification of prescreened population and reporting to an MTF;
   c. screening of donor and recipient with EldonCards (if needed; this may be omitted if prescreened for LTOWB and documented in TMDS);
   d. autologous (self-to-self) FWB transfusions; and
   e. proper documentation on Standard Form 518.
5. The PA must execute FWB transfusion as part of the DCR protocol when clinically indicated in an actual casualty.

Resuscitative Endovascular Balloon Occlusion of the Aorta

Almost 90% of all deaths in combat occur in the prehospital setting.[5] Of these deaths, the leading cause of potentially survivable death in combat is NCTH.[5] Army PAs may help reduce these deaths through the use of REBOA, first described by Lieutenant Colonel Carl W. Hughes during the Korean War. Hughes placed a balloon tipped catheter into two combat casualties,[21] and although he was unsuccessful in saving their lives, he surmised that early implementation would have better outcomes.[21] In recent years, the REBOA procedure has gained popularity as a means to gain distal hemorrhage control while increasing blood pressure and central aortic pressure until hemorrhage control can be achieved. REBOA consists of inserting a flexible catheter with a balloon tip through the common femoral artery into the aorta. Other than cessation of blood flow distal to the balloon, early use is believed to preserve cerebral perfusion and coronary filling in patients with life-threatening hypotension and hypovolemia secondary to hemorrhage.[22] The use of REBOA is not a definitive treatment, but rather a temporizing measure that may allow more time for a critically wounded casualty to receive surgical care.

Considerations for Use

REBOA insertion requires appropriate training to ensure successful implementation and use in the prehospital setting, and there is still considerable concern about the benefit and safety of prehospital REBOA placement. A statement released by the American College of Surgeons Committee on Trauma, the American College of Emergency Physicians, the National Association of Emergency Medical Services Physicians, and the National Association of Emergency Medical Technicians considered the use of REBOA in the prehospital setting inappropriate, but did not make recommendations regarding the military use of REBOA.[23] Military providers must consider who is best prepared and at what level of care this procedure should be implemented. As of 2019, Role 2 is the first level of care in which REBOA is being performed, with or without a forward surgical team (FST). Role 2 has patient resuscitation capability, accessibility to various blood products (stored or via a walking blood bank), and the ability to surgically stabilize patients when collocated with an FST element. However, with the availability of training designed for the non-surgeons and providers without critical care training, improved tools including POC ultrasound and the ER-REBOA (Prytime Medical), and changing protocols, it is feasible to use REBOA at a Role 1 facility and even at the point of injury. REBOA use and implementation are currently addressed in greater detail by the JTS Resuscitative Endovascular Balloon Occlusion of the Aorta (REBOA) for Hemorrhagic Shock CPG.[24]

Anatomy

The REBOA balloon is inflated at specific areas of the aorta to achieve desired hemorrhage control based on injury location. The aorta is divided into three zones[25]:

Zone I begins at the commencement of the left subclavian artery and extends to the celiac trunk.
Zone II begins at the celiac trunk and extends to the lowest renal artery.
Zone III begins at the lowest renal artery and ends at the bifurcation.

To impede bleeding resulting from abdominal injuries, REBOA should be placed into zone I; when trying to prevent bleeding resulting from pelvic trauma, the balloon should be inserted into zone III (however, insertion into zone III is not recommended in the prehospital setting). Zone II is the paravisceral aorta and generally accepted as a no-go zone.

Indications

REBOA offers a less invasive alternative than emergent resuscitative thoracotomy (ERT) for controlling NCTH in patients at risk for imminent cardiovascular collapse.[26] Patients with abdominal, pelvic, or junctional lower extremity bleeding are likely to benefit if hemorrhagic shock is recognized early. Precise indications for REBOA are not well studied; however, the REBOA CPG from the JTS recommends use for patients with[24]:

- blunt trauma with no major chest bleeding (negative chest radiograph, ultrasound, or bilateral chest tubes);
- a positive abdominal e-FAST exam;
- penetrating trauma to the abdomen or pelvis;
- pelvic fracture; or
- massive proximal lower extremity hemorrhage with signs of impending cardiovascular compromise (Figure 29-2).

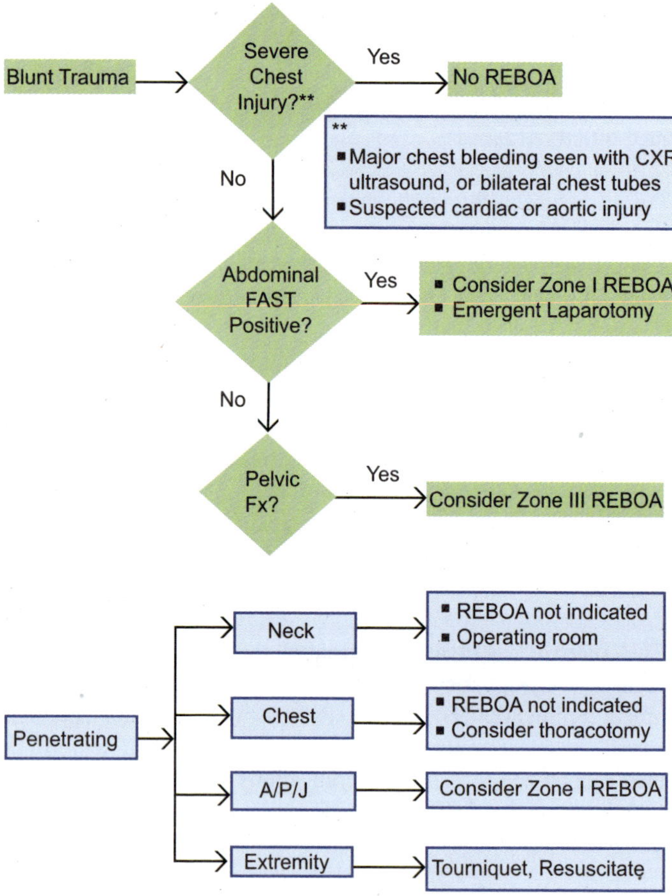

Figure 29-2. REBOA algorithm proposed by the Joint Trauma System.
A/P/J: abdominal/pelvic/junctional
CXR: chest x-ray
Fx: fracture

A more simplified approach is provided by the Committee on TCCC's ARC guidelines, which recommend use on patients with[27]:

- an injury pattern that suggests abdominopelvic non-compressible hemorrhage;

- systolic blood pressure < 90 mmHg; and
- an unsatisfactory response to the first unit of whole blood.

REBOA should not be used without proper resuscitation. The use of REBOA is still a controversial procedure and without a clear benefit for prehospital use.[28] However, combat death is a compelling motivator to implement programs and procedures that may have an unclear benefit, and REBOA may provide the temporary measure that allows adequate time to deliver severely wounded patients to a surgical capability.

Contraindications

Avoid REBOA in patients with thoracic trauma or hemorrhage.[26] These injuries should be ruled out using chest x-ray, thoracic ultrasound, or bilateral simple or tube thoracostomy. Careful planning should be done before the use of REBOA to ensure the availability of surgical resources for more definitive management.

There may be short-term and long-term sequelae to areas of the body not receiving blood flow during REBOA balloon inflation. Complications from REBOA include mesenteric ischemia and ischemia of the lower extremities; also, deployment of REBOA in thoracic aortic injury could increase hemorrhage and make the injury worse.[29] However, when compared to the more invasive emergent resuscitative thoracotomy (ERT) with aortic cross-clamping, the REBOA may be a safer and more feasible option for the Role 1 provider. ERT has its own set of complications and sequelae in addition to those outlined for REBOA; however, a detailed description of ERT is beyond the scope of a PA's practice.

Equipment and Placement

The majority of the equipment required to perform REBOA safely in the prehospital environment is available through the military logistical system. Obtaining an ultrasound may be more difficult, and PAs should purchase a handheld ultrasound device, either with unit funds or on their own. Handheld ultrasound devices are beneficial not only for use in the ARC setting, but also as a tool in the clinic.

The ER-REBOA device consists of a curled distal tip (P-tip [Prytime Medical]) and a compliant occlusion balloon. The catheter contains two lumens that run the length of the catheter and connect to extension lines with stopcocks. The balloon lumen is used to inflate and deflate the balloon. The arterial line lumen is used to monitor blood pressure. A peel-away sheath is pre-loaded on the catheter shaft to ease insertion of the catheter's P-tip into an introducer sheath hemostasis valve. The JTS Resuscitative Endovascular Balloon Occlusion of the Aorta (REBOA) for Hemorrhagic Shock CPG, listed in the Resources section of this chapter, outlines a six-step process for successful REBOA employment.[24] It also lists standard equipment needed for REBOA placement.

Initial Training

The Basic Endovascular Skills for Trauma (BEST) course at the University of Maryland's R. Adams Cowley Shock Trauma Center was the first to offer training in the use of REBOA. This training was initially for surgeons and critical care fellowship-trained emergency medicine physicians. In 2015, a physician, a PA, and a Special Operations Combat Medic (SOCM) not trained in critical care attended the BEST course as a pilot project to evaluate the possibility of performing the procedure in the prehospital setting.[30] When the ER-REBOA catheter became FDA approved, the ability to train PAs and enlisted medical personnel became more feasible. This device decreased the number of steps required to access the common femoral artery and place a REBOA catheter. Currently, the Army and the American College of Surgeons both have REBOA training programs. Additionally, the Resuscitation Adjuncts: Prehospital Transfusion & REBOA (RAPToR) course (https://www.raptocourse.com/) is specifically designed for prehospital implementation of REBOA. The 2-day course provides REBOA and FWB training in the context of ARC. The RAPToR course is sponsored by Combat Medical and Prytime Medical, and is recognized by the CoTCCC as a training option.

Sustainment Training

The military tends to offer initial training that meets standards, but often fails to offer suitable sustainment training in a quality manner. Many medical officers assigned to maneuver units have difficulties maintaining currency in various skills because of many factors, including finding time for appropriate health care coverage for their units and time to attend courses. While it is not critical for Army PAs to maintain the skill required to perform REBOA during a training cycle, it is important to attend a training course at least 60 days prior to deployment. There are several options that could allow the Army PA to successfully employ the skills required for REBOA. The most useful is training with the perfused cadaver model.[31] (Cadavers can be used for training multiple skills beyond REBOA. The use of cadavers also eliminates hospital intrusion.)

Live tissue training (LTT) is another option for sustainment training. However, any LTT requires approval from an Institutional Animal Care and Use Committee (some units have an animal use committee within their major command; others may have to check with their local MTF). The swine is the patient model of choice for REBOA sustainment training. Recently, Borger van der Burg et al described a method that allows for multiple attempts at gaining access using a swine model and placing a silicone tube next to the common femoral artery.[32]

Other sustainment options include working with the local MTF to perform arterial access, which can be as simple as ultrasound-guided radial artery access. Other options include establishing memoranda of agreement with civilian hospitals that currently use REBOA or conducting sustainment training with the Simulation Trainer for Arterial Access and REBOA (STAAR) (Prytime Medical).

Advanced Resuscitative Care/Advanced Resuscitative Care Teams

FWB transfusion and REBOA comprise the evolving concept of ARC. ARC is a momentous update to TCCC that may provide further opportunity for PAs to play a key role in reducing battlefield fatalities from exsanguination. Although TCCC has saved numerous lives since its inception in 1996, it arguably did not address the most lethal of battlefield injuries—NCTH. In an evaluation of over 4,596 battlefield fatalities from 2001 to 2011, Eastridge et al found that 87.3% of casualties die before reaching a surgeon.[5] Of these fatalities, 67% were due to NCTH (Figure 29-3).[5] This landmark study reinforced the need for a modality to address the potentially preventable deaths caused by NCTH in the prehospital setting. ARC is a concept within TCCC that specifically addresses the need to control NCTH in prehospital

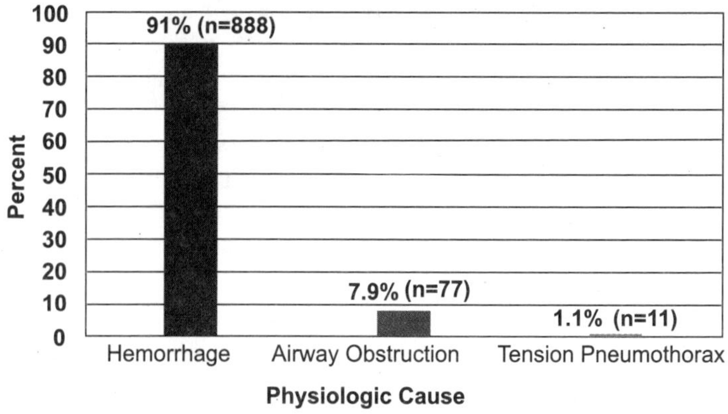

Figure 29-3. Data demonstrating non-compressible torso hemorrhage as the leading cause of death on the battlefield.
Reproduced with permission from: Eastridge BJ, Mabry RL, Seguin P, et al. Death on the battlefield (2001–2011): Implications for the future of combat casualty care. *J Trauma*. 2012;73(6 Suppl 5):S431–S437. https://journals.lww.com/jtrauma/pages/default.aspx

and Role 1 settings. ARC interventions include early and aggressive DCR with whole blood transfusions and use of the REBOA (see Figure 29-3).

Advanced Resuscitative Care Team

ARC is not meant to be performed by lone combat medical personnel, regardless of their skill level. Rather, ARC is specifically designed to be executed by an identified, well-trained, and properly equipped team. Ideally, the ARC team is composed of three or four members. The team who performs REBOA should have obtained initial training at a recognized REBOA training course and maintained their skill through an accepted means (cadaver, LTT, or STAAR).[27]

However, the official composition of teams performing ARC is yet to be determined. In the meantime, the team leader should delegate the multiple required tasks. The ARC team executes nine specific tasks: (1) ensure an adequate airway, (2) electronically monitor vital signs,

(3) establish IV or intraosseous access, (4) prepare and infuse blood products, (5) insert e-FAST and bilateral chest tubes, (6) establish common femoral artery access, (7) prepare the REBOA site, (8) perform the REBOA procedure, and (9) record the events that occur during resuscitation.[27]

As the primary medical trainer and the medical officer with the most continuity for the unit, the Army PA should lead the ARC team. PAs should seek out the appropriate training and be ready to execute this advanced resuscitative measure at the Role 1 or at the point of injury.

Training the Advanced Resuscitative Care Team

Because the ARC team is required to perform multiple tasks in a rapid and proficient manner, it is critical that the team is competent in the above listed skill sets, with particular emphasis on performing the REBOA procedure. Ideally, the ARC team would establish a baseline competency at a training course, then continue to sustain skill sets through ongoing experience with trauma patients, simulation training, or perfused cadaver-based training. At this time, there are multiple venues that can provide training in ARC: the Air Force Center for the Sustainment of Trauma and Readiness Skills (C-STARS) program, the Army Trauma Training Course, and military and civilian trauma training centers (with local training agreements).[27] As discussed above, the Army and the American College of Surgeons both have REBOA training programs. ARC was recently approved by the CoTCCC as a new component of TCCC. "TCCC Skill Sets by Responder Level,"[33] published in April 2019 by JTS and CoTCCC, includes the specific skill set that should be performed by TCCC ARC teams.[33] Although resources for ARC training are available, the CoTCCC is developing a specific ARC curriculum going forward.[34]

Unfortunately, not all casualty situations will be resolved with TCCC, DCR, and ARC due to constraints in medical evacuation or mission requirements. Therefore, Army PAs should be aware of and able to execute the principles of PFC.

Prolonged Field Care

In 2008, then Secretary of Defense Robert Gates issued a mandate that all military medical evacuation to a surgeon must occur in less than

60 minutes.[35] Although this has led to the lowest mortality rate of any conflict, providers cannot rely on 1-hour evacuations in current and future operations, and providers must plan for care over hours and even days. It should be noted, however, that findings by both Kotwal and Howard found it was not just rapid evacuation that decreased mortality, but also the ability to provide faster advanced care to the casualty.[35,36]

PFC is defined as "field medical care, applied beyond 'doctrinal planning time-lines' by a SOCM (Special Operations Combat Medic) or higher, in order to decrease patient mortality and morbidity. It utilizes limited resources and is sustained until the patient arrives at an appropriate level of care."[37] PFC was developed and became a focus of interest over the last decade in special operations and conventional forces due to the changes in deployed operations into more austere prehospital environments (Figure 29-4). PFC is an ongoing process that starts once the patient has been stabilized after initial presentation, whether in a trauma or a medical setting. It encompasses the best practices of TCCC, DCR, and continuous, assertive nursing care, and is broken down into 10 core principles. These principles have corresponding CPGs to explain and universalize medical practice (provided at www.prolongedfieldcare.org, with links to numerous articles and position papers covering the development, training, and implementation of PFC[38,39]). The JTS PFC CPGs, listed in the Resources section of this chapter, provide current recommendations on analgesia sedation management, burn management, crush syndrome, DCR, documentation, nursing care, ocular injuries, traumatic brain injury, and wound management.

Ten Core Principles of Prolonged Field Care

1. Trending vitals and documentation.
2. Resuscitation using blood products.
3. Ventilation and oxygenation.
4. Airway control.
5. Pain control.
6. Continued monitoring for potential complications.
7. Aggressive nursing care.
8. Surgical procedures (ARC).
9. Telemedicine.
10. Documentation and evacuation.[38]

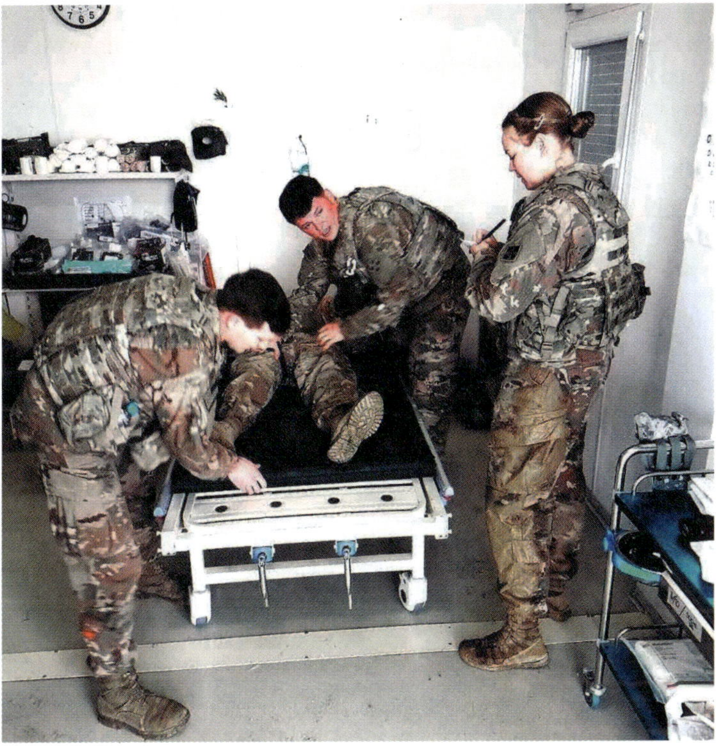

Figure 29-4. Captain Megan Smith, PA-C, with medics and soldiers at Mosul Dam, Iraq, May 2019. The unit conducted base defense drills incorporating a mass casualty exercise including evacuation of casualties from the perimeter to the Role 1. The focus was working as a team on a trauma bed with minimal medics and a single PA. The closest aeromedical evacuation asset was 1.5 hours away. The training was focused on prolonged field care and advancing 68W skills to increase medical capabilities.
Photograph courtesy of Staff Sergeant Ronald Monsen.

Training

PFC encompasses a wide spectrum of medical skills, and units may be challenged to prepare and train for situations requiring PFC skills. Situations requiring PFC can happen during stateside training events, in combat, in humanitarian deployments, and even on vacation, so it is necessary to be as prepared as possible. Limited time and resources may be obstacles, but there is no substitute for hands-on training in all components of PFC. The first things to consider are what objectives need to be accomplished to acquire a good working knowledge of PFC components. The training should be well thought out and structured to ensure all members of the team are proficient in the smallest of tasks prior to a culminating event. A short-term train-up will not sufficiently prepare a medical team to be prepared for managing a real-world PFC scenario.

Role of the Physician Assistant in Prolonged Field Care

Army PAs have a high probability of being assigned to an austere environment with limited medical resources, where they are the senior medical provider with a small team of medics. Part of a battalion PA's job is to train the medics assigned to them. Training medics to work as team is as important as training them to be competent in all medical tasks in the scope of practice. The medic team is the PA's best asset in PFC situations. PAs must therefore understand how to optimally care for a casualty if placed in a PFC scenario, and they must also understand the limitations of PFC. PAs should maintain their skills by attending medical courses that advance their capabilities; however, employing life-saving techniques on patients will always surpass simulations. The PA should be proactive in this approach by utilizing local civilian trauma centers, most of which have medical training agreements in place with MTFs that are established by MTF commanders.

Conclusion

Eliminating potentially preventable deaths on the battlefield will always be a dynamic process. As forward medical capabilities improve, the leading cause of death on the battlefield will change. However, the role of the Army PA will remain constant—implementing current medical capabilities to treat combat casualties on the front lines of the battlefield. With the implementation of FWB transfusion, REBOA, ARC, and PFC on the battlefield, the Army PA must remain educated and knowledgeable about the JTS CPGs for each of these disciplines. It is the responsibility of the Army PA to train the medical team through rehearsals that implement novel capabilities on the battlefield—well before the combat deployment. Employment of these principles will continue to reduce potentially preventable deaths on the battlefield.

References

1. Kotwal RS, Montgomery HR, Kotwal BM, et al. Eliminating preventable death on the battlefield. *Arch Surg.* 2011;146(12):1350–1358.
2. Butler FK Jr, Hagmann J, Butler EG. Tactical combat casualty care in special operations. *Mil Med.* 1996;161(Suppl:3–16).
3. Champion HR, Bellamy RF, Roberts CP, Leppaniemi A. A profile of combat injury. *J Trauma.* 2003;54(5 Suppl):S13–19.
4. Butler FK. Two decades of saving lives on the battlefield: tactical combat casualty care turns 20. *Mil Med.* 2017;182(3):e1563-e8.
5. Eastridge BJ, Mabry RL, Seguin P, et al. Death on the battlefield (2001-2011): Implications for the future of combat casualty care. *J Trauma.* 2012;73(6 Suppl 5):S431–S437.
6. Kelly JF, Ritenour AE, McLaughlin DF, et al. Injury severity and causes of death from Operation Iraqi Freedom and Operation Enduring Freedom: 2003-2004 versus 2006. *J Trauma.* 2008;64(2 Suppl):S21–S26.
7. Belmont PJ, Schoenfeld AJ, Goodman G. Epidemiology of combat wounds in Operation Iraqi Freedom and Operation Enduring Freedom: orthopaedic burden of disease. *J Surg Orthop Adv.* 2010;19(1):2–7.
8. Kragh JF Jr, Walters TJ, Baer DG, et al. Survival with emergency tourniquet use to stop bleeding in major limb trauma. *Ann Surg.* 2009;249(1):1–7.
9. Gerhardt RT, Berry JA, Blackbourne LH. Analysis of life-saving interventions performed by out-of-hospital combat medical personnel. *J Trauma.* 2011;71(1 Suppl):S109–113.
10. Lairet J, Bebarta VS, Maddry JK, et al. Prehospital interventions performed in Afghanistan between November 2009 and March 2014. *Mil Med.* 2019;184(Suppl 1):133–137.

11. Schauer SG, April MD, Simon E, Maddry JK, Carter R, Delorenzo RA. Prehospital interventions during mass-casualty events in Afghanistan: a case analysis. *Prehosp Disaster Med.* 2017;32(4):465–468.

12. Holcomb JB. Transport time and preoperating room hemostatic interventions are important: improving outcomes after severe truncal injury. *Crit Care Med.* 2018;46(3):447–453.

13. Cordova CB, Cap AP, Spinella PC. Fresh whole blood transfusion for a combat casualty in austere combat environment. *J Spec Oper Med.* 2014;14(1):9–12.

14. Cap AP, Pidcoke HF, Spinella P, et al. Damage control resuscitation. *Mil Med.* 2018;183(Suppl 2):36–43.

15. Cap AP, Beckett A, Benov A, et al. Whole blood transfusion. *Mil Med.* 2018;183(Suppl 2):44–51.

16. Fisher AD, Miles EA, Cap AP, Strandenes G, Kane SF. Tactical damage control resuscitation. *Mil Med.* 2015;180(8):869–875.

17. Strandenes G, De Pasquale M, Cap AP, et al. Emergency whole-blood use in the field: a simplified protocol for collection and transfusion. *Shock.* 2014;41 Suppl 1:76–83.

18. Strandenes G, Berseus O, Cap AP, et al. Low titer group O whole blood in emergency situations. *Shock.* 2014;41 Suppl 1:70–5.

19. Cap AP, Beckett A, Benov A, et al. Whole blood transfusion. *Mil Med.* 2018;183(suppl 2):44–51.

20. Donham B, Barbee GA, Deaton TG, Kerr W, Wier RP, Fisher AD. Risk associated with autologous fresh whole blood training. *J Spec Oper Med.* 2019;19(3):24–25.

21. Hughes CW. Use of an intra-aortic balloon catheter tamponade for controlling intraabdominal hemorrhage in man. *Surgery.* 1954;36:65–68.

22. Johnson MA, Neff LP, Williams TK, DuBose JJ, Group ES. Partial resuscitative balloon occlusion of the aorta (P-REBOA): Clinical technique and rationale. *J Trauma Acute Care Surg.* 2016;81(5 Suppl 2):S133–S137.

23. Bulger EM, Perina DG, Qasim Z, et al. Clinical use of resuscitative endovascular balloon occlusion of the aorta (REBOA) in civilian trauma systems in the USA, 2019: a joint statement from the American College of Surgeons Committee on Trauma, the American College of Emergency Physicians, the National Association of Emergency Medical Services Physicians and the National Association of Emergency Medical Technicians. *Trauma Surg Acute Care Open.* 2019;4(1):e000376.

24. Pasley J, Cannon J, Glaser J, et al. Resuscitative Endovascular Balloon Occlusion of the Aorta (REBOA) for Hemorrhagic Shock (CPG ID: 38). Department of Defense, Center of Excellence for Trauma, Joint Trauma System, CPG website. Published July 6, 2017. Accessed August 26, 2020. https://jts.amedd.army.mil/assets/docs/cpgs/JTS_Clinical_Practice_Guidelines_(CPGs)/REBOA_%20Hemorrhagic%20Shock_06_Jul_2017_ID38.pdf

25. Stannard A, Eliason JL, Rasmussen TE. Resuscitative endovascular balloon occlusion of the aorta (REBOA) as an adjunct for hemorrhagic shock. *J Trauma.* 2011;71(6):1869–1872.

26. Cannon J, Morrison J, Lauer C, et al. Resuscitative endovascular balloon occlusion of the aorta (REBOA) for hemorrhagic shock. *Mil Med.* 2018;183(Suppl 2):55–59.

27. Butler FK Jr, Holcomb JB, Shackelford S, et al. Advanced resuscitative care in tactical combat casualty care: TCCC guidelines change 18-01. *J Spec Oper Med.* 2019;18(4)37–55.

28. Bekdache O, Paradis T, Shen YBH, et al. Resuscitative endovascular balloon occlusion of the aorta (REBOA): indications: advantages and challenges of implementation in traumatic non-compressible torso hemorrhage. *Trauma Surg Acute Care Open.* 2019;4(1):e000262. doi: 10.1136/tsaco-2018-000262

29. Sato R, Kuriyama A, Takaesu R, et al. Resuscitative endovascular balloon occlusion of the aorta performed by emergency physicians for traumatic hemorrhagic shock: a case series from Japanese emergency rooms. *Crit Care.* 2018;22(1):103.

30. Teeter W, Romagnoli A, Glaser J, et al. resuscitative endovascular balloon occlusion of the aorta: pushing care forward. *J Spec Oper Med.* 2017;17(1):17–21.

31. Redman TT, Ross EM. A novel expeditionary perfused cadaver model for trauma training in the out-of-hospital setting. *J Emerg Med.* 2018;55(3):383–389.

32. Borger van der Burg BLS, Horer TM, Eefting D, et al. Vascular access training for REBOA placement: a feasibility study in a live tissue-simulator hybrid porcine model. *J R Army Med Corps.* 2019;165(3):147–151.

33. Committee on Tactical Combat Casualty Care & Joint Trauma System. Tactical combat casualty care skill sets by responder level. Published April 22, 2019. Accessed August 26, 2020. https://deployedmedicine.com/market/11/content/211/

34. Butler FK. Committee on Tactical Combat Casualty Care meeting minutes. Paper presented at: Committee on Tactical Combat Casualty Care; February 20–21, 2019; San Antonio, TX.

35. Kotwal RS, Howard JT, Orman JA, et al. The effect of a golden hour policy on the morbidity and mortality of combat casualties. *JAMA Surg.* 2016;151(1):15–24.

36. Howard JT, Kotwal RS, Santos-Lazada AR, Martin MJ, Stockinger ZT. Reexamination of a battlefield trauma golden hour policy. *J Trauma Acute Care Surg.* 2018;84(1):11–18.

37. Keenan S. Deconstructing the Definition of Prolonged Field Care. *J Spec Oper Med.* 2015;15(4):125.

38. Ball JA, Keenan S. Prolonged field care working group position paper: prolonged field care capabilities. *J Spec Oper Med.* 2015;15(3):76–77.

39. ProlongedFieldCare.org. Position paper—10 essential core capabilities for prolonged field care. Published February 9, 2015. Accessed August 26, 2020. https://prolongedfieldcare.org/2015/02/09/10-essential-core-capabilities-for-prolonged-field-care/

Additional Sources

- The CoTCCC's official website is https://www.deployedmedicine.com, and the mobile phone app is Deployed Medicine. These TCCC resources offer updates, background and supporting evidence, videos, JTS podcast information, and more.
- JTS CPGs: for TCCC, DCR, FWB, and REBOA are found at the links below.
    - TCCC Guidelines for Medical Personnel: https:/jts.amedd.army.mil/assets/docs/cpgs/Prehospital_En_Route_CPGs/Tactical_Combat_Casualty_Care_Guidelines_01_Aug_2019.pdf
    - Damage Control Resuscitation (CPG ID: 18): https://jts.amedd.army.mil/assets/docs/cpgs/JTS_Clinical_Practice_Guidelines_(CPGs)/Damage_Control_Resuscitation_12_Jul_2019_ID18.pdf
    - Whole Blood Transfusion (CPG ID: 21): https://jts.amedd.army.mil/assets/docs/cpgs/JTS_Clinical_Practice_Guidelines_(CPGs)/Whole_Blood_Transfusion_15_May_2018_ID21.pdf
    - Resuscitative Endovascular Balloon Occlusion of the Aorta (REBOA) for Hemorrhagic Shock (CPG ID: 38): https://jts.amedd.army.mil/assets/docs/cpgs/JTS_Clinical_Practice_Guidelines_(CPGs)/REBOA_%20Hemorrhagic%20Shock_06_Jul_2017_ID38.pdf
- JTS CPGs for the numerous PFC subcategories are found under the "Prehospital/En Route CPGs" header at https://jts.amedd.army.mil/index.cfm/PI_CPGs/cpgs
- Department of Defense. *Medical Readiness Training (MRT)*. DOD; March 16, 2018. DOD Instruction 1322.24.
- Department of Defense. *Joint Trauma System (JTS)*. Change 1, effective August 5, 2018. DOD Instruction 6040.47.

Chapter 30

ROLE OF THE PHYSICIAN ASSISTANT IN THE DISABILITY EVALUATION SYSTEM

Lakeshia T. Logan, PA-C, MPAS; Amy L. Jackson, PA-C, MPAS; Gail A. Martin, APA-C, MPAS; David Polston, APA-C, MPAS; Christopher H. Warner, MD; Carolynn M. Warner, MD; and Larry A. Wyatt, APA-C, MPAS

Introduction

The Disability Evaluation System is a US Department of Defense (DOD) process for determining if a wounded, injured, or ill soldier will be able to return to duty or if they will be medically separated or medically retire due to their disability. The Integrated Disability Evaluation System (IDES) is a combined process used by the DOD and the Department of Veterans Affairs (VA). The two departments work concurrently to determine the soldier's capability to continue to perform their duties and serve in the Army.

Prior to the implementation of IDES in the early 2010s, the DOD and VA disability and rating processes were completed separately. The Legacy Disability Evaluation System (LDES) process resulted in a long wait for and between evaluations, a benefits gap between soldiers' separation from the Army and when they started receiving VA benefits and disability compensation payments, and differences in the disability ratings between the Army Physical Evaluation Board (PEB) and the VA.

IDES was intended to resolve these issues by providing a simple, unified system[1,2] that resulted in consistent evaluations and ratings, and, most importantly, ensured that disabled soldiers leaving the Army were immediately linked into the VA and began receiving benefits. Although IDES streamlined the system overall, it also increased the time soldiers remained on active duty while undergoing medical evaluation and being

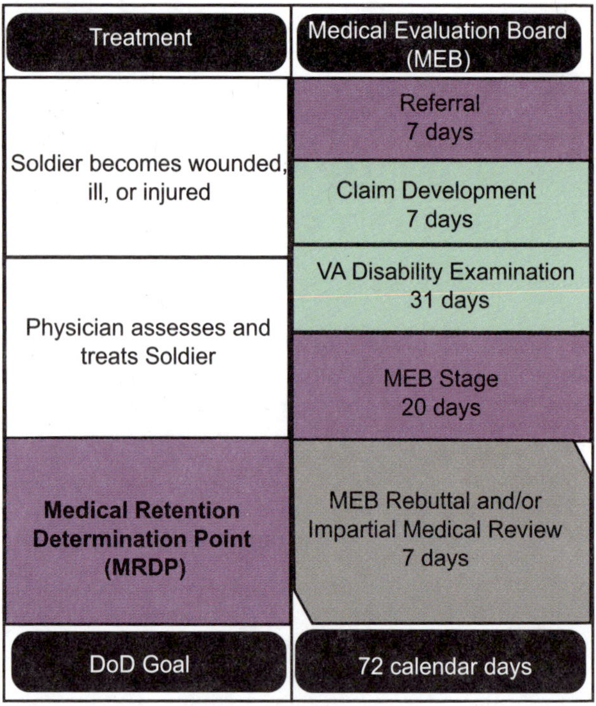

assigned disability ratings. Designed at the height of the surge of forces in Iraq and Afghanistan, the IDES process has retained its value during the more recent times of sequestration and military drawdown, helping the DOD preserve a fit and vital force and maintain military readiness.[3]

However, the LDES system allows for a DOD-led process that can be more time efficient based on the need of the soldier, the Army, or both.[3] The soldier or their commander can request that the LDES process be used instead of the IDES. The local military medical treatment facility (MTF) commander can approve the soldier's enrollment in the LDES or elect to send the soldier through IDES.

The IDES Process

The IDES process is outlined in Figure 30-1.[2] Once a soldier has reached the medical retention determination point (MRDP) and is referred to

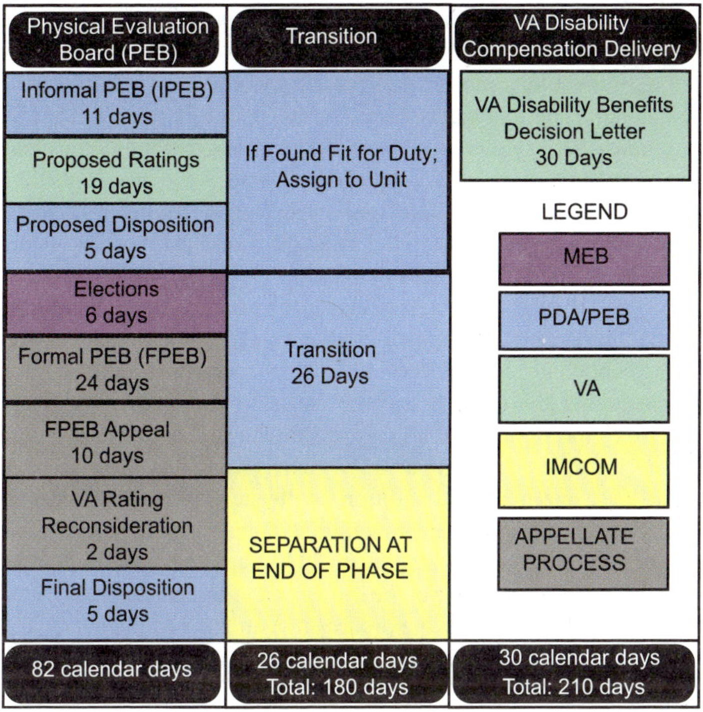

Figure 30-1 ***(left and above).*** Department of Defense/Veterans Administration Integrated Disability Evaluation System (IDES) timeliness goals.
IMCOM: Installation Management Command; PDA: Physical Disability Agency; VA: Department of Veterans Affairs
Data source: Wilkie RL. *Directive-Type Memorandum (DTM)-18-004–"Revised Timeliness Goals for the Integrated Disability Evaluation System (IDES).*" Under Secretary of Defense; July 30, 2010, Incorporating Change 2, September 19, 2019.

IDES, the process is expected to take 180 days. There are five key phases to this system, outlined below.

Treatment Phase

Once a soldier becomes injured or ill and seeks medical care, they enter the treatment phase. This will be the most common phase that physician assistants (PAs) will participate in while serving in their role as the primary care provider for the soldier. Treatment may be prescribed by the PA, or the soldier may be referred to a specialty provider. If, during the course of the treatment phase, the PA or specialty care provider determines that a soldier has at least one condition that fails to meet the medical retention standards as defined in Chapter 3 of Army Regulation (AR) 40-501, *Standards of Medical Fitness*,[4] and the soldier has reached optimal medical benefit, then the soldier has reached the MRDP and should be referred to the IDES system.

The MRDP determination and referral to a Medical Evaluation Board (MEB) and PEB must be made within 1 year of the diagnosis with the medical condition that does not appear to meet medical retention standards, but the referral may be earlier if the medical provider determines the soldier will not be capable of returning to duty within 1 year. A profile containing a "3" or more means that the individual has at least one medical condition or physical defect that requires significant limitations. The completion of the permanent 3 or 4 on the Department of the Army (DA) Form 3349, Physical Profile, with the required approval signature of the designated physician assigned by the MTF commander initiates the process transitioning to the MEB. The PA's role in this phase is further discussed below.

Medical Evaluation Board Phase

Upon referral to the IDES system, the soldier enters the MEB phase of the IDES system. This phase takes place at the local installation (or the nearest Army installation). Upon referral to the MEB, the soldier is assigned a physical evaluation board liaison officer (PEBLO), who will serve as the link to the IDES system for the soldier and the soldier's commander. The PEBLO counsels the soldier on the IDES process, assembles the soldier's case file, and gathers all necessary documents, including medical records and a nonmedical assessment from the soldier's commanding officer. The PEBLO will ensure a complete, accurate, and fully documented case file, which is the foundation for a fair and equitable disability evaluation. The PEBLO's goal is to ensure each member's case is properly documented, fairly presented, and fully considered by all elements of the disability system, with appropriate compensation.

Once the soldier's case is assembled, including a list of all potential medical conditions that require evaluation for potential disability, the soldier's medical evaluation is scheduled. Conducted by the VA, the medical examination includes both general and specialty evaluations. This evaluation is the exam of record for IDES: if there are discrepancies between the VA and any prior DOD health care provider's diagnoses or limitations, the VA exam is used for determination of disability ratings. The exam is generally completed at the nearest VA facility. Several military installations have VA clinics located on site; however, this practice varies from site to site.

Upon completion of the VA's comprehensive medical exam, the findings and evaluation are returned to the local IDES team, where the exam is reviewed by the MEB physician. The physician reviews all of the diagnoses, limitations, and conditions and applies Chapter 3 of AR 40-501[4] to determine whether the soldier meets medical retention standards. If the soldier does meet medical retention standards, the MEB is terminated at this time and the soldier is returned to duty. If the MEB physician determines that the soldier does not meet the medical retention standards, the physician must determine whether the condition existed prior to military service, if it was aggravated by the service, and whether the soldier complied with treatment recommendations and protocols. These three areas can all have an impact on the disability rating awarded for a condition. The MEB physician summarizes these findings in the narrative summary (NARSUM).

Prior to the next phase, the soldier has the opportunity to review the NARSUM and may appeal to the MEB physician or request an impartial medical review of the findings and recommendations at the local MTF. As part of the system, the soldier has access to legal counsel trained and familiar with the IDES process, who can provide recommendations on responses. Upon either the soldier's approval or disposition of the appeal, the NARSUM is forwarded to the PEB. This action completes the MEB phase of IDES. The total time for this process should not exceed 72 days. The timeline may be affected by any delays in the VA comprehensive exam, scheduled by the PEBLO, as well as the time required to address appeals of the NARSUM. It is important to note that during this phase, soldiers must be readily available for their medical evaluations and review of their NARSUM. Therefore, non-emergent leave should be discouraged.[5]

Physical Evaluation Board Phase

The PEB phase begins when the PEBLO forwards the MEB case file, including the NARSUM, to the PEB. All PEBs take place at Joint Base San Antonio. The PEB reviews the soldier's NARSUM, medical records, VA evaluation, and commander's statement about the soldier's performance, and determines whether the soldier meets fitness-for-duty standards. One of the most influential documents in this review process is the commander's statement, which provides important information about how the medical condition and any duty limitations impact the soldier's ability to perform individual tasks, and the unit's ability to complete its mission. If the soldier elects to appeal the findings of this initial review, they may request a formal hearing to present the appeal to the PEB in person.

If the PEB determines that all of the soldier's conditions render them fit for continued duty, the IDES process is complete and the soldier is returned to duty. However, if any of the medical conditions are determined to render the soldier unable to meet fitness-for-duty standards, the PEBLO forwards the soldier's case to the VA, where it is sent to the VA Disability Evaluation System rating activity site (D-RAS). D-RAS staff apply the VA Schedule for Rating Disability to assign a disability rating for each condition. Ratings are impacted by certain circumstances: when the condition began (ie, if it existed prior to service); if it was the direct result of combat service; and if it was aggravated during military service. Once D-RAS staff assign the ratings, the case is sent back to the PEB, which makes final determination on whether the soldier will be medically retired or separated as a result of their conditions.

When this process is complete, the PEB forwards the results to the soldier's PEBLO. The soldier will review the results and has the opportunity to appeal the final results. As before, the soldier is afforded opportunity for legal counsel. This stage ends when the soldier signs off on DA Form 199, Informal PEB Proceedings, which documents the findings and ratings.[1] In total, the PEB phase must be completed within 82 days; however, the time period varies significantly based on the number and type of conditions, the ongoing workload of the PEB and D-RAS, and the number of appeals submitted.

Transition Phase

After concurring with the PEB findings and D-RAS ratings, the soldier enters the transition phase. During this process, the soldier undergoes either military retirement or separation. The local installation will generate the appropriate orders, and the soldier begins the process of clearing the installation and preparing for departure from the military, including returning all required equipment, closing out evaluations, clearing housing, and shipping household goods. While the goal for this phase is 26 days, this period often does not account for any accumulated leave soldiers may take prior to their separation or retirement (leave frequently extends this timeline beyond 26 days). This phase is completed when the soldier is officially out of the military.

Reintegration Phase

Upon departure from the military, the goal of the IDES system is to ensure that the soldier becomes a VA beneficiary within 1 month. This includes receiving VA compensation payment for all service-connected medical conditions and being integrated into the VA health care system for ongoing medical care. The PEBLO and VA's medical service coordinators are integral to the success of this phase; they ensure appointments are established with the local VA wherever the soldier chooses to locate after departing the military.

Physician Assistants in the IDES

While PAs are not directly involved in the MEB process, they should be generally aware of the process and able to brief their commander on the timeframe and status of their enrolled soldiers. The soldier's assigned PEBLO will be able to provide detailed answers both to the soldier's primary care provider and directly to the chain of command. Because most PAs serve as primary care providers to soldiers, there are two key aspects in which the PA has a significant role:

1. The most important role of the PA is the initial identification and treatment of potential duty-limiting conditions and determination of the MRDP. Key parts of this process are ensuring access to care, preventing delays in care, active monitoring of soldiers

with duty limitations, and ensuring high-quality medical documentation.

2. The second key aspect is the PA's responsibility to the chain of command. Although privacy laws restrict certain aspects of what a health care provider shares with their commander, the health and welfare of a unit is one of the commander's overall responsibilities. Therefore, it is imperative for a medical officer to track medical readiness and brief the commander on the unit's deployment status.[6] Soldiers nearing MRDP will most likely be placed into the MEB process, which can affect a deploying unit. The electronic profile system provides a key mechanism for tracking medical profiles.[6] PAs should be prepared for varying levels of review to discuss duty limitations and MRDPs.

Chapter 3-3 of AR 40-502, *Medical Readiness,* defines the MRDP as "medical condition has stabilized or cannot be stabilized in a reasonable period of time for up to 12 months and impacts successful performance of duty; the ability to perform basic soldiering skills required by all military personnel and MOS [military occupational specialty] specific duties."[6] The regulation goes on to state that a referral to MEB will be made within 1 year of a soldier being diagnosed with a medical condition. However, it is more important to ensure that the soldier's medical condition has stabilized and all reasonable treatment options have been exhausted.

When working toward an MRDP with a soldier, it is important to document how any injury occurred as well as where it occurred, when applicable. Conditions noted as combat related or aggravated in a combat zone can have significant effects on a soldier's ratings and compensation. Conversely, it is also important to document any noncompliance with therapy, which may not only affect ratings, but also guide further treatment.

PAs can refer soldiers to IDES once the MRDP has been reached without the recommendation of a specialist. However, it is extremely beneficial if at least one specialist has also recommended initiation of IDES to ensure all medical care possibilities have been explored. Once it is determined that a soldier has reached the MRDP, and ideally a specialist has concurred, the soldier should be called in for a face-to-face encounter with the primary care provider to discuss the process. Soldiers should be aware that they are still under the authority of the Uniform Code of Military Justice (UCMJ)[7] and all applicable Army regulations during this phase. A permanent profile is initiated by the referring primary care manager and becomes official after the second approval signature. If the electronic profile has not been signed within 30 days, it will automatically be canceled. The MEB physician must complete a Defense Department (DD) Form 2807-1 documenting the soldier's medical history. Every prior medical complaint must be addressed to ensure that a particular complaint either meets, or does not meet, the standards of AR 40-501, Chapter 3.[4] The DD Form 2807-1 screening should be as complete as possible at the beginning to expedite the remainder of the MEB process and to reduce the number of appeals for unaddressed complaints.

Medical Care During IDES

The soldier's primary care manager remains responsible for the care of all the soldier's acute illnesses and injuries during the MEB process. Because the IDES process can take up to 210 days, it is important to maintain frequent, ongoing medical visits and coordination of care for the management of all the soldier's medical needs. Of note, once the soldier enters the PEB phase, they may undergo elective surgeries, in accordance with local policies and procedures as well as with Medical Command policy memo 13-044, *Medically Optional Surgeries for Service Members Undergoing Disability Evaluation through the Integrated Disability Evaluation System*,[8] that may impact the soldier's quality of life. The policy memo's proponent is the Medical Command's Clinical Policy Services, Health Care Delivery (G3/5/7). The approving authority for optional surgery is never a unit commander but is delegated down by the MTF commander or deputy commander of clinical services as the senior medical provider of the MTF. It is important for PAs to know these policies and procedures to prevent any unnecessary delays in the process or the soldier's medical care.

Legacy Disability Evaluation System

The LDES process is similar to the IDES, except it does not involve the VA.[3] In contrast to the IDES, the LDES should not take more than 105 days. The DOD completes the medical examinations for the qualifying conditions, processes the MEB and PEB determinations, and produces the disability ratings for the conditions that caused the service member's inability to continue service. This process has the same appeal options as the IDES. If the service member is separated or medically retired through LDES, they may apply for VA disability benefits prior to separation through VA's pre-discharge program, or they may apply after leaving the military.

Chapter Separations

As unit medical advisors, PAs must be familiar with the guidelines associated with legal actions, non-medical military separations, and IDES/LDES. In general, court martials (Article 32 of the UCMJ)[7] supersede IDES/LDES cases, while IDES/LDES supersedes administrative separation actions (involuntary separation from the service due to failure to rehabilitate or failure to meet Army standards, such as Army Substance Abuse Program participation or physical fitness and height/weight standards).[3] In most cases, if a soldier enrolled in IDES/LDES is brought up on charges and referred for a court martial, they are disenrolled from IDES/LDES, and their case is reviewed again after the conclusion of the court martial. The soldier's primary care provider will continue to provide medical care during this process.

An exception to this rule is if the soldier is recommended by their chain of command for separation in which the discharge is characterized as "other than honorable." The most common reason for this type of separation is a pattern of misconduct. In these cases, both the involuntary separation process and IDES/LDES will proceed concurrently. When the chapter separation packet (see AR 635-200, *Active Duty Enlisted Administrative Separation*[7]) is completed and the current phase of the IDES/LDES process finalized, the case will be referred to the installation's senior mission commander (the commanding general). As a unit advisor, the PA may be asked if they believe the soldier's misconduct was associated or related to their medical condition.

Conclusion

Once a soldier has reached MRDP, they are referred to IDES/LDES. PAs are generally only involved in the referral process. It is important for PAs to understand their role and how their decisions impact initiation of a MEB and ultimately the benefits a soldier may receive. Because the IDES/LDES process can take up to 210 days, a soldier can be on profile almost 2 years before the process is complete. Although it is challenging for commanders to understand the lengthy process, it is imperative that PAs explain the medical course of action, the length of time expected for the process, and the progression through each phase of IDES/LDES. This will help the commander know what to expect once a soldier is referred to IDES/LDES, and understand that due process and diligence is paramount in providing the care that soldiers deserve.

References

1. US Department of the Army. *Physical Evaluation for Retention, Retirement, or Separation*. HQDA; January 19, 2017, Administrative Revision: December 21, 2017. Army Regulation 635-40.
2. US Army Medical Command. *Integrated Disability Evaluation System Guidebook: An Overview of the Integrated Disability Evaluation System*. MEDCOM; July 2013.
3. US Department of Defense Warrior Care website. Legacy Disability Evaluation System. Accessed October 5, 2020. https://warriorcare.dodlive/mil/disability-evaluation/legacydes
4. US Department of the Army. *Standards of Medical Fitness*. HQDA; June 27, 2019. Army Regulation 40-501.
5. US Department of Defense. *Disability Evaluation System*. DOD; August 5, 2014. DOD Instruction 1332.18.
6. US Department of the Army. *Medical Readiness*. HQDA; June 27, 2019. Army Regulation 40-502.
7. US Department of the Army. *Active Duty Enlisted Administrative Separations*. HQDA; December 19, 2016. Army Regulation 635-200.
8. Headquarters, US Army Medical Command. *Medically Optional Surgeries for Service Members Undergoing Disability Evaluation through the Integrated Disability Evaluation System*. MEDCOM; March 7, 2019. OTSG MEDCOM Policy Memo 19-015.

Additional Source

US Department of the Army. *Patient Administration*. HQDA; July 8, 2014. Army Regulation 40-400.

Chapter 31

WHAT PHYSICIAN ASSISTANTS NEED TO KNOW ABOUT OPERATIONAL VIRTUAL HEALTH

Robert Cornfeld, MD, and P. Jason E.E. Auchincloss, APA-C, MPAS

Introduction

Since the invention of the telegraph, military medicine has utilized virtual health (VH) technologies to deliver health care to the point of need.[1] Digital health care delivery is a tool to assist decision-making at the point of need and address the challenges of time and distance, limited medical resources, and the requirements of immediacy in health care delivery. The multi-domain battlefield and the anti-access, area-denial future combat models demand an innovative health care delivery toolkit, including prolonged field care and VH.

Existing VH technologies offer a spectrum of modalities to provide a range of options for providers. The variety of options enables providers to utilize available bandwidth and connectivity tools depending on the military situation and their local resources. This chapter reviews existing asynchronous and synchronous technologies; highlights their innovative use by providers, both as the tools were designed and outside of their original design intent; and concludes with a view toward the future of VH.

Asynchronous Tele-Consultation

Asynchronous tele-consultation uses store-and-forward technologies to enable communication when there is no immediate timing requirement. The Pacific Asynchronous TeleHealth System (PATH) and Health Experts OnLine Portal (HELP) platforms are web-based, asynchronous, provider-to-provider tele-consultation platforms available to US government medical providers and ancillary providers to provide care for their beneficiary population. Although PATH and HELP utilize the same background technology, they cover different geographic regions: PATH is best suited to providing feedback for patients located on the West Coast and Pacific region, while HELP covers the East Coast, Europe, and Africa. Entering the patient into the appropriate site based on location can improve response times because the information does not have to be passed to the "sister" site.

Patients must have a valid Department of Defense identification number to be entered into the system. The system also accommodates military working dogs, with veterinary staff available for consultation. After the originating (patient) site provider enters pertinent patient and consultation information, consultations are answered in 8 to 72 hours by specialists at a distant Role 4 medical center. Originating site providers receive an email response when the specialist reply is available. Both systems support more than 50 specialties, are available in garrison and operational environments, and notably do not require a Common Access Card (CAC) for use (Figure 31-1). Multiple studies have validated both the requirement and benefit of asynchronous consultation on land and sea.[2,3]

There are recognized limitations to these systems, which are being addressed as the two programs are unified under a future "Global Telecommunications Portal." In the operational space, the inability to upload end-user documents from a smart phone or a tablet compromises full capabilities; a computer is needed for this function. In the austere environment, providers are unable to ask specialists about dermatologic conditions or send electrocardiograms or ultrasound images through a smart phone. However, this limitation and others should not preclude end users from adding this valuable capability to their toolkit.

In addition to provider-to-provider tele-consultation across the US European Command (EUCOM), Africa Command (AFRICOM), and Central Command (CENTCOM), the HELP platform is used by Landstuhl Regional Medical Center (LRMC) in Germany to fill clinical gaps in the Transportation Command (TRANSCOM) Regulating and Command & Control Evacuation System (TRAC2ES) program. Providers at the patient originating and distant sites typically do not have access to TRAC2ES due to knowledge, equipment, and connectivity gaps. Additionally, due to the rotational nature of their mission, deployed

Adult Medicine Specialties

Allergy/Immunology (Adult & Pediatric)
Audiology
Cardiology/ Interventional Cardiology
Clinical Pharmacy
Critical Care/ Intensivist
Concussion Clinic
Dermatology
Endocrinology
Endocrinology/ Infertility
Flight Surgeon
Gastroenterology
Gynecology
Gynecologic Oncology
Hematology Oncology
Internal Medicine
Infectious Disease
Nephrology
Nutrition (Adult & Peds)
Pain Integrative Specialty
Pathology
PM&R Specialist
Pulmonology
Rheumatology
Sleep Medicine
Sports Medicine
Vaccine Healthcare

Surgical Specialties

Breast Surgeon
Cardiothoracic Surgeon
Colorectal Surgeon
Endo-Urologist
Foot and Ankle Surgeon
Hand and Upper Extremity Surgeon
Head and Neck Surgeon
Facial Plastic and Reconstructive Surgeon
Metabolic and Advanced Laparoscopy/Bariatric Surgeon
Neuro-otologist
Neurosurgeon
Ophthalmology (Adult & Pediatric)
Refractive Surgery
Oral & Maxillofacial Surgeon
Orthopedics (Adult & Pediatric)
Orthopedics/Spine
Plastic Surgeon
Sleep Surgery
Sports Medicine Orthopedics
Surgical Oncology
Trauma & Critical Care Surgeon
Urologist (Adult & Pediatric)
Urology Oncologist
Vascular Surgeon

Pediatric Specialties

Adolescent Medicine
Cardiology
Developmental Pediatrics
Endocrinology
Gastroenterology
Genetics
Hematology Oncology
Infectious Disease
Intensive Care Medicine
Neonatologist
Nephrology
Neurology
Pulmonology
Rheumatology
Speech Language Pathology
Physical & Occupational Therapy

Radiology Specialties

Pediatric Radiology
Interventional Radiology
Nuclear Medicine
Radiation Oncology
Musculoskeletal/ Radiologist

Behavioral Health Specialties

Child & Adolescent Psychiatry
Inpatient Psychiatry
Neuropsychology
Psychology
Chemical Addictions
Pediatric Psychologist

Figure 31-1. Asynchronous specialties available for consultation. The Pacific Asynchronous TeleHealth System (PATH) and Health Experts OnLine Portal (HELP) platforms offer tremendous depth of remote specialty consultation. PM&R: physical medicine and rehabilitation providers are often unfamiliar with the medical center specialists taking care of their service members and do not have a mechanism for routine clinical updates. Finally, TRAC2ES is CAC-enabled, making mobile device use impossible.

These TRAC2ES challenges led to HELP's emergence as a medical communication platform across Eastern Europe. Originating site providers utilize the shared HELP platform to communicate directly with the LRMC's specialists taking care of their service members. Additionally, deployed service member discharge information from LRMC is entered into HELP for the originating site provider to review in order to improve continuity of care.

Synchronous Tele-Consultation

The Advanced Virtual Support for Operational Forces (ADVISOR) program provides contingency support via telephone at any time across eleven specialties (Figure 31-2). Specialty care providers are available for immediate operational support through a single, United States-based toll free phone number (+1 833-238-7756).

As do the HELP/PATH systems, ADVISOR offers a training module for originating site providers to familiarize themselves with receiving telephone-based consultation. Training and use of an ADVISOR call script is highly recommended.[4] The script provides an easy-to-follow format for providers to rapidly present information to the consultant. Consultants, in turn, are trained in the use of the script to ensure easy and error-free capture of the call details.

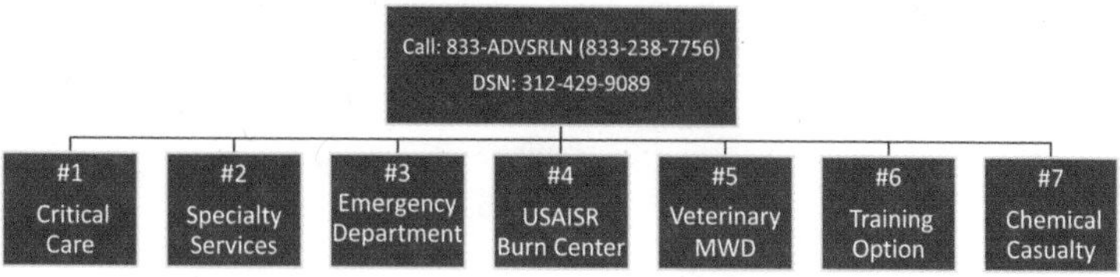

Figure 31-2. The Advanced Virtual Support for Operational Forces (ADVISOR) program line is constantly adding on-demand specialties for support of the warfighter at the point of need.
MWD: military working dog; USAISR: US Army Institute of Surgical Research

As with all communications tools, users should perform routine and deliberate verification that systems are functional. All downrange personnel should routinely confirm communications with their Theater Patient Movement Requests Center and ADVISOR to ensure clear communication prior to emergencies. This training also provides an opportunity for less seasoned providers to rehearse call scripts and ensure ease of access.[4] Testing on multiple communications platforms including Defense Switched Network (DSN), commercial dial, and satellite phone will ensure robust contingency plans.

Case Study 31-1. An active duty service member in rural Africa received an injury to his distal phalanx from use of a band saw. Medical providers utilized ADVISOR to initiate consultation with the on-call orthopedic surgeon. ADVISOR consultation progressed to use of a secure, civilian private messaging service to send images that were used to guide treatment, demonstrating that multiple modes of VH delivery are often needed.

Synchronous Video for Direct Patient Care

Military providers have leveraged existing video conferencing systems, such as Global Video Services and Cisco Jabber, for direct-to-patient care. Like traditional in-person health care, video conferencing requires patients to be scheduled when providers are available; both allow for patient privacy; and providers must be comfortable with delivering health care in both manners. Synchronous video delivery has the additional requirements of connectivity, patient presenter training, and familiarity with the technology.

The Virtual Medical Center–Europe (VMC-E) has pioneered a system called Virtual Healthcare for the Warfighter (VIEW) to address challenges of specialty health care delivery across Eastern Europe. The program enables direct-to-patient care across more than 40 specialties, building on a successful garrison-based program.[5] Technical requirements include access to the internet and a web-cam at the originating site (Figure 31-3). In contrast to commercial video platforms including Facebook and FaceTime, no software is required for download, and originating site users simply access an LRMC-hosted webpage for care delivery.

Specialty consults begin with a HELP message that initiates the care spectrum at LRMC, enables determination of whether direct-to-patient care is required, and enrolls the patient into LRMC's medical systems

Virtual Health Support for Operational Forces:
A Guide for Tri-Service Role 1 to Role 3 providers in
EUCOM, AFRICOM, CENTCOM, and SOCOM

➔ *Specialty consultative care is available via phone, email, and real-time VTC for Deployed ADSMs.*

Allergy / Immunology	**Gastroenterology**	**Nutrition**	**Rheumatology**
Army Body Comp. Prgm	**General Surgery**	**Nutrition / ABCP**	**Sleep Medicine**
Audiology	**Gynecology**	**Orthopedics**	**SUDCC**
Behavioral Health	**Hematology / Oncology**	**Pain Management**	**Speech Pathology**
Cardiology	**Infectious Disease**	**Plastic Surgery**	**TBI**
ENT	**Internal Medicine**	**Podiatry**	**Urology**
Endocrinology	**Neurosurgery**	**Pulmonology**	**Dermatology**

How to reach a Landstuhl RMC / MEDDAC-Bavaria Medical Provider:

1. Emergency Telephonic consultation (24/7/365)
- PRIMARY: ADVISOR Line: Emergency Critical Care Consultation—ICU, Medicine, Surgery Providers: +1 *Note there is frequently a pause while the computer routes your call—do not hang up.*
- ALTERNATE: LRMC Emergency Room: DSN , Comm: +49 (0)

2. Non-Emergency Care via Email or Real-Time VTC
- If able, begin with secure email consultation
  -- Health Experts on-Line Portal (HELP): Supported by LRMC and Navy Med East specialists
  -- Register at: CAC not required & registration is simple
  -- HELP will 'mini-register' the ADSM, and messages are returned within 24 hours
- "Real-time" VTC for routine specialty consultation (M-F, 0730-1600, GMT + 1)
  -- Recommend starting with a HELP consult to specialties above to determine if VTC is appropriate
  -- The specialties above support real-time, synchronous VTC
  -- Your site may / may not have VTC capabilities. Contact the RHCE Virtual Health Office at DSN , or comm. +49 to assist with scheduling your ADSM's Virtual Health appointment or establishing your site as a Virtual Health site.

Figure 31-3. Virtual health information provided to operational force providers.

to allow for patient documentation. Patient presenters ranging from specifically trained medics (military occupational specialty 68W) to unit PAs perform examinations at the direction of the distant site provider. The distant site provider documents visits in the Armed Forces Health Longitudinal Application (AHLTA), the current electronic health record, or the future Military Health System Genesis program, when available. More than 70 operational sites across EUCOM, AFRICOM, and CENTCOM are actively performing synchronous VH, receiving consultation both from LRMC and within their own units.

The VMC-E also pioneered the use of "Telehealth in a Bag" (THIAB). THIAB is a set of off-the-shelf universal serial bus (USB) devices that attach to a computer, require no native software, and leverage capabilities of Windows and Macintosh OS systems. The system enhances the capabilities of the originating site to provide greater information to distant site providers. Currently, the THIAB set includes a stethoscope and a high-definition camera for viewing the patient, including attachments for otoscopic and oronasopharyngeal examinations. The system interfaces with remote specialists and consultants using Web real-time communication.[6] PAs should contact VMC-E for guidance on obtaining a THIAB.

Case Study 31-2. The imaging capabilities of a THIAB were utilized by a unit PA to prevent medical evacuation (medevac) to LRMC. A soldier injured with a fire extinguisher during a training accident was directed to a local host nation facility for treatment, in alignment with the unit's medical concept of support. The wound was stapled closed, and over the following days developed purulence and surrounding erythema. Rather than medevac the soldier to LRMC for follow-on care, with the loss of both the soldier and an escort for an extended period, the medic (68W) utilized a THIAB and the VIEW system to demonstrate the infected wound to the unit's organic PA. The PA directed movement of the soldier to the nearby aid station in Romania, opened and packed the wound, and returned the soldier to duty, utilizing the THIAB/VIEW system for follow-on care. The use of VH maintained a vital warfighter at her place of duty for 14 days rather than having her recover at LRMC.

Synchronicity in Multiple Modalities

A recent study demonstrated the impact of the spectrum of VH modalities during a Stryker Regiment's deployment to rural Poland.[7] The availability of VH modalities for care delivery enabled individual service members to receive centralized waivers to deploy, and reduced mission days lost for health care during the unit's deployment by 213 days. Unit providers leveraged organic behavioral health assets that remained in the home station, relied on LRMC for specialty care delivery, and utilized both the HELP and VIEW platforms.

Conclusion

The VH tools described here are designed for ease of use by the end user. As in any health care procedure, frequency of use and familiarity with the modality will determine ultimate success at the time of need. Providers are encouraged to train themselves—and their care teams, including medics—on the available VH modalities prior to deployment. For example, use of the HELP/PATH platforms in garrison for tele-consultation rather than referring a service member for off-post care will develop the fluency required for use in the deployed environment.

Training for medics can incorporate use of the ADVISOR line for real-time trauma support during a prolonged field care exercise.

A spectrum of VH modalities will be a critical requirement on the future battlefield, where communication is more likely to be analogous to that on a submarine—limited, infrequent, and both synchronous and asynchronous as permitted. The benefits of virtual tele-consultation, tele-mentorship, improved medical regulating (patient movement), and direct-to-patient VH care are clear.

References

1. Zundel KM. Telemedicine: history, applications, and impact on librarianship. *Bull Med Libr Assoc*. 1996;84(1):71–79.
2. Mahnke CB, Jordan CP, Bergvall E, Person DA, Pinsker JE. The Pacific Asynchronous TeleHealth System: review of 1,000 pediatric teleconsultations. *Telemed J E Health*. 2011;17(1):35–39.
3. Lin AH, Welstead BL, Morey BL, Mahnke CB, Cole JH, Johnston MG. Return on investment analysis of Health Experts onLine at Portsmouth: A 2-year review of the Navy's newest teleconsultation system. *Mil Med.* 2017;182(5):e1696-e1701.
4. Auchincloss P, Blyth D, Nam J, et al. Fever of unknown origin in US soldier—telemedical consultation limitations in a deployment to West Africa. *J Spec Oper Med.* 2019;19(2):123–126.
5. Waibel KH, Cain SM, Hall TE, Keen RS. Multispecialty synchronous telehealth utilization and patient satisfaction within Regional Health Command Europe: A readiness and recapture system for health. *Mil Med*. 2017;182(7):e1693-31697.
6. Schermerhorn S, Auchincloss P, Kraft K, Nelson K. Pamplin J, Patella fracture in US service member in an austere location. *J Spec Oper Med.* 2018;18(1):142–144.
7. Cornfeld RJ, Cranney N, Rudy E. Operational virtual health modalities increased combat power for 1st Squadron, 2nd Cavalry Regiment During the Enhanced Forward Presence Mission. *Mil Med.* 2020. doi: 10.1093/milmed/usaa003

Chapter 32

ROLE OF THE PHYSICIAN ASSISTANT IN RESEARCH

Amelia M. Duran-Stanton, PA-C, PhD, DSc, MPAS; Brandon M. Carius, PA-C, DSc, MPAS; Owen T. Hill, PA-C, PhD, MPAS; D. Alan Nelson, PA-C, PhD, MPAS; Johnny Wayne Paul, APA-C, DMSc, MPAS; and Bradley J. Warr, PA-C, PhD, MPAS

Introduction

Army physician assistants (PAs) conduct research in both academic and clinical settings. PAs hold official research positions at the US Army Research Institute of Environmental Medicine, and they also drive investigations at other institutions, hospitals, and clinics. Regardless of setting, Army PAs should attempt to align research interests with the lines of effort designated by the Army Medical Specialist Corps (AMSC) with the intent of better serving Army soldiers. Current lines of research include:

- illness and injury prevention,
- disease and nonbattle injury management and rehabilitation,
- combat trauma management and rehabilitation, and
- health and performance optimization and reintegration.

A complete list of lines of research and their subcomponents can be obtained from the AMSC Research Committee. This committee provides support, advice, and guidance on research directly to the AMSC chief, who typically appoints the committee's head (Figure 32-1).

The onset of any research project should entail a search for similar, previously published literature. Generally, research requires a degree of originality and innovation that adds something to the current

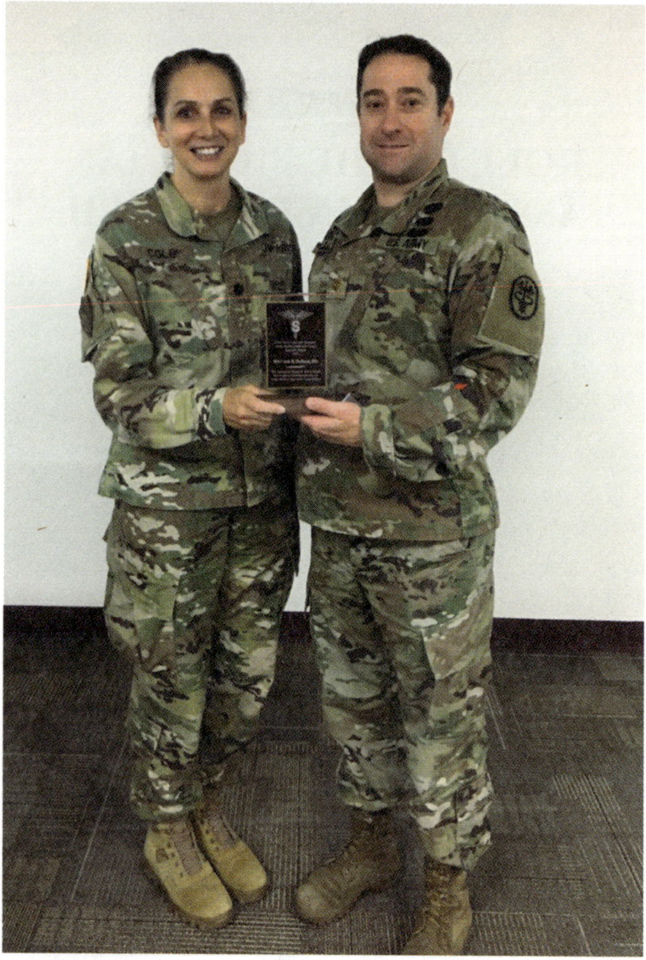

Figure 32-1. Colonel Renee Cole (left) presents the 2019 Mary Lipscomb Hamrick Research Course Lifetime Research Award to Major Seth Holland at JBSA-Fort Sam Houston, TX. Colonel Cole is currently the AMSC Research Committee lead. Major Holland is a graduate of the US Army/Baylor Doctor of Science in Physician Assistant Studies in General Surgery.
Photograph courtesy of Major Robin Cushing.

body of literature. Prior to starting any research, PAs should search online publication depositories (such as PubMed, the Army Medical Department Virtual Library, and the specific academic institution the PA is enrolled in) to ensure their idea meets this criteria.

Evaluating and Conducting Research

Evaluating and conducting research is vital to the growth and development of medical knowledge and practice, for both individual PAs and the medical community as a whole. While isolated laboratory tests provide foundational knowledge in medicine, clinical studies evaluate diagnostic and treatment hypotheses in human subjects for a more direct application to practice. When evaluating existing research and planning future research, PAs must understand the different types of studies and the hierarchy of their evidence. The levels of evidence for clinical studies and examples are provided by Elsevier at: https://www.elsevier.com/__data/promis_misc/Levels_of_Evidence.pdf.[1]

The "PICO" Approach

In developing and evaluating clinical studies and research, PA researchers should understand the goals and applications of each. Integral to this approach is the use of the "PICO" model:

P: patient or population
I: intervention (or exposure)
C: comparison (or control)
O: outcome

An example of utilizing the PICO model is a study of adult patients 18 to 65 years old complaining of a migraine headache (P), receiving 1 g of intravenous acetaminophen (I), compared to those receiving 975 mg of oral Tylenol (C), for a decrease in reported pain based on a visual rating scale (O).

A refined PICO model can be translated into a specific research question, which should include each of these four aspects. Having established these elements, PAs can start to develop and refine a research hypothesis and begin to organize a clinical study. It is important to note that, with the exception of individual case studies, case series, and expert opinions, all clinical studies require a formal submission to the institutional review board (IRB) for review and approval prior to conducting research.

Types of Studies

The different types of analytic and descriptive studies vary in strength based on the scientific rigor of their respective designs, as outlined in Exhibit 32-1. They are briefly described below.

Metaanalyses

- Metaanalyses systematically group multiple clinical trials, generally with similar characteristics, to test for a shared hypothesis with a larger sample population.
- A popular meta-analysis resource is the Cochrane Reviews database, which contains over 7,500 systematic reviews of literature.
- Strengths: establish a larger sample population for enhanced testing power; draw more diverse populations for enhanced comparison and broader application.
- Weaknesses: strength of evidence depends on strength of sampled

Exhibit 32-1. Study types, from strongest to weakest, based on the scientific rigor of their respective designs.

1. Analytic studies
    a. metaanalysis
    b. experimental: randomized clinical controlled trial
    c. observational
        i. cohort study
        ii. case-control study
        iii. cross-sectional study
2. Descriptive studies
    a. aggregate: ecologic study
    b. individual
        i. cross-sectional study
        ii. case series
        iii. case report
3. Other: expert opinions

trials; time consuming; heterogeneity of sampled studies may confound results; possible selection bias in choice of studies included.

Randomized Clinical Controlled Trials

- In clinical trials, the exposure is determined by the investigator.
- "Randomized" means that differential confounding factors are removed by randomly assigning the exposure.
- Strengths: provide strongest evidence for causality because of clear temporality, cause and effect, and control for unknown confounding factors.
- Weaknesses: expensive; time consuming; possibility of selection bias; potential lack of generalizability to the population of interest.

Cohort Studies

- Cohort studies are prospective studies in which individuals with an exposure are identified and compared to individuals without the exposure with respect to future outcomes of interest. They are longitudinal studies (conducted over time) in which outcome incidence is compared between exposed and unexposed groups.
- Yields: cumulative incidence relative risk ratios and incidence density relative risk ratios.
- Strengths: clearly defined temporality because the exposure occurred before the outcome.
- Weaknesses: time consuming; costly; loss to follow-up is common.

Case-Control Studies

- Case-control studies are retrospective studies in which individuals with a condition (cases) are identified and compared to individuals without the condition (controls) with respect to prior exposures.
- Yields: odds ratios and prevalence ratios.
- Strengths: efficient use of time; less costly; can study rare diseases; statistically efficient.
- Weaknesses: temporal ambiguity; recall bias; selection bias.

Cross-Sectional Studies

- Cross-sectional studies can be seen as "snapshots" in which individuals are selected without regard to outcome or exposure status. Data is collected at one point in time at the individual level. Often these are the first analytic studies to be conducted, because if a causal relationship is not identified, no further studies are needed.
- Yields: odds ratios and prevalence ratios.
- Strengths: relatively inexpensive and efficient.
- Weakness: temporality (because data on exposure and outcome is captured at one point in time, the exposure could have occurred after the outcome of interest).

Ecologic Studies

- In ecologic studies, the units of measurement are captured at the population level (as opposed to the individual level). These studies use group data to describe correlations between conditions and exposures in various populations.
- Yields: correlation ratios.
- Strengths: quick; efficient; yields multinational and multiorganizational comparisons.
- Weaknesses: no direct linkage between exposures and outcomes at the individual level; risk of ecologic fallacy (the correlation identified at the population level does not necessarily represent a relationship at the individual level).

Case Series

- Case series consist of multiple patients who have a similar pattern of presentation, evaluation, or diagnoses, providing a theme for reader learning. These studies are essential for the early identification of problematic exposures, but are not analytic in nature like the studies listed above.
- Yields: illness characteristic and treatment themes.
- Strengths: provide insight into patient populations too small, diverse, or dispersed (in time or place) to effectively conduct proper trials.
- Weaknesses: largely retrospective in nature; small populations; no explicit comparison group.

Case Reports

- Case reports (Figure 32-2) consist of a single patient who has a unique presentation, evaluation, or diagnoses, providing notable insight into an illness. They are essential for reference of rare cases, but are not analytic in nature and cannot establish definitive trends for diagnosis and treatment.
- Yields: illness characteristics and anecdotal treatments.
- Strengths: provide insight into patient populations that are too small, diverse, or dispersed (in time or place) to effectively conduct proper trials.
- Weaknesses: retrospective in nature; isolated cases; no explicit comparison group.

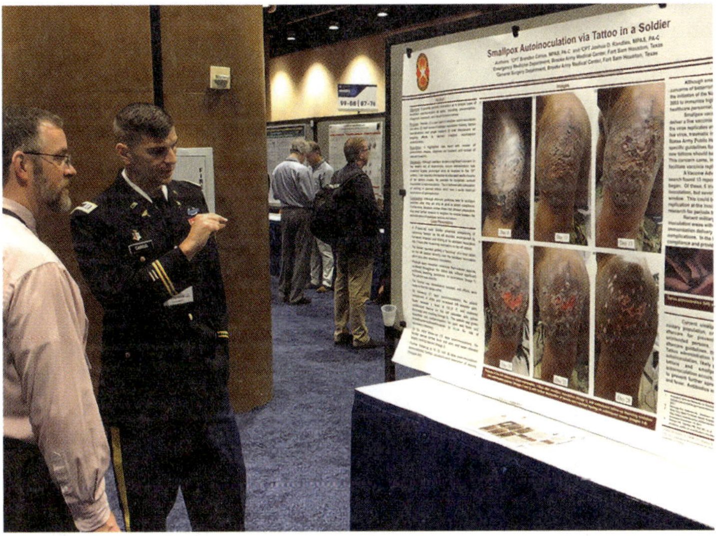

Figure 32-2. Then-Captain Brandon Carius presents a poster on a case report during the Military Health System Research Symposium in Kissimmee, Florida, in August 2018. Major Carius is a graduate of the US Army/Baylor Doctor of Science in Physician Assistant Studies in Emergency Medicine program. Photograph courtesy of Major Brandon Carius.

Expert Opinions

- Expert opinions are statements on the diagnoses or treatment of illness by a prominent member or several members of a specific or overlapping medical specialties, who may or may not refer to published studies for support of their position.
- Yield: an opinion.
- Strengths: provide guidance and insight into the diagnosis and treatment of conditions in the absence of published literature.
- Weaknesses: largely uncited/otherwise unsupported positions.

Collaboration

Current scientific research is expected to include complexity and in-depth analysis. It follows that a substantial range of resources must be marshaled to conduct a research project, particularly in terms of individual talents. Collaboration has therefore been seen as integral to modern research, ensuring that each project is a productive endeavor, with input from multiple perspectives.[1] Research collaboration represents more than the simple involvement of many people, however. Collaboration is a complex process that is not easily defined or assessed,[2] although the presence of differing talents and perspectives is a key component. Collaborations can be established among individuals, departments, or institutions. As providers accustomed to practicing in and leading collaborative medical teams, PAs are well suited to lead this process. In this era of evidence-based medicine, their foundation in clinical science ensures the critical perspective needed for productive medical research.

The recognized benefits of collaboration in research[3] each apply to PAs. Collaboration promotes the effective use of individual talents, while providing PAs an opportunity to employ clinical experience in addition to research-related training (Figure 32-3). Research allows the transference of knowledge. PAs may therefore find that collaboration provides a new mechanism to impart wisdom, both to partner researchers and to readers of publications. Their involvement in collaborative research allows critical experiences and lessons learned to be incorporated into evidence-based practice standards. Collaboration is also a source of intellectual stimulation and companionship as well

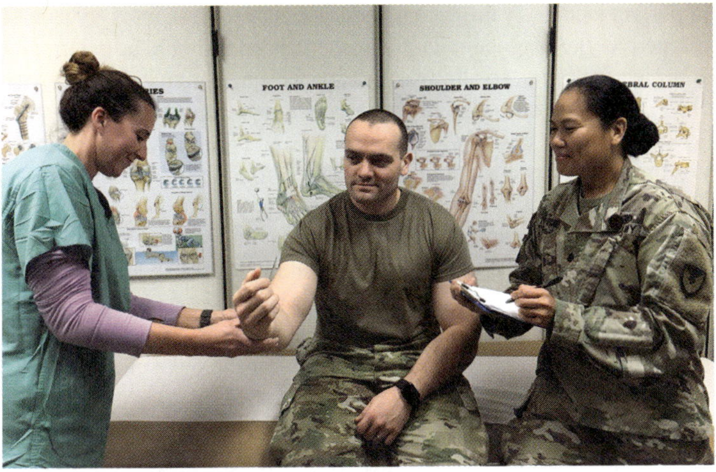

Figure 32-3. Major Meghan Joyce (left) and Lieutenant Colonel Amelia Duran-Stanton (right) validate goniometer elbow measurements on Captain David Korb (center), a physician assistant student during his orthopedics rotation at the Brooke Army Medical Center in March 2020. Lieutenant Colonel Duran-Stanton and Major Joyce are graduates of the US Army/Baylor Doctor of Science in Physician Assistant Studies in Clinical Orthopedics program. Lieutenant Colonel Duran-Stanton also earned a Doctor of Philosophy in Postsecondary and Adult Education through Capella University.
Photograph courtesy of Lieutenant Colonel Amelia Duran-Stanton.

as professional networking. PAs may find these benefits refreshing after prior clinical experience involving relatively limited interaction with other professionals.

Balancing Research with Clinical Duties

Research is detail-oriented and requires a significant time investment. While interactions with subjects may occur in the course of normal clinic duty, work for research is often completed outside of these times. It is important to establish a schedule and remain disciplined throughout the research process, which will allow for effective management of multiple requirements. In the beginning of the research process, it is important to identify the primary and associate investigators (PI and AI, respectively). Assigned roles and responsibilities should be determined at project initiation so all investigators can appropriately balance their clinical responsibilities with the research requirements.

The PI should devise a project timeline and routinely schedule team meetings, whether virtual or face-to-face, to establish accountability. A realistic schedule must be developed to minimize conflict with clinical duties. Backward planning from an agreed-upon end goal is key. Incremental goals and metrics should be established and divided among the research team. Setbacks are inevitable, making it imperative for team members to remain flexible. Time management is a cornerstone to successful research, particularly for those who have clinical duties, required professional development, or travel.

Programs Requiring Research

Currently, the Doctor of Science (DSc) in emergency medicine, general surgery, and orthopedics residency programs, as well as the Doctor of Medical Science (DMSc) degree, require Army PAs to complete a research project. The research may include primary data collection and analysis, secondary data analysis, or metaanalysis. Army PA residents should choose a topic that interests them and solicit feedback from staff along the way. Army PA residents are also required to choose a staff advisor for their topic and routinely meet with the advisor to discuss progress. It is also important to get explicit guidance from the program director on all research requirements. Residencies are generally 18-month programs, and residents must dedicate adequate time to completing their research while managing clinical and didactic responsibilities. All DSc residents are required to defend their research project at the end of the program to university and residency faculty.

When an Army PA is selected for funding to pursue a PhD at a civilian school of choice, they must meet the research requirements of the selected program. Earning a PhD requires completing a dissertation project, which usually includes primary data collection and analysis. Most military schools also require research skills, so it is important to hone research skills as early as possible. During the Interservice Physician Assistant Program, for example, students are required to conduct a literature review for their master's paper.

Captains Career Course students must research and write an analysis of command principles applied to a historical battle. The Command and General Staff College requires students to submit defense papers that include research. The Senior Service College requires students to complete, at minimum, a strategy paper and a research project. The earlier a PA learns how to conduct research, finds out how to format papers depending on the academic or publication requirements, and understands the basics of technological research tools and resources, the better the quality of their work will be as they progress throughout their career.

Institutional Review Board Process

Most types of research involve review and oversight by a third party in order to ensure safe conduct and protections for participants. Military and civilian institutions utilize an IRB as an impartial third party to assess the safety of proposed research prior to its initiation. Before starting an IRB submission, potential investigators should familiarize themselves with the latest requirements, although several have remained consistent. These include an updated curriculum vitae (CV) and completion of Collaborative Institutional Training Initiative (CITI) instruction. CITI course certification, which is good for 3 years, provides potential investigators with a thorough background on the Human Research Protections Office, its purpose, and the paramount need for human protection and safety in conducting scientific research. In the military, IRB organization is generally aligned with the regional health command structure. Using templates, prospective research is submitted to the IRB, where it is first administratively reviewed for proper packet completion, and then categorized for one of three stratified levels of review:

Exempt

- Studies that are deemed to have less than minimal risk to participants, and fit into one of several categories, such as being conducted in an educational setting.
- Examples include anonymous surveys, laboratory studies not involving human samples, or comparing two different educational curricula.

Expedited

- Studies that involve only minimal risk to participants, defined as not being "greater in and of themselves than those ordinarily encountered in daily life or during the performance of routine physical or psychological examinations or tests"[4]; that do not involve vulnerable populations (such as prisoners or military trainees); and that fit into one of several categories, such as data obtained through noninvasive means routinely employed in clinical practice (such as radiographic imaging), or blood samples collected by venipuncture from healthy volunteers.
- Examples include examination of human specimens (such as a blood sample study) or a records review of identifiable patient information.

Full Board Review

- Studies deemed to involve more than minimal risk to participants, or that involve certain categories such as vulnerable populations (eg, persons under age 18, prisoners, military trainees); procedures that might cause physical harm; or collection of information that could seriously harm the participant legally, socially, or financially if other people could identify them.
- Examples include physical exertion testing after blood donation; comparing ketamine to acetaminophen for intravenous pain relief; testing a new type of endotracheal tube for emergent intubation.

Potential investigators must maintain perspective and patience when approaching their local IRB for review and approval of a study. While exempt studies can be returned with approval within weeks, those involving full review, or even expedited review, can take many months or even over a year for approval. IRB panels generally meet on a monthly basis to conduct reviews, and often require multiple revisions and additional input (generally referred to as "stipulations") prior to approval.

Upon approval, investigators should ensure that they understand future requirements from the IRB, including potential ongoing reviews on a scheduled basis (such as annually). Deviations from the approved protocol necessitates notification to IRB office personnel and potentially halting study execution until further review. This is generally outlined in the IRB approval packet.

Upon completion of data collection, IRB procedures must be followed to successfully "close" a study. After a study is closed, investigators must either maintain or destroy paper copies of data as specified in their protocol. Investigators should work with a statistician, either local or easily accessible through electronic communication, to verify their data for statistical analysis. Upon completion of data analysis, investigators create a draft manuscript, presentation, or both, which must be submitted to the IRB public affairs office prior to submission to any conference or journal.

Writing and Publishing

Research is conducted for the primary purpose of increasing medical knowledge, but its effect is limited if not effectively disseminated. Publishing research is the best method to reach the greater medical community. Journal themes range from general practice (eg, the *Journal of the American Academy of Physician Assistants*) to various medical specialties. It is important that PAs have target journals in mind from the outset to ensure compliance with the publisher's requirements (see a partial list of journals under Tools and Resources at the end of this chapter). Formatting guidelines are found on most journals' websites. Strictly following these guidelines, in addition to striving for effective writing (keeping the article as short and succinct as possible), will ensure the best chance of a smooth submission process and, ultimately, article acceptance. Additionally, when conducting a literature review, Army PAs should consult local and online resources available through the military prior to purchasing any references. These are most easily accessed by consulting the local hospital or regional medical center librarian.

The AMSC has recently added publications, presentations, and civilian organization involvement as part of the requirements to earn the 9A proficiency designation (discussed in the attachment to Chapter 1 of this handbook). Additionally, PAs should attend the AMSC's annual Mary Lipscomb Hamrick (MLH) Research Course, taught by subject matter experts, even when they are not in academic programs (Figure 32-4). The earlier PAs attend this course, the earlier they can learn the basics of research and begin networking and collaborating with fellow researchers, while earning continuing medical education and military school credit. (Additional details about the MLH course are available

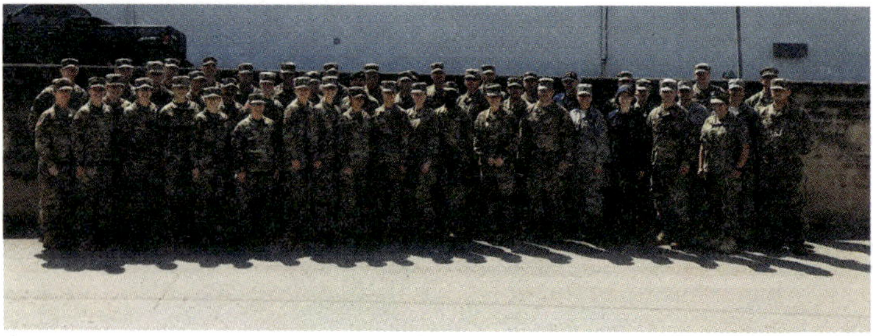

Figure 32-4. Army Medical Specialist Corps faculty and attendees during the 2019 Mary Lipscomb Hamrick Research Course.
Photograph courtesy of Major Robin Cushing.

on the AMSC's MilSuite page at https://www.milsuite.mil/book/groups/army-medical-specialist-corps. See other chapters in this handbook for additional course listings, as well as information on PAs who have earned MLH research awards.)

Mentoring in Research

There are many opportunities for mentorship within the research community, both supervisor-subordinate and peer-to-peer.

Academic Settings

Army PAs pursuing an advanced graduate degree benefit from mentorship, not only by their academic advisors, but also by fellow Army PAs who have previously earned an advanced degree. Particularly when studying in a civilian school, guidance on how to maneuver through the program in a timely fashion as an active duty PA is imperative. Earning a PhD requires planning and execution of very specific steps, including didactic studies, comprehensive exams, research proposals, and dissertation defense. Similar key events may be present in master's-level programs as well. Failing to complete or meet the standards at every step can result in significant delays or failure to complete the program. Army PA mentors can help provide the guidance necessary to stay on track throughout these programs.

Research Institutes

Army PAs may serve in a research institute, including the US Army Research Institute of Environmental Medicine, where the focus of their duties is to plan, execute, and analyze research (Figure 32-5). These positions may or may not require an advanced or specific degree. Peer-to-peer mentorship while working in these settings can be very useful: learning the steps to getting a research protocol approved by an IRB,

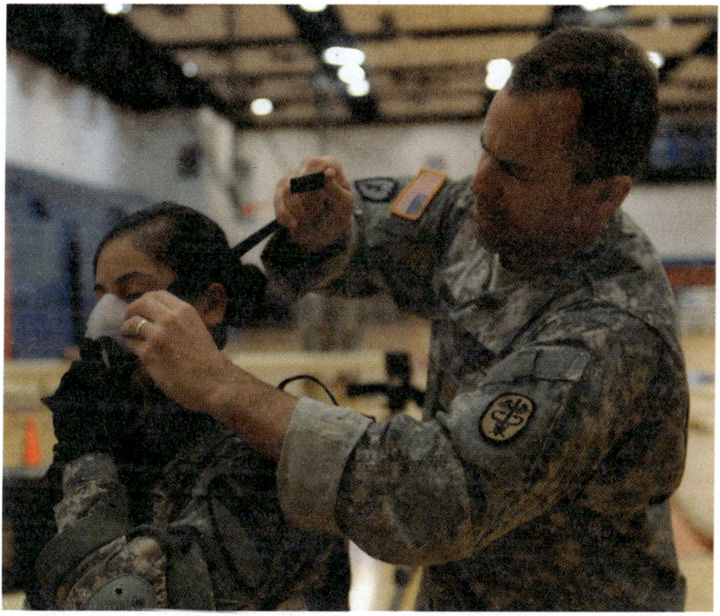

Figure 32-5a. Major Bradley Warr, research physician assistant and chief of the Military Performance Branch of the US Army Research Institute of Environmental Medicine in Natick, Massachusetts, prepares a soldier for measurement of oxygen consumption while carrying 25-mm ammunition cans at Fort Hood, Texas, as part of the Training and Doctrine Command Physical Demands Study in December 2013. Major Warr earned his Doctor of Philosophy in Physical Activity, Nutrition and Wellness from Arizona State University. Photograph courtesy of Major Bradley Warr.

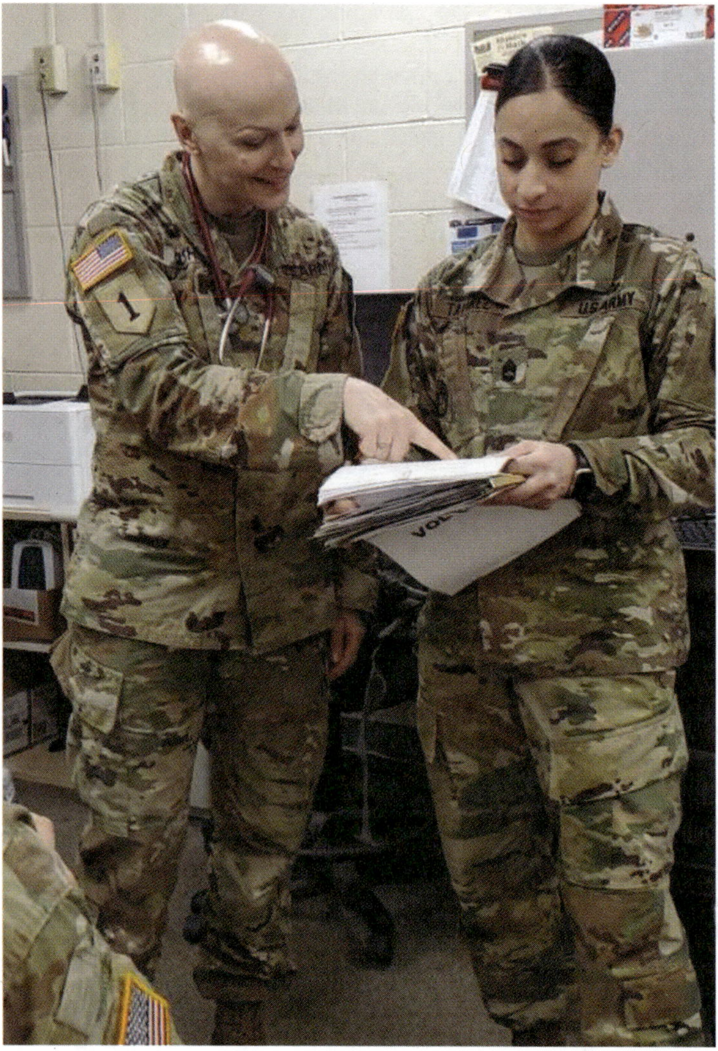

Figure 32-5b. Major Robin Cushing and Sergeant First Class Eileen Tavarez discuss drug research protocols with human volunteers. This double-blind experimental study evaluated the effects of cocoa flavonoids on blood circulation in February 2020. Major Robin Cushing earned her Doctor of Philosophy in Public Health from the University of Hawaii.
Photograph courtesy of Major Robin Cushing.

evaluating the scientific rigor of a proposal, efficiently using available resources, and reviewing manuscripts are all topics that can be discussed among peers. Finding a mentor with significant experience in these processes is appropriate and will contribute to successful research.

Lessons Learned

The following lessons learned will help PAs in navigating the world of research as well as in pursuing other endeavors. PAs should:

- begin with the end in mind—determine when a product or project is due and backwards plan from that goal;
- collaborate early and often—it is important for a researcher to identify their resources and network;
- discuss projects frequently with mentors, especially those who can assist in moving them forward; and
- involve statisticians early in the project, not just when needed.

Tips for Success

Along with lessons learned, the following tips for success will help PAs maximize their opportunities in research. PAs should:

- maintain an updated CV for all authors and collaborators;
- review the IRB requirements and follow them (when in doubt, ask for clarification);
- meet with a senior researcher or researchers in the beginning of the research endeavor, which will save a lot of time and missed steps, especially for junior researchers;
- utilize all the research platforms available in streamlining the project (see Tools and Resources at the end of this chapter);
- attend a research course at the earliest possible time and before it is required, particularly if planning to attend a long-term health education and training program;
- manage time wisely and know all the deadlines required to complete a project; and
- take the time to identify past and current literature that supports the project. A strong literature review is the foundation of the research project.

Conclusion

The ability to conduct research is important for all PAs. Conducting research helps PAs improve their clinical practice while contributing to the body of existing medical literature. All PAs, regardless of educational background, can learn new skills and use them in their current environment. PAs do not need doctorate-level education to conduct research; they require only willingness, fortitude, and interest; time-management skills; and eagerness to learn, especially from senior researchers.

References

1. Elsevier. Levels of evidence for clinical studies. Accessed March 19, 2020. https://www.elsevier.com/__data/promis_misc/Levels_of_Evidence.pdf
2. Bozeman B, Lee S. The impact of research collaboration on scientific productivity. Presentation given at: American Association for the Advancement of Science Annual Meeting; February 11, 2003; Denver, CO. Accessed March 1, 2020. http://gtresearchnews.gatech.edu/newsrelease/Collab.pdf
3. Katz JS, Martin BR. What is research collaboration? *Res Policy.* 1997;26(3). Accessed March 19, 2020. https://doi.org/10.1016/S0048-7333(96)00917-1
4. Loan-Clarke J, Preston D. Tensions and benefits in collaborative research involving a university and another organization. *Stud Higher Ed.* 2002;27(2):169–185. Accessed March 1, 2020. http://www.tandfonline.com/doi/pdf/10.1080/03075070220120001

Tools and Resources

Reference Management Tools

- EndNote: https://endnote.com/
- Mendeley: http://www.mendeley.com (also a collaboration tool)
- Microsoft Word: https://support.office.com/en-us/article/create-a-bibliography-citations-and-references-17686589-4824-4940-9c69-342c289fa2a5

- Paperpile: http://www.paperpile.com
- RefWorks: https://www.refworks.com
- Zotero: http://www.zotero.org (also a collaboration tool)

File Sharing

- DoD SAFE: https://safe.apps.mil/
- Box: http://www.box.com
- Google Drive: https://www.google.com/drive
- Dropbox: https://www.dropbox.com

Statistical Tools

- Power and Sample Size Calculator: http://powerandsamplesize.com/
- Statistical Package for the Social Sciences: https://www.ibm.com/analytics/spss-statistics-software
- MiniTab https://www.minitab.com
- Survey Monkey
- Poll Everywhere

Online Publication Depositories

- PubMed: https://www.ncbi.nlm.nih.gov/pubmed
- AMEDD Virtual Library: https://medlinet.amedd.army.mil/
- Research Gate: https://www.researchgate.net/
- Army Public Health Center: https://phc.amedd.army.mil/topics/discond/ptsaip/Pages/References.aspx
- ProQuest: https://www.proquest.com

Collaboration Tools

- Skype
- Zoom
- Facebook Messenger
- Google
- MilSuite
- Trello
- Blackboard Collaborate
- Adobe Connect

Journals

- *American Journal of Emergency Medicine*
- *Cureus*
- *Journal of the American Academy of Physician Assistants*
- *The Medical Journal* (US Army Medical Center of Excellence)
- *Journal of Orthopaedics for Physician Assistants*
- *Journal of Special Operations Medicine*
- *Journal of Trauma and Acute Care Surgery*
- *Military Medicine*
- *Prehospital Emergency Care*
- *Transfusion*
- *Visual Journal of Emergency Medicine*

Research Resources

- Army Human Resource Protection Office
- Army Medical Research Development Command: https://mrdc.amedd.army.mil/index.cfm/collaborate/research_protections/irbo
- Brooke Army Medical Center Department of Clinical Investigation: https://www.bamc.health.mil/staff/research/dci/
- Collaborative Institutional Training Initiative: https://www.citiprogram.org

Chapter 33

ROLE OF THE PHYSICIAN ASSISTANT IN GLOBAL HEALTH ENGAGEMENT

Christopher G. Metcalf, PA-C, MPAS, and Erin Stibral, APA-C, MPAS

Introduction

Global health engagement (GHE) comprises a very rewarding, and often challenging, mission set. GHE activities are diverse and support numerous strategic goals that support the Department of Defense (DOD) and advance US security objectives. US military medical personnel may participate in GHE activities at many levels. Most often Army physician assistants (PAs) will be involved in GHE at the tactical level; however, they may also have opportunities to participate at the operational level, while serving at an Army service component command (ASCC), or on a strategic level within the combatant commands (COCOMs). PAs involved in GHE work within the US government and military systems and also work closely with other entities, including nongovernmental organizations and partner nation (PN) military systems. Individuals working in GHE at the tactical or operational level will be part of a command surgeon's staff.

Background

Department of Defense Instruction (DODI) 2000.30 provides a framework for DOD GHE activities and delineates how GHE activities support US National Security Policy and defense security cooperation strategy.[1] Because of the linkage of GHE and national security it is imperative that all individuals planning and conducting GHE activities have a basic understanding of military GHE principles and underlying purposes, country-specific security cooperation (SC) objectives, and the overarching National Security Strategy.

Security Cooperation

SC is a means by which the combatant commander can achieve their objectives as laid out in the theater campaign plan. SC activities are engagements that build defense relationships while also promoting US security interests and can span all phases of military operations. The broad US objectives from which campaign plans are derived are outlined in the National Security Strategy.

GHE activities are a subset of SC and should directly support the ASCC or CCMD security cooperation plan, US embassy integrated country plan, and National Security Strategy objectives. Detailed information on security cooperation can be found in DA Pamphlet 11-31, *The Army Security Cooperation Handbook*.[2]

Global Health Engagement

DOD GHE activities are used to enhance stability and support medical capacity development within PNs. GHEs are an important tool for maintaining influence and building trust with US allies and PNs. A key consideration for any DOD GHE activity is that it must benefit the US military in addition to supporting the PN. This benefit can include improving military-to-military relationships, increasing interoperability, enhancing security, and providing readiness opportunities for US personnel.[1]

The directive that DOD GHE must provide a benefit to the DOD as well as the PN is a key discriminator between how nongovernmental organizations (NGOs) and governmental organizations, including the military, approach these types of engagements. NGOs abide by four humanitarian principles. One of these principles, the humanitarian imperative directs engagements based solely on providing humanitarian assistance wherever it is needed. Medical providers, including military providers, often view these activities from a humanitarian perspective, but the main purpose behind military GHE activities is supporting defense and security objectives.[3] NGOs, on the other hand, participate in GHE events solely for the humanitarian goal of improving global health and health systems.

GHE in the broadest sense is any health engagement between military members of different nations. Planned GHE events may be distinct engagements that are coordinated with a country, or they may be events embedded within an exercise. GHE events include but are not limited to subject matter expert exchanges (SMEEs), disaster relief exercise and exchange (DREE), medical conferences, and medical seminars (MEDSEMS). GHE can also be medical personnel from both nations working side by side to provide direct care as part of a subject matter expert exchange. GHE includes not only human health care, but also veterinary medicine, preventive medicine, and medical operations planning. Figure 33-1 is an example 5-year health engagement plan. Examples of individual GHE events are shown by year and line of effort (LOE). This well-developed plan demonstrates how distinct GHE events can be coordinated across organizations and LOEs to support both PN and US objectives.

Implementation Considerations

Concerns have been raised from both within and outside the DOD regarding the way DOD GHE activities are conducted. Common concerns include the risks of providing short-term solutions to chronic problems and undermining PN health care systems. DOD GHE activities also have the potential to undermine nonmilitary GHE activities.[4] For this reason, GHE activities should never be stand-alone medical events. GHE activities should tie into a health security cooperation strategy designated by the ASCC or CCMD surgeon's office. They should attempt to support the needs of both the US military and the PN by developing a long-term, sustainable medical capability or capacity. To ensure the GHE activities are having the desired effect, a system for assessment, monitoring, and evaluation must be part of the SC plan.[5]

Roles and Duties

Tactical Level

At the tactical level (corps and below), PAs assigned as staff officers usually participate in GHE as planning team members or by conducting GHE activities as part of an exercise. For successful GHE planning and exercising, it is important to understand the higher headquarters

Strategic Enablers, Tools, and Resources
Pacific Pathways, Disaster Response Exercise Exchange (DREE), PACIFIC ANGEL, Joint Chief of Staff Exercises, Global Health Security Agenda Phase 1 Country (CDC Liaison), National Guard SPP, Uniformed Services University Center for Global Health Engagement (USU CGHE), APMHE, AFRIMS, USAID, APCSS, CFE-DM, NEPMU

Line of Effort	2018 Engagement	2019 Engagement	2020 Engagement
Health System Support (Shape)		PKO L2H Trauma SMEE (ASCC) AVN Patient Movement SMEE; PACIFIC ANGEL (AF, ASCC)	Med Spt to PKO Clinical/ Functional SMEE (ASCC) Site visit to TCCC training center (ASCC)
Health Service Support (Posture)	BioPrep/ Emergency response SMEE Phase 2 (RHC/ CDC/AFRIMS); GPOI FHP Multi-Lat with a 3rd nation	BioPrep/Emergency response TTX Phase 3 (RHC/CDC/ AFRIMS/AF)	Clinical Laboratory Infectious Borne Diseases SMEE (MEDCEN/ AFRIMS)
Force Health Protection (Ready)	Used GPOI funding and integrated into the BioPrep/Clinical Lab SMEE	PH/PM Capacity Building (Navy/AF/ PHC/AFRIMS) DREE	Preventive Med Deployment OEHSA Phase I SMEE (Navy/AF/ PHC/AFRIM)
Strategic Leadership (Communicate)	• Land Forces Talks (annual) • Bilateral Defense Dialogues • Senior Leader Engagement (ASCC 2017/2019/2021) • APMHE		
Priorities	PARTNER NATION-HMA, HADR, PKO COCOM-HA/DR, PKO, Defense Professionalization ASCC-HA/DR, PKO, Counter Improvised Explosive Devices (CIED), Mil-Mil Relationships		

Figure 33-1. Example of a 5-year health engagement plan. Examples of individual global health engagement events are shown by year and line of effort. AF: Air Force; AFRIMS: Armed Forces Research Institute of Medical Sciences; APMHE: Asia Pacific Military Health Exchange; APCSS: Asia Pacific Center for Security Studies; ASCC: Army service component command; AVN: aviation;

2021	2022	2023
Engagement	**Engagement**	**End State**
Med Spt to PKO Med Ops TTX (ASCC)	Med Spt to PKO Med Ops TTX (ASCC)	Improved operational military medical training from individual to collective skills, with a trauma focus (Supports HA/DR, PKO) Increased capability to detect and respond to emerging infections/ pandemics (Supports HA/DR, GHSA) Improved ability to evaluate environmental threat during HADR/ PKO events (supports HA/DR, PKO)
Clinical Laboratory Disposal of Haz Waste SMEE (MEDCEN)	Five-Year Evaluation Biopreparedness and PKO SMEEs (ASCC/HHS/ CDC)	
PH/PM ISO deployment operations SMEE (ASCC)	PH/PM ISO deployment operations SMEE (ASCC)	

CDC: Centers for Disease Control and Prevention; CFE-DM: Center for Excellence in Disaster Management and Humanitarian Assistancc; COCOM: combatant command; FHP: Force Health Protection; GHSA: global health security agenda; GPOI: global peace operations initiative; HA/DR: humanitarian assistance/disaster response; HHS: Department of Health and Human Services; HMA: Humanitarian Mine Action Program; L2H: level 2 hospital; MEDCEN: Medical Center; NEPMU: Navy Environmental Preventive Medicine Unit; OEHSA: Occupational and Environmental Health Site Assessment; PKO: peace-keeping operations; RHC: Regional Health Command; SMEE: subject matter expert exchange; SPP: State Partnership Program; TCCC: Tactical Combat Casualty Care; TTX: table-top exercise; USAID: US Agency for International Development country plan and underlying purpose of the activity (Figures 33-2 and 33-3). If at all possible, PN medical personnel should be included in the event. To plan or execute a successful engagement, the following items must be considered:

- country health context (determinants or variables that effect the health of the local population including social, political, cultural, and economic issues);
- the CCMD or ASCC health security cooperation plan;

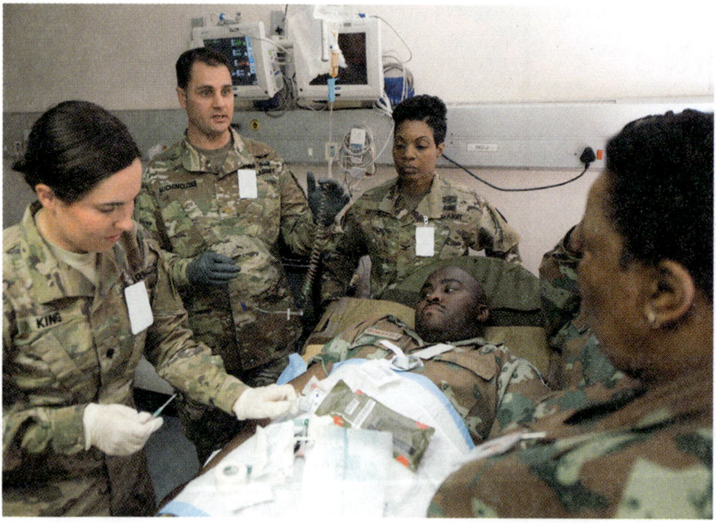

Figure 33-2. Specialist Kassandra King (left front), a combat medic with US Army Africa, performs an intravenous procedure. Major Paul "Jason" Auchincloss (left rear), a senior physician assistant with US Army Africa, discusses Army treatment techniques with South African soldiers during a training session for the Shared Accord exercise at the South African Army Combat Training Center in Lohatla, July 26, 2017. Photograph by Sean Kimmons.
Reproduced from Kimmons S. South African exercise becomes homecoming for USA Army physician assistant. US Army Africa website. Published August 16, 2017. Accessed May 27, 2020. https://www.usaraf.army.mil/media-room/article/28355/south-african-exercise-becomes-homecoming-for-us-army-physician-assistant

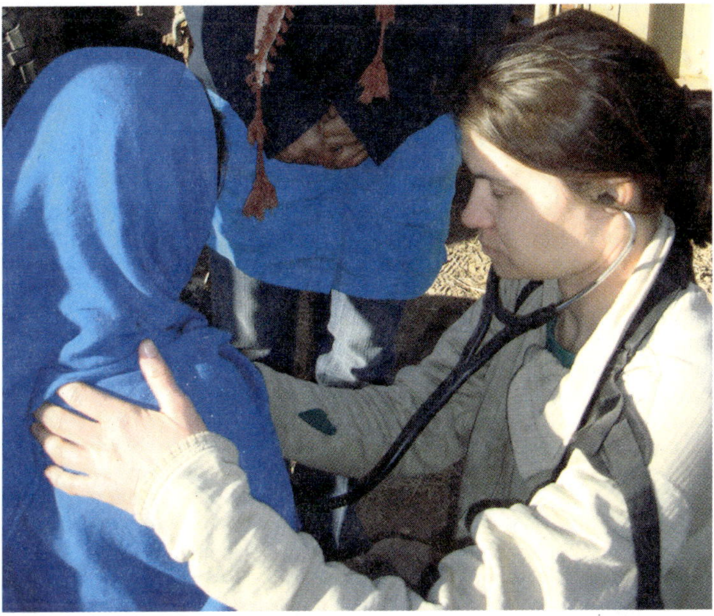

Figure 33-3. Then-Captain Erin Stibral examines a local Afghan child during a Medical Civilian Assistance Program (MEDCAP) visit in 2009, Kandahar Province, Afghanistan.

- overall security cooperation country plan and LOEs;
- coordination with the US embassy country team for approval, PN contacts, and other planning considerations; and
- general knowledge of PN military and military medical systems.

These considerations are complex and may involve intricate coordination among US and PN stakeholders, as well as approval from appropriate DOD and embassy authorities. GHE are multifaceted operations with established systematic procedures that must be followed by all planners and participants.

Operational Level

PAs working in GHE at the operational level may be assigned to the ASCC or regional health command. They usually have GHE as a primary duty and work closely with SC teams. If the primary duty of an individual is GHE, they are part of the SC workforce and are required to have some level of SC training. These PAs often participate in bilateral (Army-to-Army) talks and provide input to the overall SC plan and country plans. A PA serving as the GHE officer develops a GHE strategy and specific health engagement plans for any country where GHE is being conducted. This plan should be developed with medical input from bilateral talks, COCOM, and ASCC SC guidance (see Figure 33-1).

Another important consideration is that GHE has no dedicated funding stream. GHE events compete against other requirements for SC and COCOM funding, so it is very important to understand funding authorities to ensure they meet the legal requirements.

Some of the key tasks for an operational-level job are listed below.

- Develop ASCC GHE strategy.
- Develop 5-year country plans to ensure activities support specific health LOEs that aim to develop sustainable capacity.
- Coordinate with US embassy country teams for engagement planning.
- Ensure subordinate units conducting GHE activities understand the overall GHE strategy and country-specific health engagement plans.
- Provide oversight to subordinate units and track GHE activities to ensure they support the GHE plan.
- Submit engagement proposals for funding in accordance with appropriate authorities.
- Review and validate all GHE efforts submitted for funding within the ASCC.
- Coordinate with CCMD and sister services to ensure GHE strategies are mutually supportive and to prevent duplication.

Strategic Level

Currently, PAs are less likely to find themselves in key strategic billets executing GHE activities at CCMD or higher levels. However, many GHE activities at both the tactical and operational level can have lasting strategic implications.

PAs working in GHE at CCMD or higher levels should have a thorough understanding of the National Security Strategy and other US government strategic documents that support and direct DOD GHE activities. They must work closely with their respective SC sections and have a well-developed CCMD GHE strategy (see Figure 33-1) that synchronizes the activities of the services. A few of the key tasks for this position are listed below.

- Participate in bilateral military-to-military talks.
- Develop CCMD-level GHE strategy and country plans.
- Provide guidance in areas of expertise.
- Deconflict GHE activities among the services.
- Look for opportunities to conduct synergistic activities with other units and services.
- Coordinate with US Agency for International Development (USAID) and nongovernmental organizations working in the operational area to share resources and deconflict engagements.
- Review and validate all GHEs submitted for funding within the COCOM.

Desired Skills and Attributes

The following attributes are helpful for someone desiring to work in the GHE arena:

- ability to travel frequently;
- enjoy travel to foreign countries;
- ability to work independently;
- strong work ethic;
- knowledge of US military capabilities and military medical planning;
- ability to work well with both military and civilian organizations;
- cultural sensitivity;
- excellent written and verbal communication skills;
- civilian global health or public health training;
- interest in international relations; and
- diverse operational experience including deployment experience, preferably in multiple roles of care.

Training

The Air Force and Navy both have developed a pathway to train their medical personnel on global health competencies. These programs are specifically designed to train individuals to work within the GHE arena. The Air Force International Health Specialist program was established in 2000 to develop health professionals to provide global health expertise to the major commands, component commands, and CCMD.[6] The Navy established the Office of Global Health Engagement in 2012. In 2017 a Global Health Specialist Program was established to facilitate the growth of global health knowledge and skills within Navy medicine to support SC through GHE.[7] Both of these programs confer a skill identifier to individuals who complete the training. Currently, the Army does not have a formalized GHE training program for medical personnel. However, it is essential that those working at the operational and strategic levels have both GHE and SC training. These training opportunities are important to effectively support a professional SC workforce and ensure GHE activities are embedded with the overall SC plan.

Despite the lack of a formal training program for Army GHE, courses are available. The two primary organizations that offer training are the Uniformed Services University (USU) Center for Global Health Engagement (CGHE), and the Defense Security Cooperation Agency Defense Security Cooperation University (DSCU). To professionalize the entire SC workforce, including GHE, these two organizations are updating training and materials designed to support the workforce. DSCU opened its doors in September 2019 with the goal of ensuring that everyone working in an SC position has a basic understanding of how SC links to the National Security Strategy and is certified at the basic level by 2020. For this purpose, an SC position is defined as one in which 50% or greater of assigned duties are SC related.[8] The courses include both online and resident training options. USU CGHE holds several courses that are tailored toward understanding GHE. Additionally, they are in the process of developing a GHE handbook that will help individuals working in GHE positions.

PAs participating in GHE events at the tactical level should have a general understanding of GHE and how it is nested within the larger SC plan. They should communicate with their ASCC and ensure all events support the ASCC GHE strategy. They would benefit from attending the USU CGHE Fundamentals of Global Health Engagement course, and having access to USU CGHE resources, but do not require the formalized SC courses offered by DSCU.

Fundamentals of Global Health Engagement Course

This 3-day course administered by the USU CGHE is intended to provide a basic understanding of strategic, operational, and civil–military considerations during GHE activities. The course provides an understanding of the processes involved from planning to assessment, monitoring, and evaluation. This course is recommended for anyone participating in GHE activities, especially those involved in planning. The course is taught by a mobile training team to classes of approximately 30 students.[9]

Global Health Strategies for Security Course

GHSS is a 1-week graduate-level certificate course offered through USU's CGHE. This course focuses on the strategy behind military GHE and the interactions between the military and other organizations within this space. This course is designed for DOD line and medical personnel who are involved in the planning assessment, implementation, and evaluation of DOD GHE activities. The USU CGHE Fundamentals of Global Health Engagement course is a prerequisite for this course.[9]

Introduction to Security Cooperation

This DSCU course is a 12-hour distance learning course for personnel who perform SC duties. The overview covers the full range of SC activities including policy, planning, execution, and evaluation. The course website is https://www.discs.dscu.mil/_pages/courses/course.aspx?id=SC-101.[10]

Intermediate Security Cooperation Planning, Oversight, and Execution

This DSCU course includes 16 hours of distance learning and 4 days of in-residence training. It is designed to provide students with the skills to plan, oversee, and execute SC at a COCOM level. The course includes discussion on authorities, funding, and interagency coordination. Introduction to Security Cooperation is a prerequisite for this course. The course website is https://www.discs.dscu.mil/_pages/courses/course.aspx?id=POE-201.[10]

Development in Vulnerable Environment Course

This USAID Office of Civilian-Military Cooperation course provides an overview of USAID structure, mission, and policies. The intent of the course is to enhance collaboration and planning between DOD and USAID.[11]

Department of Defense Regional Security Cooperation Centers

There are five DOD regional centers that host region-specific SC courses that are extremely beneficial for familiarizing PAs to the region and region-specific challenges. These centers offer orientation and more in-depth SC courses[12]:

- George C. Marshall European Center for Security Studies, Garmisch, Germany
- Daniel I. Inouye Asia-Pacific Center for Security Studies, Honolulu, HI
- William J. Perry Center for Hemispheric Defense Studies, Washington, DC
- Africa Center for Strategic Studies, Washington, DC
- Near East-South Asia Center for Strategic Studies, Washington, DC

Evaluation

PAs serving in staff positions at the tactical or operational level are most often rated by either the deputy surgeon or command surgeon. The senior rater will either be one of the general officers in the command or the surgeon, depending on the rater. Either of these rating schemes will allow the PA to have a physician within their rating chain.

Lessons Learned and Tips for Success

Working in GHE is both rewarding and challenging. At the tactical level, a PA will get experience working alongside PN forces, building relationships that can be drawn upon during times of crisis or during GHEs. PAs will experiences challenges in planning within the framework of another nation's timeline, and might have both language and cultural barriers to overcome.

At the operational and strategic level, PAs will have the opportunity to meet with senior military leaders, and work with PN counterparts to develop a joint GHE plan that provides long-lasting benefits for both the PN and the US military. A strong understanding of the region involved is extremely important, and the following tips will also increase success:

- Develop a close relationship with SC counterparts. They can provide invaluable country information. At the operational or strategic level, PAs will likely spend just as much, if not more time, working with them as with other surgeon section staff.
- The PA will be seen as the subject matter expert in GHE and should seek out training opportunities to develop their knowledge base.
- Every opportunity to learn about the GHE region or country should be exploited.
- Tie in with the embassy team early and frequently during planning.
- Ensure the GHE engagement is part of the overall SC plan and supports the theater campaign plan.

One of the challenges of being a PA serving as a staff officer is ensuring enough clinical hours to meet credentialing and privileging requirements. PAs in these types of positions must seek out clinic opportunities to work in a clinic that meets their unique requirements.

Conclusion

The role of GHE will continue to evolve and grow in importance for SC plans. Medical activities can be considered a "soft" initial entry operation to establish military-to-military relationships. These relationships can evolve to encompass virtually all warfighting functions to further the SC and theater campaign plans.

In order for GHE to be an effective tool, activities must nest within the overall SC plan. It is imperative that the workforce has sufficient training and resources to effectively plan and manage GHE activities. PAs currently participate in GHE at the tactical level whether they realize it or not. As GHE becomes a more formalized part of SC, PAs with proper preparation and training are capable of executing a larger role as GHE planners at both the operational and strategic levels.

References

1. US Department of Defense. *Global Health Engagement (GHE) Activities*. DOD; 2017. DOD Instruction 2000.30.
2. US Department of the Army. *Army Security Cooperation Handbook*. DA; 2015. DA PAM 11-31.
3. Michaud J, Moss K, Licina D, et al. Militaries and global health: peace, conflict, and disaster response. *Lancet*. 2019;393:276–286.
4. Quinnan G. The future of Department of Defense global health engagement. *Joint Force Quarterly*. 2016;80.
5. US Department of Defense. *Assessment, Monitoring, and Evaluation Policy for the Security Cooperation Enterprise*. DOD; 2017. DOD Instruction 5132.14.
6. Air Force Medical Service website. Accessed June 26, 2020. https://www.airforcemedicine.af.mil/About-Us/Global-Health-Engagement/International-Health-Specialist/
7. Navy Medicine Office of Global Health Engagement website. Accessed June 26, 2020. https://www.med.navy.mil/Pages/InfoViewPage.aspx?ItemID=15
8. Lopez C. New defense school to certify security cooperation workforce. US Department of Defense website. Published September 26, 2019. Accessed June 26, 2020. https://www.defense.gov/Explore/News/Article/Article/1971845/new-defense-school-to-certify-security-cooperation-workforce/
9. Uniformed Services University Center for Global Health Engagement website. Accessed June 25, 2020. https://www.usuhs.edu/cghe
10. Defense Security Cooperation University website. Accessed June 26, 2019. https://www.dscu.mil/
11. US Agency for International Development website. Accessed June 26, 2020. https://www.usaid.gov/dive
12. Defense Security Cooperation Agency website. Accessed June 26, 2020. https://www.dsca.mil/programs/dod-regional-centers

Additional Sources

- Department of Defense. Defense Security Cooperation Agency website. Accessed June 26, 2020. https://www.dsca.mil/
- Uniformed Services University. Center for Global Health Engagement website. Accessed June 26, 2020. https://www.usuhs.edu/cghe

Chapter 34

ROLE OF THE CIVILIAN PHYSICIAN ASSISTANT IN A MILITARY MEDICAL TREATMENT FACILITY

Christine C. Cabal, PA-C, MPAS

Introduction

The primary role of a civilian physician assistant (PA) in a military medical treatment facility (MTF) is to serve as a health care provider in the capacity they are credentialed in. Civilian PAs also provide continuity of operations and expertise when there are provider shortages and problems with patient access. Uniformed PAs often leave for deployments and field training exercises, resulting in understaffing in both tactical and clinical settings. Uniformed PAs also have a high turnover rate due to permanent change of station cycles, the expiration of term of service, or retirement. By filling valid authorizations and serving as augmentation, civilian PAs optimize the health and readiness of service members, the retired community, and their families, ultimately adding to the overall strength of the US Army. Civilian PA positions are filled by prior service military personnel as well as civilian trained personnel.

Mission

The Army civilian PA supports service members, retirees, and families during times of peace, conflict, and war. The Army Civilian Corps Creed is very similar to the Soldier's Creed. Army civilians share the same values and overall mission as the Army enlisted and officer personnel (Figure 34-1).

Army Civilian Corps Creed

I am an Army Civilian – a member of the Army Team.
I am dedicated to our Army, our Soldiers and Civilians.
I will always support the mission.
I provide leadership, stability, and continuity during war and peace.
I support and defend the Constitution of the United States and consider it an honor to serve our Nation and our Army.
I live the Army values of Loyalty, Duty, Respect, Selfless Service, Honor,
Integrity, and Personal Courage.
I am an Army Civilian.[1]

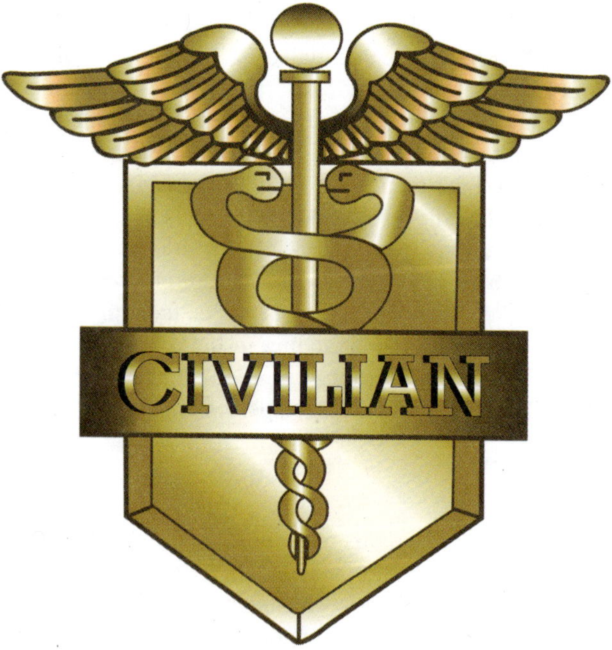

Figure 34-1. The Army Civilian Corps crest.

Supervision

The civilian PA is supervised by a physician, who ensures the practice remains within recognized medical standards. The PA is usually self-directed and has the autonomy to apply evidence-based clinical practice guidelines and engage patients actively in their health care. The extent and nature of supervision varies with the setting and patient problems.[2]

Duties and Responsibilities

Civilian PAs are responsible for the examination, diagnosis, and treatment of pediatric, adult, and geriatric populations within personal credentials and privileges delineated by the MTF. The civilian PA works collaboratively with a physician in patient evaluation, management, and creating an integrated plan of care that the patient understands and can comply with.[2]

Civilian PAs must be competent leaders to effectively manage others. They must possess fundamental capabilities such as understanding Army culture, developing a team, building trust, and supporting the commander. As an Army civilian PA, it is essential to have an understanding of Army culture, including terminology, customs, values, and ranks. Understanding customers is the key to delivering high-quality health service support. Civilian PAs need to know the MTF's organizational processes and procedures to manage expectations. Investing time and energy in learning the system produces better outcomes. MTFs follow high-reliability organization (HRO) principles that help develop and sustain the organizational objectives. The five principles of HRO are:

1. Sensitivity to operations.
2. Reluctance to simplify.
3. Preoccupation with avoiding failure.
4. Deference to expertise.
5. Commitment to resiliency.[3]

Civilian PAs have the opportunity to teach, coach, and mentor the next generation of PAs and medics. They can inspire, encourage, and develop a team of soldiers, health care professionals, leaders, and administrators (Figure 34-2). Trust is necessary to create a strong bond among Army professionals. A civilian PA must embrace team practice by not only focusing on their empanelment, but also striving to help other staff members. Expect to be another provider's surrogate due to high turnover. Expect to see Army, Air Force, Navy, and Marine patients, including reserve component and National Guard members. Civilian PAs must support the priorities, initiatives, and requirements of the MTF commander.

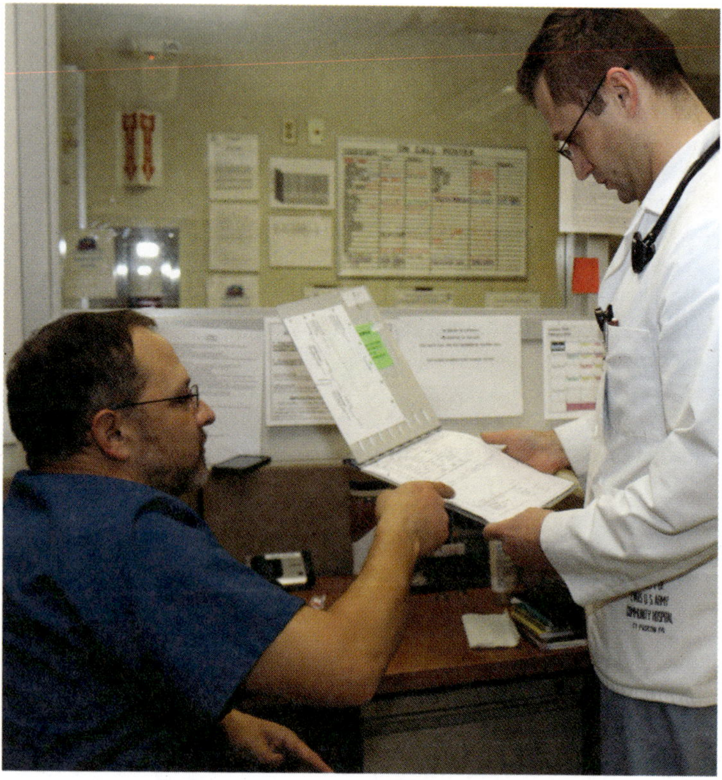

Figure 34-2. Mr. Andrew Flores precepts an Interservice Physician Assistant Program Phase 2 student, Officer Candidate Joshua Lane, at Evans Army Community Hospital Emergency Room in Fort Carson, Colorado.
Reproduced from: Troth JL. Evans trains future physician assistants. US Army website. Published January 19, 2016. Accessed May 15, 2020.
https://www.army.mil/article/161103/evans_trains_future_physician_assistants

Desired Skills and Attributes

The following skills and attributes are beneficial:

- Reviewing, documenting, and updating patient care through the electronic health record systems such as the Armed Forces Health Longitudinal Technology Application (AHLTA), Military Health System GENESIS, Composite Health Care System, and Essentris.
- Appropriately completing DD Form 689, Individual Sick Slip, or DA Form 3349, e-Profile (if applicable), to communicate to the chain of command patients' physical limitations to prevent further harm.
- Navigating through web-based applications for management of individual medical readiness such as the Army Medical Protection System (MEDPROS), the Air Force Aeromedical Services Information Management System (ASIMS), and the Navy Medical Event Reporting (MER) system.
- Being an ideal team player by having a strong work ethic and by motivating other staff members to do the same.
- Initiative and innovative thinking to improve policies, processes, and practices.
- Demonstrating flexibility by maintaining productivity, quality of work, and morale while adapting to changing conditions or unexpected obstacles.
- Providing excellent customer service through active listening, spoken and email communication, and telephone etiquette.
- Communicating effectively, both orally and in writing, and providing consultation, teaching, and coordination with patients and their family members regarding medical care. Establishing ongoing information exchange with leaders and subordinates promotes individual and organizational transparency in all actions and decision making.

Education and Training

A civilian PA must graduate from an accredited PA program, become certified by passing the Physician Assistant National Certifying Examination (PANCE), and maintain certification through the National Commission on Certification of Physician Assistants (NCCPA) by (*a*) taking a recertification exam every 10 years, (*b*) earning 100 continuing medical education (CME) credits every 2 years, and (*c*) paying a certification maintenance fee every 2 years. Civilian PAs utilize the three training domains of the Army leader development model: operational, institutional, and self-development. [4]

Operational Training

Civilians gain experience from operational assignments at current positions, different organizational levels, specialty areas, and various geographical sites. The operational training environment will challenge Army civilians to excel in positions of higher responsibility. The Defense Health Agency (DHA) incorporates standardized medical trauma training to support current initiatives, such as tactical combat casualty care (TCCC) and prolonged field care. In the operational setting, TCCC prioritizes triage, treatment, and management of the most common preventable deaths resulting from combat.[5,6]

Institutional Training

- Army civilians complete Civilian Education System (CES) courses by registering through the Civilian Human Resources Training Application (CHRTAS), a portal of the Army Training Requirements and Resources System (ATRRS). CES includes five levels of courses to provide leadership education for Army civilians throughout their careers, depending on their general schedule (GS) grades [7]:
- Foundation Course (level 1) for GS 1–15.
- Basic Course (level 2) for GS 1–9.
- Intermediate Course (level 3) for GS 10–12.
- Advanced Course (level 4) for GS 13–15.
- Continuing Education for Senior Leaders (level 5) for GS 14 and 15.

Self-Development Training

Civilian PAs must maintain knowledge of changing treatment protocols and procedures; self-development is their own responsibility. There are many ways to strengthen competencies to maintain or improve performance. These include but are not limited to the following:

- professional reading or self-study;
- attending conferences or seminars (web-based training, classroom training, or international events);
- independent research;
- community leadership positions that support development goals;
- individual study or practice;
- volunteer opportunities (search and rescue, medical volunteer abroad);
- off-duty academic schooling to acquire an advanced degree;
- earning certifications (fellowship in wilderness medicine, diploma in mountain medicine, tactical emergency casualty care);
- mentoring or being mentored; and
- professional mobility—civilian PAs can often change specialties and receive on-the-job training.[2]

Performance Management

Army civilians create an individual development plan (IDP) to outline development objectives, training opportunities, and career goals. Army civilians can refer to the Army Career Tracker for specific professional developmental models with key assignment lists.[8] The IDP is an instrument to help project a professional path and establish a timetable to achieve short-term and long-term career goals. The IDP should be completed annually in conjunction with the annual performance plan. Just as uniformed PAs have the officer evaluation report (OER) to monitor career progression, civilian PAs use the Department of Defense Performance Management and Appraisal Program (DPMAP) to discuss performance expectations with supervisors. Performance management helps civilians grow into competent leaders who can potentially advance to higher levels of personal fulfillment and professional achievement.[9-11]

Sample IDP

Short-Term Goal (1-Year Plan)

- CES Foundation Course no later than 90 days after in-processing.
- Attend Emergency Medicine Boot Camp.
- Listen to monthly EM:Rap videos.

- Read 1 professional book per month.
- Self-study.
- Conduct team briefings/group presentations.

Long-Term Goal (5-Year Plan)

- CES Intermediate Course (distance learning and resident instruction).
- Take college or university classes.
- Participate in professional organizations (NCCPA, Wilderness Medical Society).
- Perform volunteer work (search and rescue, Army Ten Miler).
- Networking.

Sample DPMAP Performance Element and Standards for a Civilian PA

- **Objective 1:** Meet Medical Command (MEDCOM) efficiency standards for a PA in a community hospital setting.
- **Standard:** Achieve a combined 75% of established MEDCOM standards for Joint Outpatient Experience Survey (JOES), relative value unit (RVU), and Practice Management Revenue Model (PMRM) values.
- **Objective 2:** Maintain current licensure, CME benchmarks, and required certifications.
- **Standard:** Maintain current and active NCCPA licensure.
- **Standard:** Earn the required 100 hours per 2 years of CME to maintain current NCCPA licensure.
- **Standard:** Maintain current certification in Basic Life Support (BLS), Advanced Life Support (ALS), and Pediatric Advanced Life Support (PALS) disciplines.
- **Objective 3:** Train students across multiple disciplines in emergency medicine.
- **Standard:** Work with PA students, nurse practitioner students, medical students, and student medics to ensure at least 80% pass rate for emergency department rotations in their respective fields.
- **Objective 4:** Complete charting and mandatory training in a timely manner.
- **Standard:** Work with emergency department coders to ensure 75% of patient encounter charts are completed during initial patient encounter.

- **Standard:** Maintain 75% currency of mandatory Swank Health Training, both online and face to face.
- **Objective 5:** Complete assigned additional duties.
- **Standard:** Complete assigned additional duties as designated to meet 75% of suspense dates established by the department chief or appropriate committee chair.[10]

Continuing to Serve

Civilian PAs with a military background have the advantage of familiarity with policies and procedures that enable them to excel in the MTF environment. They have unique skill sets in operational medicine and staff briefings that allow them to relate to most of the patient population and have confidence in delivering high-quality health care regardless of the circumstances. Expertise gained through military training and remote conditions allows these PAs to practice medicine by using effective communication, leading by example, and being highly adaptable in constantly changing situations.

Many prior armed forces personnel hang up their uniform before military retirement but continue to serve the country by becoming civilian employees in the federal government. Those who performed honorable active military service have additional benefits under the Federal Employees Retirement System (FERS). To allow creditable military service to be used toward retirement eligibility, for example, GS employees can make military service deposit (MSD) payments to their civilian retirement fund prior to separation from federal employment. The MSD amount is a sum equal to 3% of military basic pay during the period of military service, plus interest (which starts accruing after 2 years of federal employment). The deposit may be paid to the Defense Finance and Accounting Service in a lump sum or through payroll deduction. Those who are eligible can also apply their active duty service time toward both Guard and Reserve retirement and FERS retirement.[12]

Lessons Learned

The following are lessons learned for civilian PAs:

- A team is only as strong as its weakest link. Identify deficiencies in the organization and focus on improving these shortfalls to enhance staff motivation and work ethic. Common operational problems include interpersonal conflict, stress, lack of motivation, poor teamwork, lack of trust, lack of accountability, and poor communication.

- Medics and nurses should be extensions of the civilian PA's capabilities. The more competent the health care staff, the more efficient the PA will become as a member of a cohesive team. Leaders have the ability to influence people, and that's one of the keys to success (Figure 34-3).

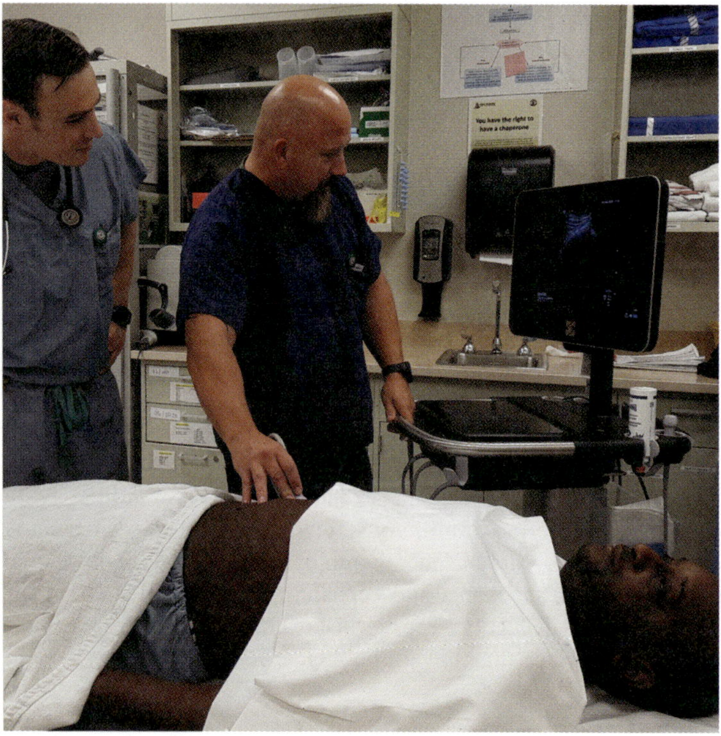

Figure 34-3. Mr. Arne E. Oas teaches bedside ultrasound techniques on a simulated patient (Sergeant Jason Williams) as a physician assistant student, Officer Candidate Daniel W. Matthes, learns how to conduct a focused assessment with sonography in trauma (FAST) exam.
Photograph courtesy of Christine C. Cabal.

- Learn to humanize medicine. See patients as people and not as objects. The PA must treat patients as if they are their own family. Recognize that no one likes to go to the hospital. Patients are there to get help from the PA and their staff. Some may require more education than others; therefore, part of the job is having patience with patients. The PA will never know if that "chronic knee pain" is a superficial reason for a rape victim to seek help. The PA will never know when that "STD check" is actually testicular cancer in a 21-year-old soldier. The PA is going to come into contact with people who are at their absolute breaking point in their MTF. If patients are angry and have an attitude, the PA should not take it personally (this may be the saddest, most stressful, loneliest time for that patient). The PA has the privilege of being able to take care of the nation's finest soldiers, families, and civilians. The PA must take care of them like they were their own.

Tips for Success

Along with lessons learned, these tips for success will help future civilian PAs succeed beyond expectations:

- Focus on outcomes. Develop a strategy for the team and the overall health care system to meet desired results with measurable targets and standards. When there is a goal in mind, it is easy to know which priorities and initiatives to support. Consistently holding others accountable to a high standard (as opposed to waiting for the annual evaluation) raises the performance level of each team member. Ultimately, organizations and team members without growth and purpose do not flourish and have low job satisfaction.
- Do not strive to make everyone happy. Some patients or customers will disapprove of their plan of care (eg, they cannot get the magnetic resonance imaging they want or the pain medication they prefer). All the PA has to do is ask themselves, "Did I meet the standard of care?" If the answer is "YES," do not lose sleep over the negative interactive customer evaluation comments and move on. If the answer is "NO," then conduct a self after-action review and determine how the PA can make the situation better next time, learn from it, and then move on.
- The PA is in charge of their career and life goals. Maintain discipline to consistently work for professional and personal growth. Attend

seminars, read journals, and use podcasts. Most importantly, the PA must take care of themselves (not just their physical fitness, but also their emotional, spiritual, social, and family fitness).

Conclusion

The civilian PA contributes tremendously to the MTF by providing high-quality care to service members, the retired community, and their families. They serve as teachers and mentors to medics, as an augmentation to uniformed providers on tactical missions, and as leaders who inspire devotion and hard work. Civilian PAs enhance the overall readiness of the armed forces through effective leadership, skilled management of expectations, continuous learning, and embracement of team practice.

References

1. Department of the Army. Army Civilian Corps Creed. Accessed May 15, 2020. https://www.army.mil/values/corps.html
2. Civilian Personnel On-Line (CPOL) portal. Accessed May 15, 2020. https://acpol.army.mil/
3. Weick K, and Sutcliffe K. *Managing the Unexpected: Sustained Performance in a Complex World.* 3rd ed. John Wiley & Sons; 2015.
4. US Army Combined Arm Center. Army Leader Development Strategy. DA; 2013. Accessed May 11, 2020. https://Usacac.army.mil/Sites/Default/Files/Documents/Cal/Alds5june%20202013Records.Pdf
5. US Department of Defense. *Medical Readiness Training (MRT)*. DOD; 2018. DOD Instruction 1332.24.
6. US Department of Defense. *Joint Trauma System (JTS)*. DOD; 2016. DOD Instruction 6040.47.
7. US Department of the Army. *Army Training and Leader Development.* DA; 2017. Army Regulation 350-1, Subchap 4-3.
8. Army Career Tracker website. Accessed May 15, 2020. https://actnow.army.mil/

9. US Department of Defense. *DOD Civilian Personnel Management System: Performance Management and Appraisal Program*. DOD; 2016. DOD Instruction 1400.25, vol 431.

10. DOD Performance Management and Appraisal Program (DPMAP) website. Accessed March 23, 2020. https://www.dcpas.osd.mil/LER/DPMAP

11. Office of Personnel Management (OPM) website. Accessed March 23, 2020. https://www.opm.gov

12. US Office of Personnel Management. *Federal Employees Retirement System (FERS) Transfer Handbook; a Guide to Making Your Decision.* OPM; 2008: 7-13. Federal Personnel Manual Accessed May 15, 2020. https://www.opm.gov/retirement-services/publications-form/pamphlets/ri90-3.pdf

Chapter 35

THE INDEPENDENT MEDICAL OPINION PROCESS AND THE PHYSICIAN ASSISTANT'S ROLE

Leah Bucholz, PA-C, MPAS, and Maura Lappin, DO

Introduction

The Department of Veterans Affairs (VA) disability process is a benefits program available for veterans who have become sick or injured while serving, or who may have had an injury or illness worsened by their service on active duty while serving their country. The process can be complex and even overwhelming for any soon-to-be-exiting service member as well as for the current veteran population. The military clinician has a dual role as a veteran entitled to benefits and as a potential health care practitioner involved in the process. A new and inexperienced physician assistant (PA) is generally focused on current mission requirements and may not comprehend the importance of their position for patients they evaluate and treat. On the other hand, a seasoned PA nearing retirement likely understands the importance of documentation and the impending likelihood that a patient may enter the VA disability process. It is the goal of this chapter to help the junior PA as well as the seasoned PA understand the independent medical opinion process, as well as how the PA can impact the lives of disabled service members in their transition to veteran status.

Preparation for Service Members

Active Duty

Active duty PAs can best prepare veterans by encouraging them to seek medical care for all ailments and by ensuring these complaints are thoroughly documented in their service treatment record. The

Department of Defense (DD) Form 2807, Report of Medical History, and the DD 2808, Report of Medical Examination, are especially crucial during the separation process. These medical appointments and reports may be the only opportunity service members have to discuss some of the conditions they have suffered over their years of military service. Many transitioning service members, especially those with over 20 years of active duty service, may require several visits to comprehensively document their medical histories.

Army National Guard and Army Reserve

Army National Guard and Army Reserve service members may experience more difficulty obtaining evidence of disability than active duty service members. For National Guard and Reserve service members during periods of inactive duty service, documentation of an injury incurred in the line of duty (LOD) is generally helpful when applicable. This can be a formal or informal process and should start with the completion of a Department of the Army (DA) Form 2173, Statement of Medical Examination and Duty Status, which describes the incident and injury and is signed by the unit commander and the attending physician or patient administrator. Of note, LOD investigations can be performed for active duty, National Guard, and Reserve components. Information on this type of investigation can be found in Army Regulation 600-8-4, *Line of Duty Policy, Procedures, and Investigations.*[1]

Independent Medical Opinion Letters

Independent medical opinion letters, often referred to as "nexus letters," illustrate a link or nexus between an in-service injury and the veteran's current disability. They may demonstrate that a condition occurring during service is still affecting the veteran or link a service-connected condition to another condition that developed more recently. These letters can be helpful, especially after a veteran has exited service, if there is a lack of clear contemporaneous medical documentation in the active duty record.

What to Include

The best nexus letters are brief, yet comprehensive enough to include all pertinent material and medical evidence that may apply.

There are several main components to writing a quality nexus letter. First, the author of the expert opinion should substantiate their credentials, which will help the reader understand that the content is the author's best clinical judgment, made with the guidance and knowledge from all their accumulated training and experience, and not merely a random statement. It is also vital to inform the reader that appropriate documentation and evidence has been reviewed in order to reach the letter's conclusion. Including specific references to the facts in the reviewed medical records will affirm that the author has evaluated available medical and service records provided by the veteran.

A persuasive nexus letter will also provide ample evidence to back up the opinion. Merely stating that in the author's opinion, condition A is connected to condition B, garners some weight if the appropriate credentials and qualifications have been included, but it is often not enough. Including an explanation of why or how the conclusion has been reached based on facts in the patient's medical records and references to the medical literature will strengthen the letter and opinion immensely. To be valuable to the VA, the nexus letter must be based on the medical records and the applicable literature.

Quantifying the Opinion

A critical part of a nexus letter is quantifying the opinion on the link between the two conditions. The author has told the reader who they are (why the author is qualified to present an opinion) and what evidence has been considered (the veteran's medical and service records as well as evidence from medical literature); the reader should then attempt to quantify how likely the connection is between conditions. This may be achieved by several different statements that convey different levels of certainty, as follows:

- "is due to" conveys the author believes with 100% certainty the conditions are linked (as with all things in medicine, there are few certainties, and this is not a frequently used statement);
- "more likely than not" communicates there is a greater than 50% chance the conditions are linked;
- "at least as likely as not" expresses the author believes the conditions are linked with equal to or greater than 50% certainty based on the author's expertise and literature;

- "not at least as likely as not" conveys a less than 50% certainty of linkage; and
- "is not due to" states that in the author's opinion, there is a 0% chance the conditions are linked (this not a commonly used statement since full certainty is rare in medicine, and this statement would negate any previous information in the letter about the connection; the lack of a causal link would also be a reason not to provide a letter).

Conclusion

In closing, it is essential to remember there is no greater honor than caring for service members on and off the battlefield. Continuing to care for them after separation is a choice PAs can make—to further care for veterans in the VA disability process. It is an extremely complex process, often difficult to navigate, even for experienced PAs with a wealth of medical knowledge. The process can be even more difficult to navigate and overwhelming for separating service members and veterans. The medical documentation in each service member's record is vital to the claims they may ultimately file. All injuries and illnesses may become the basis for a future disability claim. For these reasons among many others, it is important that PAs operating in the military health system or providing care to service members and veterans make a concerted effort to not only provide outstanding care, but also to ensure quality documentation is established within the record.

Acknowledgements

The authors would like to acknowledge Alan Bucholz, PA-C, MPAS, and Kory McCullah, PA-S, MSLA, for their assistance in reviewing and editing this chapter.

Reference

1. US Department of the Army. *Line of Duty Policy, Procedures, and Investigations*. DA; March 15, 2019. Army Regulation 600-8-4.

Additional Sources

- US Department of Veterans Affairs. *Summary of VA Benefits for National Guard and Reserve Members and Veterans*. VA; 2012. Accessed August 26, 2020. https://www.benefits.va.gov/BENEFITS/benefits-summary/SummaryofVANationalGuardandReserve.pdf
- 38 CFR, Part 3, § 3.317.
- US Department of Veterans Affairs. *M21-1 Adjudication Procedures Manual*. Accessed August 26, 2020. https://www.knowva.ebenefits.va.gov/system/templates/selfservice/va_ssnew/help/customer/locale/en-US/portal/554400000001018/topic/554400000004049/M21-1-Adjudication-Procedures-Manual
- US Department of the Army. *Military Occupation Classification and Structure*. DA; July 19, 2018. DA Pamphlet 611-21.
- US Department of the Army. *Standards of Medical Fitness*. DA; June 27, 2019. Army Regulation 40-501.

Epilogue:
The Future of the Army Physician Assistant

The Army Physician Assistant (PA) profession was established for a noble purpose—to provide more accessible health care for soldiers in a turbulent world. Today, PAs have eclipsed that purpose, and are advancing medicine in ways never before envisioned. PAs serve as legislators, health system CEOs, hospital commanders, city officials, medico-legal experts, professors, education system leaders, and advisors to heads of state. The future of the profession is in adapting to an ever-changing health care industry.

The vision for the Army PA profession is to reinforce the spirit of innovation and performance in medical and readiness systems embodied by PAs to improve the deployability and survivability of our soldiers. PAs have too long been relegated to an obsolete force structure that does not encourage professional growth or validate the great breadth and depth of capability and experience our PAs bring to Army Medicine and commanders. Great opportunities have opened for PAs to collaborate and lead at all levels of Army Medicine. We must bolster Army Medicine by mentoring outstanding PAs to provide leadership and expertise throughout the Army and the Defense Health Agency. With great opportunity also comes great responsibility, and we must recognize that responsible mentorship and enforcement of quality and professional standards must be reinforced wherever PAs are posted. Army PA's training and credentialing must prepare and support them for the inevitable autonomy necessitated by the dispersed and multi-domain nature of current and future deployments. That autonomy must always be tempered with adherence to standards of care, scope of practice, self-restraint, and consultation to ensure PAs and Combat Medics have robust capabilities that meet the needs of commanders.

PAs serve as the face of Army Medicine. Together with Combat Medics, PAs are many times the first professional medical officers that Soldiers seek for medical readiness and care. The PA profession offers an avenue for outstanding combat medics and soldiers to become PAs, and we must always improve pathways to recruit Medics to the Interservice PA Program (IPAP) to retain the "From the Line, For the Line" character of the Army PA. As a product of that pathway, I charge all Army PAs to seek out excellent candidates for IPAP and direct commissioning, and to facilitate their preparation to build a force of PAs with the depth of operational experience the Army, Department of Defense, and the world need for the future.

The *US Army Physician Assistant Handbook*, First Edition, collated the writings of the thought leaders of the Army PA profession. Only 2 years later, Army Medicine and the world have changed immensely. Because of all who have contributed to the first edition, we now have a snapshot in time of the opinions, challenges, and successes of those authors. Now, as the Military Health System continues to reform at a blistering pace along with the US civilian health system, current PA leaders continue to develop, lead, and share their hearts and opinions in this new addition. You are the real engine behind our positive energy! Thanks to all of you who enhance the PA profession and help others in the military and civilian communities. This publication is a true testament to all who have contributed and shared.

To all the individuals I have had the opportunity to serve with, be led by, or watch their leadership from afar, I want to say thank you for being the inspiration and foundation for the second edition of the *US Army Physician Assistant Handbook*. Without the experiences and support from peers and our teams, which touch on every aspect of military and civilian medicine, this book would not exist. You have given us all the opportunity to be surrounded by a great group of individuals. To be a leader among other great leaders is an honor. Thank you and special acknowledgements to COL Amy Jackson and LTC Amelia Duran-Stanton for their leadership, tenacity, and sustained unconditional support for the second edition of the *Physician Assistant Handbook*.

The associated dynamics of DOD and the recent organizational changes have presented many opportunities. The readiness growth and development experience is both internally challenging and rewarding as we continue to grow in support of our forces. I especially want to thank the individuals who helped make this happen and mentor those who will publish the next editions.

Colonel David Hamilton
The 9th Army Physician Assistant Consultant
to the Army Surgeon General

ABBREVIATIONS AND ACRONYMS

A

A: Airborne
AAC: Army Acquisition Corps
AAPA: American Academy of Physician Assistants
AATS: ARNG Aviation Training Site
ABLS: Advanced Burn Life Support
ABN DIV: airborne division
ABSITE: American Board of Surgery In-Training Examination
ACAT: acquisition category
ACE: ask, care, escort
ACEP: American College of Emergency Physicians
ACFT: Army Combat Fitness Test
ACGME: Accreditation Council for Graduate Medical Education
ACM: Army Capability Manager
ACR: armored cavalry regiment
ACU: Army combat uniform
AD: active duty
ADDIE: analysis, design, develop, implement, evaluate
ADP: AMEDD Distribution Plan
ADSO: active duty service obligation
ADTMC: algorithm-directed troop medical care
AFAB: assigned female at birth
AFRICOM: Africa Command
AFSCP: Army Flight Surgeon Course–Primary
AGR: Active Guard Reserve
AHA: American Heart Association
AHLTA: Armed Forces Health Longitudinal Technology Application
AHO: allied health officer
AHS: Army health system
AHSMS: Allied Health Sciences Military School
AI: associate investigator
AIM.2: Assignment Interactive Module Version 2
AIT: advanced individual training

ALARACT: All Army Activities message
ALP: accepted list position
ALS: Advanced Life Support
ALSE: Aviation Life Support Equipment (course)
AMA: American Medical Association
AMAB: assigned male at birth
AMEDD: Army Medical Department
AMEDDB: Army Medical Department Board
AMH: Army Medical Home
AMHRR: Army Military Human Resource Record
AMP: aviation medicine program
AMSC: Army Medical Specialist Corps
AMSMS: Army Medicine Secure Messaging Service
AMT: aviation medicine team
AO: action officer
AOC: area of concentration
AOR: area of responsibility
APA: aeromedical physician assistant
APA: American Psychiatric Association
APM: assistant program manager
APMC: AMEDD Professional Management Command
APPD: Army Medicine Personnel Proponent Directorate
AR: Army regulation
ARC: advanced resuscitative care
ARC: American Red Cross
ARC-PA: Accreditation Review Commission on Education for the Physician Assistant
ARMEDCOM: Army Reserve Medical Command
ARMS: Aviation Resource Management Survey
ARNG: Army National Guard
ARSOAC: Army Special Operations Aviation Command
ARSOF: US Army Special Operations Forces
ARTB: Airborne and Ranger Training Brigade
ASA: Assistant Secretary of the Army
ASAB: assigned sex at birth
ASAP: Alcohol Substance Abuse Program
ASBP: Armed Services Blood Program
ASBS: Army Selection Board System
ASCC: Army service component command

ASD: AMEDD Student Detachment
ASI: additional skill identifier
ASIMS: Aeromedical Services Information Management System
ASL: Army senior leader
ATAAPS: Automated Time and Assistance Production System
ATLS: Advanced Trauma Life Support
ATP: Aircrew Training Program
ATP: Army techniques publication
ATRRS: Army Training and Requirements Resources System
AUSA: Association of the US Army
AWC: Army War College

B

BAMC: Brooke Army Medical Center
BAS: battalion aid station
BCP: Board Certified Pay
BCT: brigade combat team; basic combat training
BCT3: Brigade Combat Team Trauma Training
BDD: Benefits Due at Discharge
BDE: brigade
BDE CDR: brigade commander
BDE SURG: brigade surgeon
BEST: Basic Endovascular Skills for Trauma (course)
BLS: Basic Life Support
BN: battalion
BOG: Boots on Ground
BOLC: Basic Officer Leader Course
BRS: blended retirement system
BSM: Bachelor of Science in Medicine

C

C2P2: Credentials Certification and Privileging Preparation
C4: Combat Casualty Care Course
C4I: command, control, communication, computers, and intelligence
CAC: common access card
CACO: congressional affairs contact officer
CAD: course administrative data
CAF: competency assessment file
CAMP: Career Acquisition Management Portal

CAPPMIS: Career Acquisition Personnel and Position Management Information System
CAQ: Certificate of Added Qualifications
CASEVAC: casualty evacuation
CASPA: Central Application Service for Physician Assistants
CATC: Combat Advisor Training Course
CBMH: Community-Based Medical Home
CBRNE: chemical, biological, radiological, nuclear, and explosive
C/B/T: company/battery/troop
CC: clinical coordinator
CC: corps chief
CCC: Captains Career Course
CC-DL: Common Core distance learning
CCMD: combatant command
CDID: Capabilities Development Integration Directorate
CENTCOM: Central Command
CES: Civilian Education System
CG: commanding general
CGHE: Center for Global Health Engagement
CGSC: Command and General Staff College
CGSOC-CC: Command and General Staff Officer Course–Common Core
CHCS: Composite Health Care System
CHRTAS: Civilian Human Resources Training Application
CIMPT: Center for Initial Military Training
CITI: Collaborative Institutional Training Initiative
CJCS: chairman of the Joint Chiefs of Staff
CJPA: Council of Junior Physician Assistants
CLINOPS: clinical operations
CLL: chief of legislative liaison
CLS: Combat Lifesaver
CME: continuing medical education
COCOM: combatant command
CoE: center of excellence
CONUS: continental United States
COP: combat outpost
CoS: chief of staff
CoTCCC: Committee on Tactical Combat Casualty Care
COVID: coronavirus disease

CP: continuation pay
CPD: citrate phosphate dextrose
CPG: Clinical Practice Guideline
CPI: continuous process improvement
CPP: Combat Paramedic Program
CPR: cardio pulmonary resuscitation
CR2C: Community Ready and Resilient Council
CR2I: command ready and resilient integrator
CSA: chief of staff of the Army
CSBPO: corps-specific branch proponency officer
CSHT: cross-sex hormone therapy
CSL: command selection list
CSM: command sergeant major
CSP: Consolidation of Special Pay (program)
CST: civil support team
C-STARS: Center for the Sustainment of Trauma and Readiness Skills
CTC: combat training center
CV: curriculum vitae
CWS: Certified Wound Care Specialist

D

DA: Department of the Army
DAC: Defense Acquisition Corps
DACM: Director of Acquisition Career Management
DA Pam: Department of the Army pamphlet
DAU: Defense Acquisition University
DCAM: DMLSS Customer Assistance Module
DCC: deputy corps chief; Direct Commission Course
DCCS: deputy commander for clinical services
DCG: deputy commanding general
DCG (M): deputy commanding general for maneuver
DCG (S): deputy commanding general for support
DCMT: Department of Combat Medic Training
DCR: damage control resuscitation
DCR: DOTMLPF-P change recommendation
DCSM: division command sergeant major
DD: Defense Department
DD: deployment director
DDT: dichlorodiphenyltrichloroethane

DEA: Drug Enforcement Agency
DEERS: Defense Enrollment Eligibility Reporting System
DFAS: Defense Financing and Accounting Service
DHA: Defense Health Agency
DHA-IHB: Defense Health Agency–Immunizations Healthcare Branch
DIV PA: division senior physician assistant
DIV SURG: division surgeon
DL: deployment-limiting
DMAIC: define, measure, analyze, improve, control
DMHRSi: Defense Medical Human Resources System internet
DMLIIS: Defense Medical Logistics Item Identification System
DMLSS: Defense Medical Logistics Standard Support
DMO: directed military overstrength
DMO: diving medical officer
DMRTI: Defense Medical Readiness Training Institute
DOD: Department of Defense
DODI: Department of Defense instruction
DODVPR: DOD Veterinary Pathology Residency
DOM: Directorates of Management
DoOM: Department of Operational Medicine
DOTD: Directorate of Training and Doctrine
DOTMLPF-P: doctrine, organization, training, materiel, leadership, personnel, facilities, and policy
DPAA: Defense Prisoner-of-War/Missing-in-Action Accounting Agency
DPMAP: Defense Performance Management and Appraisal Program
D-RAS: Disability Rating Activity Site
DREE: disaster relief exercise and exchange
DS: Department of Defense self-service
DSc: Doctor of Science degree
DScPAS: Doctor of Science in Physician Assistant Studies
DScPAS-EM: Doctor of Science in Physician Assistant Studies–Emergency Medicine
DScPAS-GS: Doctor of Science in Physician Assistant Studies–General Surgery
DScPAS-O: Doctor of Science in Physician Assistant Studies–Orthopedics
DSCU: Defense Security Cooperation University
DSM: Diagnostic and Statistical Manual of Mental Disorders
DSS: deputy state surgeons

DTIC: Defense Technical Information Center
DTM: directive-type memorandum
DTMC: DiLorenzo Troop Medical Clinic
DUI: driving under the influence

E

EBC: education branch chief
ED: emergency department
e-FAST: extended focused assessment with sonography in trauma
EHR: electronic health record
EIA: exercise-induced asthma
eMMPS: Electronic Medical Management Processing System
EMPA: emergency medicine physician assistant
EMR: electronic medical record
EMT: emergency medical technician
EMT-B: Emergency Medical Technician–Basic
ERT: emergent resuscitative thoracotomy
EUCOM: US European Command

F

FAST: focused assessment with sonography in trauma
FDA: Food and Drug Administration
FEB: flight evaluation boards
FEMA: Federal Emergency Management Agency
FERS: Federal Employees Retirement System
FHP: force health protection
FM: field manual
FMS: foreign military sales
FMSWeb: Force Management System website
FORSCOM: US Army Forces Command
FRAGO: fragmentation orders
FS: flight surgeon
FST: forward surgical team
FTE: full-time equivalent
FTX: field training exercise
FWB: fresh whole blood

G

GEARS: Global Electronic Approval Routing System
GEM: graduate education manager

GHE: global health engagement
GID: gender identity disorder
GME: graduate medical education
GOSC: General Officer Steering Committee
GRE: Graduate Record Examination
GS: general schedule
GSPA: general surgery physician assistant
GTMO: Guantanamo Bay Naval Base

H

H2F: Holistic Health and Fitness (program)
HAZMAT: hazardous materials
HBT: hospital-based training
HCD-CPS: healthcare delivery–clinical policy and services
HC-ITAB: Health Care Interservice Training Advisory Board
HELP: Health Experts OnLine Portal
HHBn: headquarters and headquarters battalion
HIPAA: Health Insurance Portability and Accountability Act
HLD: House Liaison Division
HMO: hyperbaric medical officer
HN: host nation
HPLRP: Health Professions Loan Repayment Program
HPO: health professions officer
HPOBCP: health professions officer board certification pay
HPOIP: health professions officer incentive pay
HPORB/IP: combined retention bonus/incentive pay
HQ: headquarters
HQDA: Headquarters, Department of the Army
HQ IMCOM: Headquarters, Installation Management Command
HR: human resources
HRC: US Army Human Resources Command
HRO: high-reliability organization
HSD: Health Services Division

I

IAW: in accordance with
ICD: International Classification of Diseases
ICTB: interfacility credentials transfer brief
ICTL: individual critical task list
ICU: intensive care unit

IDES: Integrated Disability Evaluation System
IDP: individual development plan
IET: initial entry training
IFAK: Individual First Aid Kit
IG: inspector general
IGAR: inspector general action request
ILE: Intermediate Level Education
IMCOM: Installation Management Command
IMT: initial military training
IP: incentive pay
IPAP: Interservice Physician Assistant Program
IPAT: integrated process action team
iPERMS: interactive Personnel Electronic Records Management System
IPPS-A: Integrated Personnel and Pay System–Army
IRB: institutional review board
ISAP: individual student assessment plan
ISOS: International SOS
ITRO: Interservice Training Review Organization
IUD: intrauterine device
IV: intravenous
I/W: instructor/writer

J

JBSA-FSH: Joint Base San Antonio–Fort Sam Houston
JC4I: Joint Command, Control, Communications, Computer and Intelligence
JCIDS: Joint Capabilities Integration and Development Systems
JDG: joint detention group
JIATF-S: Joint Inter-Agency Task Force–South
JMAR: Joint Medical Asset Repository
JMAU: Joint Medical Augmentation Unit
JMOC: Joint Medical Officer's Course
JOES: Joint Outpatient Experience Survey
JOPES: Joint Operation Planning and Execution System
JP: joint publication
JPEO: Joint Program Executive Office
JPME: joint professional military education
JRC-PA: Joint Review Committee for Educational Programs for the Assistant to Primary Care Physician

JRTC: Joint Readiness Training Center
JSAP: Joint Staff action process
JSOC: Joint Special Operation Center
JSOC: Joint Special Operations Command
JTDI: Joint Technical Data Integration
JTF: joint task force
JTIMS: Joint Training Information Management System
JTS: Joint Trauma System

K
KBAS: Kittery Beach Aid Station

L
LAHC: Lyster Army Health Clinic
LD: line of duty
LDB: Leader Development Branch
LDES: Legacy Disability Evaluation System
LDM: Lean Daily Management
LES: leave and earnings statement
LIN: line item number
L/MER: Labor/Management Employee Relations office
LOD: line of duty
LOE: line of effort
LRMC: Landstuhl Regional Medical Center
LSS: Lean Six Sigma
LTHET: long-term health education and training
LTOWB: low-titer group O whole blood
LTT: live tissue training

M
M3PT: Medical Materiel Mobilization Planning Tool
MAP: MTOE Assigned Personnel
MAR2: MOS administrative retention review
MARCORSYSCOM: Marine Corps Systems Command
MASCAL: mass casualty
MBB: Master Black Belt
MC: US Army Medical Corps
MCAHC: McDonald Army Health Clinic
MCDS: Medical Command Deployment Support

MCRW: Medical Contingency Requirements Workflow
MD: medical director
MDMP: military decision-making process
MDRE: medical dental readiness event
MEB: Medical Evaluation Board
MEDCoE: US Army Medical Center of Excellence
MEDCOM: US Army Medical Command
MEDDAC: Medical Activity
MEDEVAC: medical evacuation
MEDEX: medicine extension
MEDLOG: Medical Logistics Division
MEDO: medical operations officer
MEDOPS: medical operations
MEDPROS: Medical Protection System
MER: Medical Event Reporting
MES: medical equipment set
METC: Medical Education and Training Campus
MHA: Master of Healthcare Administration
MHA: Medical Health Assessment
MHS: military health system
MILPER: military personnel message
MLH: Mary Lipscomb Hamrick (research course)
MMAS: Master of Military Art and Science
MMC: Medical Master Catalog
MNG: Saudi Arabian Ministry of the National Guard
MoC: member of Congress
MODS: Medical Operating Data System
MOS: military occupational specialty
MOU: memorandum of understanding
MP: military police
MPAS: Master of Physician Assistant Studies
M&RA: Manpower and Reserve Affairs
MRB: medical recruiting brigade
MRBn: medical recruiting battalion
MRC: medical recruiting center
MRDC: Medical Research and Development Command
MRDP: medical retention determination point
MRO: medical regulating officer
MRS: medical recruiting station

MS: Medical Service Corps
MSAT: Medical Situational Awareness in the Theater
MSD: military service deposit
MSTC: Medical Simulation Training Center
MTF: medical treatment facility
MTOE: modified table of organization and equipment
MTT: mobile training team
MWDE: MEDPROS Web Data Entry
MWR: morale, welfare, and recreation

N

NARSUM: narrative summary
NATO: North Atlantic Treaty Organization
NBME: National Board of Medical Examiners
NC: Nurse Corps
NCCPA: National Commission on Certification of Physician Assistants
NCO: noncommissioned officer
NCOIC: noncommissioned officer-in-charge
NCQA: National Commission on Quality Assurance
NCR: National Capital Region
NCTH: noncompressible torso hemorrhage
NDAA: National Defense Authorization Act
NDS: National Defense Strategy
NGO: nongovernmental organization
NMS: National Military Strategy
NOVA: National Organization for Victim Assistance
NPDB: National Provider Databank
NREMT: National Registry of Emergency Medicine Technicians
NRP: Neonatal Resuscitation Program
NSN: national stock number
NSS: National Security Strategy
NTC: National Training Center

O

OCLL: Office of the Chief, Legislative Liaison
OCONUS: outside the continental United States
OC/T: observer controller/trainer
ODA: operational detachment alpha
OER: officer evaluation report

OHPA: occupational health physician assistant
OIC: officer-in-charge
OISD: operational, institutional, and self-development
OJSS: Office of the Joint Staff Surgeon
OML: order of merit list
OPA: orthopedic physician assistant
OPMD: Officer Personnel Management Directorate
OPM-SANG: Office Program Manager–Saudi Arabian National Guard
OPORD: operations orders
OR: operating room
ORB: officer record brief
OSHA: Occupational Safety and Health Administration
OSUT: one-station unit training
OT&E: operational testing and evaluation
OTSG: Office of the Surgeon General

P

PA: physician assistant
PA-C: physician assistant-certified
PACKRAT: Physician Assistant Clinical Knowledge Rating and Assessment Tool
PACU: post-anesthesia care unit
PAEA: Physician Assistant Education Association
PALS: Pediatric Advanced Life Support
PANCE: Physician Assistant National Certifying Exam
PANRE: Physician Assistant National Recertifying Exam
PATH: Pacific Asynchronous TeleHealth System
PCC: Pre-Command Course
PCF: practitioner's credentials file
PCMH: Patient-Centered Medical Home
PCS: permanent change of station
PD: program director
PEB: physical evaluation board
PEBD: pay entry basic date
PEBLO: physical evaluation board liaison officer
PETD: Professional Education and Training Department
PFC: prolonged field care
PFCCS: Pediatric Fundamentals of Critical Care Support
PI: performance improvement; primary investigator

PICO: patient or population, intervention or exposure, comparison or control, outcome
PME: professional military education
PMRM: Practice Management Revenue Model
PN: partner nation
POC: point of care
POG: Psychological Operations Group
POI: program of instruction
POW: prisoner-of-war
PPO: personnel proponency officer
PPRW: Program and Positions Requirement Worksheet
PROFIS: Professional Filler System
PRT: physical readiness training
PSR: patient safety report
PSV: primary source verification
PULHES: physical, upper, lower, hearing, eyes, psychiatric

Q

QA: quality assurance
QM: quality management

R

R2: Ready and Resilient
R2I: R2 Integration
RAPToR: Resuscitation Adjuncts: Prehospital Transfusion & REBOA (course)
RASP: Ranger assessment and selection program
RC: reserve component
RCMS: Reserve Component Manpower System
RDMS: Registered Diagnostic Medical Sonographer
REBOA: resuscitative endovascular balloon occlusion of the aorta
RIAT: Rapid Impact Assessment Team
RIMS: Reserve Incentives Management Sub-System
ROI/ROII: report of investigation or report of investigative inquiry
RSLC: Reconnaissance and Surveillance Leaders Course
RTB: Ranger training brigade
RTBn: Ranger training battalion
RVU: relative value unit

S

SA: self-assessment
SAAM: School of Army Aviation Medicine
SAB: Strategic Advisory Board
SAFM-BUL: secretary of the Army for financial management–budget liaison
SAPA: Society of Army Physician Assistants
SARC: sexual assault response coordinators
SATTOC: Security Assistant Team Training Orientation Course
SAV: Staff Assistance Visit (program)
SCMH: Soldier-Centered Medical Home
SEA: senior enlisted advisor
SECARMY: secretary of the Army
SERE: survival, escape, resistance, and evasion
SES: Senior Executive Service
SF: special forces
SFA: security force assistance
SFAB: Security Force Assistance Brigade
SFAC: Security Force Assistance Command
SFG: special forces group
SGL: small group leader
SGT: sergeant
SHPE: Separation History and Physical Examination
SKOs: sets, kits, and outfits
SMDR: structure manning decision review
SME: subject matter expert
SMEE: subject matter expert exchange
SMOG: Standard Medical Operating Guidelines
SMS: Soldier Management System
SMTS: Soldier Medic Training Site
SOAR: special operations aviation regiment
SOATB: Special Operations Aviation Training Battalion
SOC: special operations command
SOCM: Special Operations Combat Medic
SOF: US Army Special Operations Forces
SOP: standard operating procedure
SP: Army Medical Specialist Corps
SPMGTF: Special Purpose Marine Ground Task Force
SPPM: suicide prevention program manager

SQN: squadron
SRP: soldier readiness processing
SSC: Senior Service College
STAAR: Simulation Trainer for Arterial Access and REBOA

T

TAIR: Total Army Involvement in Recruiting
TAMMIS: Theater Army Medical Management Information System
TASS: Total Army School System
TCCC: tactical combat casualty care
TCMC: Tactical Combat Medical Care course
TCS: temporary change of station
TDA: table of distribution and allowances
TDY: temporary duty
TEWLS: Theater Enterprise-Wide Logistics System
TMDS: Theater Medical Data Store
TMO: tactical medical officer
TMT: Task Management Tool
TOC: tactical operations center
TOD: tour of duty
TOE: table of organization and equipment
TOMS: TRADOC Organic Medical Structure
TOPMIS: Total Army Personnel Management Information System
TPMRC: Theater Patient Movement Requirements Center
TQM: total quality management
TR: TRADOC regulation
TRAC2ES: Transportation Command Regulating and Command & Control Evacuation System
TRADOC: Army Training and Doctrine Command
TRANSCOM: Transportation Command
TRAP: training resource arbitration panel
TSG: the surgeon general
TSG-PARA: The Surgeon General Physician Assistant Recognition Award
TSOC: Theater Special Operations Command
TTD: transfusion-transmitted disease
TTPs: tactics, techniques, and procedures
TWI: training with industry
TXA: tranexamic acid

U

UAC: unit assemblage code
UCMJ: Uniform Code of Military Justice
UIC: unit identification code
UMR: unit medical readiness
UNMC: University of Nebraska Medical Center
USAACE: US Army Aviation Center of Excellence
USAFRICOM: US Africa Command
USAG: US Army garrison
USAMMA: US Army Medical Materiel Agency
USAMMDA: US Army Medical Materiel Development Activity
USAR: US Army Reserve
USARAF: US Army Africa
USARC: US Army Reserve Command
USAREC: US Army Recruiting Command
USARIEM: US Army Research Institute of Environmental Medicine
USASAM: US Army School of Aviation Medicine
USASOC: US Army Special Operations Command
USNH-GB: US Naval Hospital–Guantanamo Bay
USSOCOM: US Special Operations Command
USU: Uniformed Services University

V

VA: Department of Veterans Affairs
VC: Veterinary Corps
VH: virtual health
VVR: vasovagal reaction

W

WAATS: Western ARNG Aviation Training Site
WAMC: Womack Army Medical Center
WHINSEC: Western Hemisphere Institute for Security Cooperation
WHMO: White House Military Office
WHMU: White House Medical Unit
WHO: World Health Organization
WMDs: weapons of mass destruction

X

XO: executive officer

INDEX

A

B

C

D

G

H

K

L

M

N

O

Q

R

U

X

Y

Z